LEUKEMIAS - UPDATES AND NEW INSIGHTS

Edited by **Margarita Guenova** and **Gueorgui Balatzenko**

Leukemias - Updates and New Insights
http://dx.doi.org/10.5772/59646
Edited by Margarita Guenova and Gueorgui Balatzenko

Contributors

Khalid Al-Anazi, Eduardo Mansilla, Sandra Loydover Peña Luengas, Gustavo H. Marin, Luis Rivera, Gustavo Roque, Adrian Tarditti, Kimberly Payne, Sinisa Dovat, Chandrika Gowda, Olivia Francis, Yali Ding, Parveen Shiraz, Olga Blau, Bo Yuan, Isabel González-Gascón Y Marín, José-Ángel Hernandez, María Hernández-Sanchez, Ana Eugenia Rodríguez-Vicente, Takayuki Takahashi, Hiroko Tsunemine, Brian Wigdahl, Betty Condran, Lorena Loarca, Rositsa Vladimirova, Dora Popova, Elena Vikentieva, Margarita Guenova, Branimir Spassov, Gueorgui Balatzenko, Georgi Mihaylov

Published by InTech

Janeza Trdine 9, 51000 Rijeka, Croatia

Publishing Process Manager Iva Lipovic

Technical Editor InTech DTP team

Cover InTech Design team

First published November, 2015

Printed in Croatia

Additional hard copies can be obtained from orders@intechopen.com

Leukemias - Updates and New Insights, Edited by Margarita Guenova and Gueorgui Balatzenko

p. cm.

ISBN 978-953-51-2202-9

For EU product safety concerns:
IN TECH d.o.o., Prolaz Marije Krucifikse Kozulić 3, 51000 Rijeka, Croatia,
info@intechopen.com or visit our website at intechopen.com.

Meet the editors

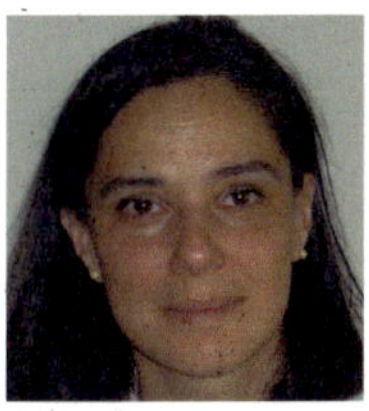

Professor Dr. Margarita Guenova received her medical training at the Medical University of Sofia and her PhD degree at the National Center of Haematology in 2000. She is employed as Head of the Laboratory of Haematopathology and Immunology and Professor of Hematology and Blood Transfusion at the National Specialised Hospital for Active Treatment of Haematological Diseases, Sofia, Bulgaria, teaching both undergraduate and graduate studies at the Sofia Medical University. She specializes in the field of leukemia and lymphoma diagnostics. In regard to her scientific interests, she worked on the elucidation of critical mechanisms of leukemia pathogenesis and progression, investigation of clinically relevant biomarkers and potential targets for therapy in leukemias and lymphomas, characterization of leukemic stem cell populations, minimal residual disease, and implementation of a multifaceted approach in oncohematology. Dr. Guenova has authored and coauthored many abstracts, articles in peer-reviewed journals, and book chapters. She serves on several editorial boards and is the President of the Bulgarian Society of Hematology as well as a member of several professional societies, such as the Bulgarian Society of Pathology, the Bulgarian Association of Clinical Immunology, the European Hematology Association, the European Association of Haematopathology, and the International Society of Haematology.

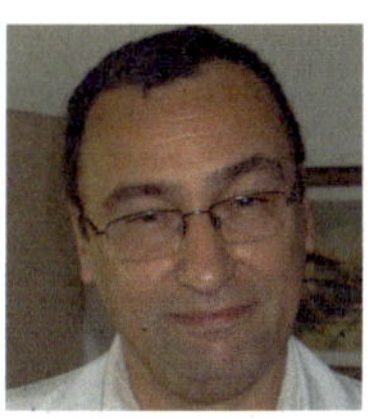

Professor Dr. Gueorgui Balatzenko received his medical training at the Medical University of Sofia and his PhD degree at the National Center of Haematology in 2002. He obtained additional qualifications at the Red Cross Blood Bank, Groningen-Drenthe, the Netherlands; Institute Paoli-Calmettes, Marseille, France; and Necker-Enfants Malades, Paris, France. He is Professor of Hematology and Blood Transfusion at the Laboratory of Cytogenetics and Molecular Biology at the National Specialised Hospital for Active Treatment of Haematological Diseases, Sofia, Bulgaria, teaching both undergraduate and graduate studies at the Sofia Medical University. His major interest is in the field of molecular investigations in leukemias. In regard to his scientific achievements, he worked on the elucidation of the incidence and clinical relevance of molecular biomarkers in chronic and acute leukemias as well as on the molecular monitoring of treatment response. Dr. Balatzenko has authored and coauthored many articles in peer-reviewed journals and book chapters. He is a member of several professional societies, such as the Bulgarian Society of Hematology, the Bulgarian Society of Genetics, and the European Hematology Association; a life member of the UICC; and a referee for international journals.

Contents

Preface

Leukemias are a heterogeneous group of clonal diseases of different cell lineages that originate from a cell of the hematopoietic and lymphatic tissues with diverse incidence, etiology, pathogenesis, and prognosis. A significant progress in the clinical management has been achieved, but despite that current therapeutic approaches often produce prolonged survival, the therapeutic responses are often partial, brief, and unpredictable. However, hematology has constantly been advancing in parallel with technological developments that have expanded our understanding of the phenotypic, genetic, and molecular complexity and extreme clinical and biological heterogeneity of leukemias. This in turn allowed for developing more effective and less toxic alternative therapeutic approaches directed against critical molecular pathways in leukemic cells.

The continuous and rather extensive influx of new information regarding the key features and underlying mechanisms as well as treatment options of leukemias requires frequent updating of this topic. The primary objective of this book is to provide the specialists involved in the clinical management and experimental research of acute and chronic leukemias with comprehensive and concise information on some important theoretical and practical developments in the biology, clinical assessment, and treatment of patients with leukemias as well as on some molecular and pathogenetic mechanisms and their respective translation into novel therapies. Specific clinical scenarios such as pregnancy and age are also within the scope of the book. An international panel of experts provide novel insights into various aspects of leukemias and contribute their experience to updates in the field.

Classically, leukemias have been classified according to their cellular origin, as myeloid or lymphoid, or according to their course, as acute or chronic.

Acute lymphoblastic leukemia (ALL) remains among the greatest challenges in hematology, even if the road to curing most children with ALL, the most common childhood cancer, may be the greatest success story in the history of cancer. Approximately 80% of children with ALL are now cured however, for those children with unfavorable features, defined either by disease biology or by response to treatment, the outcomes remain poor. The first chapter addresses the great strides that have been made in effectively treating pediatric leukemia and presents data on the contribution of risk stratification combined with intensified therapies. The authors focus on role of the increasingly more precise genomic studies for defining specific subtypes of high-risk leukemia and identifying druggable targets in aberrant pathways complemented with the development of relevant preclinical models which are expected to fuel rapid advances in the future. Recent genomic and immunophenotypic studies underlie the identification of new clinically relevant ALL subtypes, such as the early T-cell precursor ALL (ETP-ALL), which has been recently recognized as a form with poor prognosis and reviewed in the second chapter. Recent advances in the biology, genetics, and clinical features of this aggressive disease are presented in a comprehensive summary of the major characteristics and scoring systems in the reported series, further contributing with two clinical cases with a particular clinical presentation. Various viruses have been claimed to be associated with lymphoid neoplasms, including HTLV-1 and HIV. The third chapter reviews the interaction of these two retroviruses within the immune system and more specifically examines the impact of HIV-1 infection on the leukemogenic process induced by HTLV-1 in coinfected individuals as well as the impact of HTLV-1 infection on HIV-1 disease.

Acute myeloid leukemia (AML) accounts for approximately 80% of cases of acute leukemia in adults. It is characterized by clonal proliferation of myeloid precursors and accumulation of leukemic blasts in the bone marrow, ultimately resulting in hematopoiesis failure. Although nowadays AML is cured in 35–40% of adult patients who are 60 years of age or younger and in 5–15% of patients who are older than 60 years of age, the outcome in a significant proportion of patients who are unable to receive intensive chemotherapy without unacceptable side effects remains dismal. The cytogenetic and the enormous molecular heterogeneity of the disease have become increasingly apparent over the past years. The recent large-scale sequencing of AML genomes is now providing opportunities for patient stratification and personalized approaches to treatments that are based on individual mutation profiles. The fourth chapter addresses recent knowledge on genetic and molecular aberrations in AML, describing the incidence, prognostic influence, and association with other molecular markers of the most important recurrent mutations in AML. It is followed by a comprehensive update on non-M3 AML etiology, classification, risk stratification, emergencies, complications, disease in special circumstances, and current and future therapeutics provided in the fifth chapter of the book.

The unsatisfactory clinical outcomes of a significant proportion of AML patients urged the development of **new anti-AML therapy strategies**, one of which includes the implementation of new nucleoside analogs. The sixth chapter summarizes the available data in regard to clofarabine, which has offered new promising perspectives within induction and consolidation therapies. This chapter evaluates the efficacy and tolerability of the drug as a single agent and in combination therapy, including hematopoietic stem cell transplantation, for AML patients. On the other hand, the treatment of most cases of acute promyelocytic leukemia differs from the usual AML treatment. Initial treatment includes the non-chemotherapy drug all-trans-retinoic acid (ATRA), which is most often combined with chemotherapeutic drugs. Another option is to include another differentiating drug called arsenic trioxide (ATO). This is often used in patients who cannot tolerate an anthracycline drug, but it is an option for other patients as well. The seventh chapter highlights the pharmacokinetics of ATO and the detailed mechanisms underlying the cytocidal effects of arsenic compounds. A detailed insight into potential future clinical applications of those promising candidates endowed with potent antitumor activities in view of combination with arsenic compounds is provided.

In regard to chronic leukemias, **B-cell chronic lymphocytic leukemia (B-CLL)** is the most common type of leukemia in adults. CLL displays immense clinical heterogeneity, as many patients have an indolent disease that will not require intervention for many years, while others will present with an aggressive and symptomatic leukemia. While clinical staging systems have been used to stratify patients into risk categories, they lack the ability to predict disease progression or response to therapy. Therefore, the significant interest in identifying additional prognostic markers that can be used to distinguish those patients who may have an aggressive form of CLL and might benefit from early intervention has pushed research toward unraveling the biology of the disease. Numerous cellular and molecular markers with potential prognostic and therapeutic significance have been identified. In parallel, an increasing number of therapeutic compounds and new targeted therapies are under development with promising results. The eightth chapter presents a concise overview of the new prognostic markers of CLL, the relationship they have with each other to build prognostic scores, the role they have in guiding treatment decisions, and the novel therapies that have emerged recently with immunologic, biochemical, and genetic targets. However, conventional treatments are still not directed to the interactions between CLL cells and their microenvironment. The existence of a complex network of antiapoptotic and prosurvival molecules, including cell adhesion, proinflammatory, angiogenic, and proto-oncogenic molecules, is responsible for supporting the infiltrating malignant cells and for the maintenance of the neoplastic tissue in CLL. Many prosurvival signaling pathways potentially sustaining CLL cell maintenance interact with one another. Thus, it appears that developing new classes of drugs affecting simultaneously various signaling pathways, and therefore abrogating signaling redundancy-associated chemoresistance to classical drugs, is feasible. Based on these concepts, the ninth chapter comprises a review of recent studies on key biomarkers of intercellular interactions of the leukemic population, which enable clarification of key processes in the development of the disease and can be the basis for defining a separate risk patient group to optimize the therapeutic approach. It is essential to have new treatment modalities in order to increase the anti-B-CLL effects, providing greater biological activity and much more specificity for the disease. However, in general, in most anti-neoplastic therapies, the side effects are also frequent and the development of resistance or relapse is usually inevitable. The achieved efficiency might be associated with unacceptable toxicity. Therefore, current scientific research efforts are focused on the development of anti-neoplastic agents, which might achieve maximum effect and also decrease the potential damage on normal cells. The tenth chapter presents a novel therapy using zinc oxide nanoparticles and photodynamic therapy for the treatment of CLL, claiming that this new therapeutic approach is a very specific one with very low toxicity for non-leukemic cells and probably very useful not only for B-CLL but also for all the other indolent lymphomas as well as for all types of cancer.

Besides the specific characteristics of various leukemias, a diagnosis of a **blood cancer during pregnancy** is a rare and traumatic experience which poses unique challenges for the mother and the unborn baby, as well as for the treating medical team in managing both the pregnancy and the blood disorder. The last chapter covers the available data about the consequences of maternal and fetal exposures to cytotoxic chemotherapy, radiotherapy, and targeted therapies; a detailed description of coexistence between various types of leukemia and pregnancy; and the specific data obtained from the major studies and important case reports on pregnancy in different types of leukemia.

Each chapter is a separate publication that reflects each author's views and concepts. However, the book presents an update and introduces novel insights into our current understanding of the biology and clinical presentation, the risk assessment, and therapeutic challenges in patients with leukemias.

Prof. Dr. Margarita Guenova, MD, PhD
Laboratory of Haematopathology and Immunology,
National Specialised Hospital for Active Treatment of Haematological Diseases, Sofia, Bulgaria

Prof. Dr. Gueorgui Balatzenko, MD, PhD
Laboratory of Cytogenetics and Molecular Biology,
National Specialised Hospital for Active Treatment of Haematological Diseases, Sofia, Bulgaria

Chapter 1

Pediatric High Risk Leukemia — Molecular Insights

Chandrika Gowda, Olivia L. Francis, Yali Ding, Parveen Shiraz, Kimberly J. Payne and Sinisa Dovat

Additional information is available at the end of the chapter

http://dx.doi.org/10.5772/61247

Abstract

Acute leukemia comprises of 31% of all cancers in children making it the most common childhood malignancy. Significant strides have been made in treatment, partly through risk stratification and intensified therapy. A number of subtypes remain at high risk for relapse and poor outcome, despite current therapies. Here we describe risk stratification and molecular diagnosis used to identify high risk leukemias and guide treatment. Specific cytogenetic alterations that contribute to high risk B and T cell acute lymphoblastic leukemia (ALL), as well as infant leukemia are discussed. Particular attention is given to genetic alterations in IKZF1, CRLF2, and JAK, that have been identified by whole genome sequencing and recently associated with Ph-like ALL. Ongoing studies of disease mechanisms and challenges in developing pre-clinical patient-derived xenograft models to evaluate therapies are discussed.

Keywords: Acute lymphoblastic leukemia, Pediatric Leukemia, high risk leukemia, Ikaros, IKZF1, CRLF2

1. Introduction

Acute leukemia comprises 31% of all cancers in children, making it the most common childhood malignancy. Acute lymphoblastic leukemia (ALL) makes up 80% of these cases and the remaining are leukemias of the myeloid lineage. Among the lymphoblastic leukemias, there are two immunophenotypic groups: B cell precursor ALL (B-ALL, 80% of all ALL) and T cell ALL (T-ALL, 20%). In the following sections, the further classification of each of these subtypes of leukemia, based on their molecular characteristics, is discussed. Also discussed are the clinical importance, prognosis, and new therapies available for each subtype.

2. Overview of classification of pediatric leukemia

2.1. Definition of standard and high risk leukemias

The National Cancer Institute (NCI) has classified acute lymphoblastic leukemia in children based on age at diagnosis, initial white blood count, and the presence of extra medullary disease.

- Standard risk: initial WBC count less than 50,000/μL and age 1 to younger than 10 years
- High risk: initial WBC count 50,000/μL or greater and/or age 10 years or older

The Children's Oncology Group (COG) has classified acute leukemia into four risk groups using prognostic factors that are strongly predictive of outcome such as: 1) age; 2) initial white count; 3) gender; 4) presence of extra medullary disease at diagnosis (CNS or testicular disease); and 5) blast cytogenetic findings and ploidy, and 6) response to induction therapy [1, 2].

Based on these factors, the four risk groups for COG classification of newly diagnosed B-ALL for the AALL08B1 study are low risk, average risk, high risk, and very high risk. In T-ALL, high white count does not have a prognostic significance. The above classification applies to B cell phenotype cases. The presence of CNS or testicular disease, age <1 year, and trisomy 21 are considered high risk. The importance of tumor cell characteristics will be discussed in the following sections.

2.2. Molecular diagnosis and its importance

Immunophenotyping is used to classify leukemia into B-ALL and T-ALL [3, 4].

B-ALL: comprises 80% of ALL. B-ALL cells express cytoplasmic CD79a, CD19, HLA-DR. Surface CD10 (formerly known as common ALL antigen or CALLA) is seen in 90% of these cases. Subtypes are as follows:

- Common Precursor B Cell ALL (75% of cases): These cells are CD10 positive and express no surface or cytoplasmic Ig. This group has the best prognosis.
- Pro B ALL (5% of cases): Commonly seen in infants with MLL rearrangement. These cells are CD10 negative and express no surface or cytoplasmic Ig.
- Pre B ALL (20% of cases): These cells express cytoplasmic Ig.

T-ALL: These cells express cytoplasmic CD3, with CD7 plus CD2 or CD5 on leukemic blasts. T-ALL is associated with older age, male gender, high initial white count, and mediastinal mass.

Cytogenetic alterations: The presence of recurrent numerical and structural chromosomal abnormalities in both ALL and AML are very common and are associated with prognostic significance. Hence, cytogenetic characteristics are now used for risk stratification of patients with ALL [5, 6].

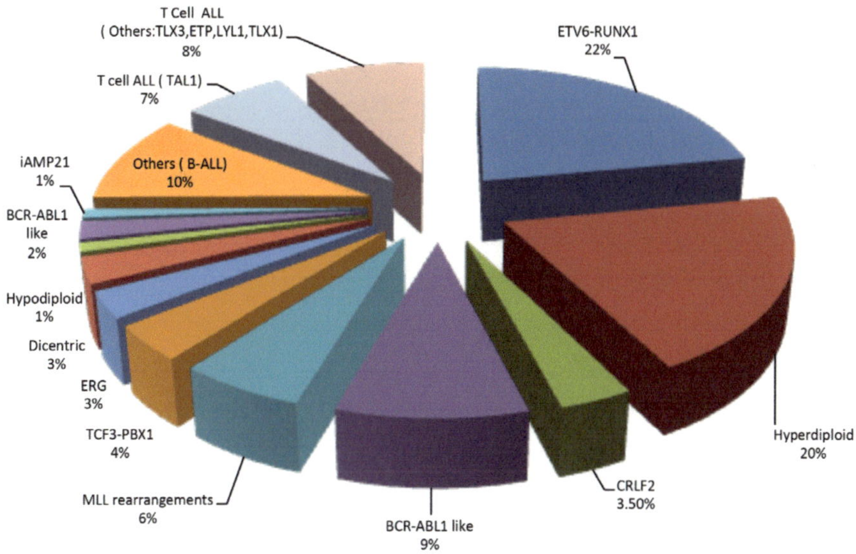

Figure 1. Frequency of Cytogenetic Abnormalities in ALL

Subtype	Frequency (%)	Clinical Significance
Hyperdiploid (>50 Chromosomes)	20-30	Good prognosis
t(12;21)(p13;q22)ETV6-RUNX1	15-25	Good prognosis; expression of myeloid antigens
t(1;19)(q23;p13)TCF3-PBX1	2-6	Good prognosis; associated with CNS relapse; more frequent in African American
CRLF2 rearrangements	5-7	55% OF Down Syndrome ALL; poor prognosis in non-DS ALL; IKZF1 and JAK1/2 alterations common
ERG deletion	7	Good outcome
t(9;22)(q34;q11.2)BCR-ABL1	2-4	Improved outcome with TKI and intensive chemotherapy
ABL1, PDGFRB, JAK2 rearrangements	2-5	'BCR-ABL1 like' ALL; high WBC count; associated with IKZF1 alteration
MYC rearrangement	2	Good outcome with short term intensive chemotherapy
PAX5	2	Unknown prognostic significance
t(4;11)(q21;q23) MLL- AF4	1-2	Infant ALL ; poor prognosis specially in <6 month age
Hypodiploid (<44 chromosomes)	1-2	Poor Prognosis; associated with IKAROS gene family and RAS pathway mutations

Table 1. Common Genetic Alterations and Clinical Significance B-ALL.

Risk stratification based on cytogenetic characteristics has revealed many subgroups of NCI standard and high risk groups that are now treated differently. Many treatment strategies using targeted therapies directed at specific genetic alterations in the tumor cells have opened up a new era of leukemia therapy. Figure 1 and Table 1 show cytogenetic abnormalities seen in ALL [6, 7].

3. Infant leukemia and leukemia with MLL rearrangement

3.1. Overview of infant leukemia

Infant leukemia comprises only 1–2 % of childhood ALL. The cells often show an immature pro-B phenotype. They present with very high WBC count and large extra medullary disease burden which confer poor prognosis in this subset of children [8].

3.2. Biology of infant leukemia

Rearrangements of the *KMT2A* (also known as mixed lineage leukemia (MLL)) gene located on chromosome 11q23 are seen in more than 80% of infant ALL, with increased frequency in patients under 6 months of age. They are also seen in ~50% of infant AML [8] and a majority of adults with therapy-related leukemia secondary to topoisomerase II inhibitors. Balanced translocations result in the fusion of *MLL* to a number of different partner genes, leading to the production of novel chimeric proteins with t(4;11)(q21;q23) *MLL-AFF1* (also called *MLL-AF4*) being the most common. Other rearrangements are t(11;19)(q23;p13.3) *MLL-/ELN*; t(6;11)(q27;q23) *MLL/MLLT4, also called MLL/AF6*; t(9;11)(p22;q23) *MLL/MFT3*, also called *MLL-AF9*; and t(10;11)(p12;q23) *MLL/MLLT10*, also called *MLL/AF10*. The *MLL gene product* plays a critical role in hematopoiesis by regulating the *HOX* group of genes, which sequentially influence hematopoietic stem cell renewal and leukemogenesis [9, 10].

3.3. Risk stratification, current therapeutic approaches and outcome in infant leukemia

Infant ALL is considered high risk for many reasons. The factors that confer poor prognosis are age younger than 6 months, extreme hyperleukocytosis (>300,000 white blood cells/μL), CD10 negativity, and the presence of *MLL* rearrangement. The type of the partner gene fused to *MLL* does not seem to influence outcome [9, 11, 12]. Studies by the BFM group and the international ALL protocol Interfant-99 have shown that patients who were early good responders to prednisone therapy had a better outcome [13, 14].

Infant ALL is currently treated with intensive chemotherapy including high dose cytarabine – "AML-like" therapy. The prednisone poor responders are classified as high risk and require intensification of therapy. Hematopoietic stem cell transplantation for infants with ALL in first remission remains controversial [15, 16].

http://dx.doi.org/10.5772/61247

4. FLT3 mutations in ALL

4.1. Incidence of *FLT3* alterations in ALL and its prognostic significance

Constitutive activation of FMS-like tyrosine kinase 3 (FLT3) plays an important role in the pathogenesis of hematopoietic malignancies. *FLT3* activating mutations, internal tandem duplications (ITD), and kinase domain (KD) mutations were initially discovered in acute myeloid leukemia (AML) and are associated with poor prognosis in both adult and pediatric AML. However, in lymphoblastic leukemia, FLT3 ITD did not cause significant change in overall survival and event free survival [17]. Recently, FLT3 overexpression has been seen in two types of ALL: 18% of infant ALL with *MLL* rearrangement and 21–25% of hyperdiploid ALL and in relapsed ALL samples [18, 19]. Studies have shown that high *FLT3* expression mutation identifies MLL-AF4+ (also called *MLL-AFF1+*) ALL patients at very high risk of treatment failure and poor survival, emphasizing the value of ongoing/future clinical trials for FLT3 inhibitors [20–23].

4.2. FLT3 inhibitors in the treatment of leukemia with FLT3 alterations

Recent gene expression studies have shown that in *MLL*-rearranged leukemia, FLT3, a receptor tyrosine kinase that plays a role in promoting cell proliferation and transformation is overexpressed. This has led to the pursuit of FLT3 inhibitors as targeted therapy for this disease [22]. Currently, Lestaurtinib (CEP-701™), an oral, highly selective small-molecule FLT3 inhibitor, is being used in COG - phase III trial wherein infants with *MLL*-rearranged ALL are being randomized to intensive chemotherapy with or without Lestaurtinib.

5. BCR-ABL positive leukemia

5.1. Incidence, current therapy, and outcome in BCR-ABL+ (Ph+) leukemia

Chimeric BCR–ABL1 protein is encoded by *BCR-ABL1* fusion gene created by reciprocal t(9;22)(q34;q11) translocation on chromosome 22, also known as the Philadelphia chromosome. The *BCR–ABL1* fusion gene is generated by joining most of the coding region of the *ABL1* tyrosine kinase gene (Abelson murine leukemia) on chromosome 9 to the breakpoint cluster region (*BCR*) gene on chromosome 22. The molecular consequence of all BCR–ABL1 fusion proteins is a hyperactive ABL1 kinase domain and aberrant phosphorylation of a variety of targets [23, 24]. There are two gene product variants: p190, which is seen in >90% of Philadelphia+ (Ph+) ALL in children, and p210, which is seen in CML.

Ph+ ALL comprises 3–4% of pediatric ALL, and about 25% of adult ALL cases. Prior to tyrosine kinase inhibitors, these patients had dismal outcomes despite the use of intensive chemotherapy and hematopoietic stem cell transplant in the first remission was the best available option [24].

5.2. Tyrosine kinase inhibitors in BCR-ABL+ (Ph+) leukemia and current challenges

Imatinib was the first generation of tyrosine kinase inhibitors that changed the face of treatment for Ph+ ALL and CML. The addition of Imatinib to intensive chemotherapy in childhood BCR-ABL1–positive ALL results in a 4-year event-free survival rate of 84%, more than double that of historical controls [25]. About 40% of the newly diagnosed Ph+ ALL patients carry point mutations within the kinase-binding domain of BCR-ABL that confers resistance to Imatinib.

Dasatinib and Nilotinib are second-generation tyrosine kinase inhibitors. Dasatinib is a multikinase inhibitor targeting several tyrosine kinases, including BCR-ABL and SRC kinases. It is 325 times more potent than Imatinib, binds to the active and inactive forms of BCR-ABL, and has excellent CNS penetration. These are effective in patients resistant to Imatinib, except those with the *T315I* mutation [26].

Currently, allogeneic hematopoietic stem cell transplant (HSCT) is the standard of care in second remission for patients with Ph+ ALL. It has been observed that most of the patients treated with tyrosine kinase inhibitor (TKI)-based therapy will eventually relapse without HSCT. However, benefits of allogeneic HSCT in first remission, after intensive chemotherapy and TKI therapy, has to be considered based on donor availability, minimal residual disease (MRD) status, and clinical status of the patient [27]. Recent studies in both adults and children have failed to prove clear benefit of allogeneic HSCT in the first remission for this group of patients mainly because of the small sample size [23, 28, 29].

6. *Ikaros*-altered ALL

6.1. Overview of *Ikaros*

Ikaros is a DNA-binding zinc finger protein encoded by the *IKZF1* gene. Ikaros is a transcription factor that functions as a regulator of gene expression and chromatin remodeling [30]. Ikaros regulates the development and function of the immune system and acts as a master regulator of hematopoietic differentiation. Genomic profiling studies identified *IKZF1* as an important tumor suppressor in ALL, particularly in ALL that is associated with poor prognosis [31, 32]. The mechanism by which Ikaros suppresses malignant transformation and the development of ALL is largely unknown. In the past few years, experiments by several groups have shown that Ikaros regulates expression of its target genes by recruiting them to pericentromeric heterochromatin, resulting in their activation or repression [33, 34].

6.2. Clinical importance of Ikaros deletion

IKZF1 has been established as one of the most clinically relevant tumor suppressors in high-risk ALL. Genome wide analysis studies have shown that 15% of all cases of pediatric B-cell ALL show deletion of a single *IKZF1* allele or mutation of a single copy of *IKZF1*, resulting in haploinsufficiency of *IKZF1*. Haploinsufficiency occurs with expression of a functionally inactive Ikaros splice form that acts as a dominant negative. Genetic inactivation of *IKZF1* is more rare in T-ALL where *IKZF1* alterations occur in ~5% of cases [35]. Over 80% of BCR-ABL1

ALL and 66% of chronic myeloid leukemia (CML) patients during lymphoid blast crisis show mutation or deletion of an *IKZF1* allele. One-third of BCR-ABL1 negative ALL patients also show *IKZF1* deletion or mutation. This group of patients is at increased risk of poor outcome with more than threefold increase in relapse rate [30]. Poor outcome associated with *IKZF1* alteration is frequently independent of age, sex, white cell count, and level of minimal residual disease – factors which are commonly used for risk stratification. Testing for *IKZF1* status at the time of diagnosis is now being explored in prospective trials. In recent genome profiling studies, *IKZF1*-altered high risk pediatric ALL cases have shown marked similarity to BCR-ABL positive ALL giving rise to a new subset of cases now called "Ph-like " or "BCR-ABL-like" ALL. This will be discussed further later in the chapter.

6.3. Regulation of Ikaros function in T cell leukemia

The role of Ikaros in normal T cell development is demonstrated by evidence that Ikaros regulates the expression of key genes in T cell differentiation. T cell differentiation is significantly impaired in Ikaros-deficient mice. Terminal deoxynucleotide transferase *(DNTT)* is a gene product critical for thymocyte differentiation that is regulated by Ikaros. Ikaros also regulates the expression of CD4, CD8, and IL-2 and plays a critical role in T cell differentiation [36, 37].

6.3.1. Regulation of Ikaros function

Casein kinase has been shown to phosphorylate Ikaros at multiple sites, and indeed, CK2 kinase is responsible for the majority of Ikaros phosphorylation. Studies by the Dovat group showed that a single phosphomimetic mutation at amino acid 13 or 294 caused the redistribution of Ikaros protein in the nucleus from pericentromeric localization to a diffuse nuclear staining pattern, while phosphoresistant mutations produced no changes in the subcellular localization of Ikaros. These data suggest that targeting of Ikaros to pericentromeric heterochromatin is regulated by its phosphorylation at specific amino acids [34, 38].

6.3.2. CK2 mediated phosphorylation of Ikaros impairs Ikaros function

Recent studies have demonstrated that CK2-mediated phosphorylation of Ikaros controls essential functions of Ikaros including DNA-binding, subcellular localization, and chromatin remodeling, as well as the level of Ikaros protein in cells (via ubiquitination and degradation). Phosphorylation of Ikaros by CK2 kinase also regulates cell cycle progression and Ikaros function in T cell differentiation [39, 40]. Since the overexpression of CK2 kinase and the loss of Ikaros function have been strongly associated with leukemogenesis, it is proposed that increased CK2 kinase activity leads to impaired function and/or degradation of Ikaros, which results in malignant transformation and the development of leukemia.

6.4. Inhibition of CK2 as a potential therapeutic approach to treat high risk leukemia

Casein Kinase II inhibition has been an attractive therapeutic strategy in several malignancies. A specific CK2 inhibitor, CX-4945, orally bioavailable small molecule is in Phase I clinical trial for solid tumors. The role of CK2 inhibitor as an antileukemic drug in ALL needs to be explored.

7. Hypodiploid ALL

7.1. Subclassification and treatment outcome of hypodiploid ALL

Hypodiploid ALL comprises 1–2% of all B-ALL cases and confers poor prognosis. Hypodiploid ALL is a chromosome number abnormality in the leukemic cells that results in 45 chromosomes or less. Hypodiploid ALL has been subdivided in various ways. In general, Hypodiploid ALL may be subclassified into the following four groups:

- near-haploid cases – 24–31 chromosomes
- low-hypodiploid cases – 32–39 chromosomes
- high-hypodiploid cases – 40–43 chromosomes
- near-diploid cases – 44–45 chromosomes

Patients with 44 or 45 chromosomes have a much better outcome than patients with fewer than 44 chromosomes [41].

7.2. Genomic profiles of hypodiploid ALL

Recently, a large group of 124 pediatric patients with hypodiploid ALL were analyzed using microarray profiling of gene-expression and copy-number alteration, and next-generation sequencing. These analyses indicate that near-haploid and low-hypodiploid ALL are distinctive from each other and from other types of ALL. In near-haploid ALL, genetic alterations target RTK (receptor tyrosine kinase) signaling, Ras signaling, and the lymphoid transcription factor gene *IKZF3,* while in low-hypodiploid ALL, genetic alterations involve *TP53, RB1,* and *IKZF2* [42].

RTK and Ras signaling alterations were present in more than two-thirds (70.6%) of near-haploid ALL cases, while they were much less common in low-hypodiploid (8.8%) and near-diploid ALL (31.8%). The RTK and Ras signaling alterations involve deletion, amplification, and/or sequence mutation of *NF1, NRAS, KRAS, MAPK1, FLT3*, or *PTPN11.*

The *TP53* alterations were present in 91.2% of low-hypodiploid ALL, but less than 5% of non-low-hypodiploid ALL. Meanwhile, *TP53* alterations are also present in non-tumor cells in 43.3% of the mutation-carrying cases, suggesting that the *TP53* mutations are inherited and the low-hypodiploid ALL might be a manifestation of Li-Fraumeni Syndrome (LFS).

The *Ikaros* gene family is very important for lymphoid development and differentiation. *IKZF2* is highly expressed in common lymphoid progenitors and pre-pro-B cells, while *IKZF3* is mainly expressed in more mature lymphoid precursors. *IKZF2* and *IKZF3* alterations occur in low-hypodiploid and near-haploid ALL, respectively, suggesting that low-hypodiploid ALL may arise from the transformation of a lymphoid progenitor that is a less mature lymphoid than those from which near-haploid ALL arises. More importantly, both low-hypodiploid and near-haploid leukemic cells show activation of Ras-signaling and PI3K-signaling pathways. In addition, PI3K and mTOR inhibitors can inhibit proliferation of both low-hypodiploid and near-haploid leukemic cells ex vivo, which indicates that these drugs should be further investigated as a new therapeutic strategy for hypodiploid ALL [42].

8. Leukemias involving the *E2A-PBX1* translocation

8.1. Introduction: Wild type E2A and PBX1

The *TCF3* gene (also known as *E2A)* encodes two proteins, E12 and E47, which are generated by differential splicing events. Both proteins contain a C-terminal basic helix-loop-helix (bHLH) domain and two activation domains called AD1 and AD2. E2A proteins function as transcriptional activators by binding to E-box DNA sequence and recruiting histone acetyltransferase complexes. E2A proteins contribute to various aspects of lymphocyte differentiation and development. In E2A deficient mice, B cell development is arrested at the early pro-B stage [43].

PBX1 was first described through its involvement in the translocation t(1; 19) [44]. *PBX1* itself is not expressed in lymphoid cells, though its related genes, *PBX2* and *PBX3*, are expressed in lymphocytes [45]. PBX1 contains a homeodomain involved in DNA binding and protein-protein interaction. It can cooperate with other homeodomian containing proteins of HOX and MEINOX classes to regulate the transcription of target genes [46].

8.2. Structure and function of the *E2A-PBX1* translocation

The chromosomal translocation between chromosomes 1 and 19 results in a fusion event between *TCF3* and *PBX1*, which is detected in 3–5% of all pediatric pre-B cell ALL cases [47, 48]. The E2A-PBX1 fusion proteins contain two-thirds of the N-terminal of E2A proteins (which retain the AD1 and AD2 domain, but lose the bHLH domain) and most of the PBX1 protein. Two forms of E2A-PBX1 proteins are detected, E2A-PBX1a and E2A-PBX1b, which differ at the C-terminus of PBX1 [49].

The E2A-PBX1 fusion protein is capable of transforming various cell types. Enforced expression of E2A-PBX1 induces lethal lympho-proliferative diseases in transgenic mice and aggressive myeloproliferative diseases in a murine bone marrow transplantation model [50].

8.3. Target genes of E2A-PBX1

Many efforts have been made to find the mechanisms by which E2A-PBX1 mediates transformation of pre-B cells. One important way is try to find potential target genes or pathways that are regulated by E2A-PBX1. Using ChIP-chip assay, Diakos et al. found 108 direct E2A-PBX1 targets [51]; however, few targets have been studied in detail. *Wnt16* and *EB-1* are two target genes of E2A-PBX1 that are well studied. Wnt16 belongs to the Wnt family, a group of signaling factors that plays important roles in many developmental processes including cell differentiation, proliferation, polarity, and migration [52]. Wnt16 is normally expressed in peripheral lymphoid organs but not in bone marrow. In contrast, Wnt16 is highly expressed in bone marrow and cell lines that are derived from pre-B ALL patients carrying E2A-PBX1 [52]. *EB-1* expression was much lower in marrow from pre-B ALL patients without t(1; 19) than marrow from pre-B ALL patients and pre-B cell lines that contain the t(1; 19). EB-1 is a signaling protein containing a phosphotyrosine binding domain, and may play a role in the regulation of cell proliferation. [53].

8.4. Clinical treatment and outcome for E2A-PBX1 ALL

For pediatric B-ALL patients with the E2A-PBX1 fusion protein, the prognosis has been controversial. It was initially associated with poor outcome when treated with antimetabolite-based therapy [54, 55], but the recent development of intensified chemotherapy has much improved the outcome of this subgroup. However, in a trial conducted by St. Jude Children's Research Hospital, although patients with the t(1; 19) had an overall favorable outcome with intensified chemotherapy, this group had a significantly higher incidence of CNS relapse, suggesting intensive CNS-directed therapy is needed to further improve the outcome in this group of patients [56].

9. Ph-like ALL

9.1. Description and prevalence of Ph-like ALL

Ph-like (BCR-ABL1-like) ALL defines a distinct subtype of high risk ALL that is characterized by a gene expression profile similar to that of Ph+ ALL but lacking the characteristic t(9;22) translocation. This subtype represents about 15–20% of all cases of ALL [57, 58]. The prevalence of Ph-like ALL increases with age: 10–13% of ALL in children and 21–27% of ALL in adolescents and young adults. Patients with Ph-like ALL have higher leukocyte counts at presentation and are more likely to have minimal residual disease at the end of induction chemotherapy. The survival rates of patients with Ph-like ALL is significantly lower when compared to non-Ph-like ALL among all age groups, adults faring worse than children [58]. Genes that are involved in B cell development, including *IKZF1* (Ikaros), are deleted more frequently in Ph-like ALL as compared to non-Ph-like ALL (82% vs. 36%) [57, 58]. Genomic alterations involving kinase signaling have been observed in >90% of Ph-like ALL. These include alterations involving *ABL1, JAK, EPOR, CRLF2, IL7R, FLT3*, Ras, and others [58]. Subtypes of Ph-like ALL are shown in Figure 2.

9.2. Translocations involving ABL1 in Ph-like B-ALL

The *BCR-ABL1* translocation and the resulting Ph+ leukemia was described in Section 4. Other translocations involving the *ABL1* gene have been demonstrated in B-ALL as well as T-ALL. The *ETV6* gene encodes an Ets family transcription factor that is essential for hematopoiesis and vascular growth. The *ETV6-ABL1* fusion, t(9;12)(q34;p13) is a rare event that has been reported in 22 cases of hematological malignancies including 6 cases of B-ALL and one case of T-ALL [59]. The *RCSD1-ABL1* fusion, t(1;9)(q24;q34), has been identified in 3 cases of B-ALL

[60]. One case of B-ALL with *SFPQ-ABL1* fusion, t(1;9)(p34;q34), and another case of B-ALL with *ZMIZ1-ABL1* fusion, t(9;10)(q34;q22.3) have been reported [61, 62].

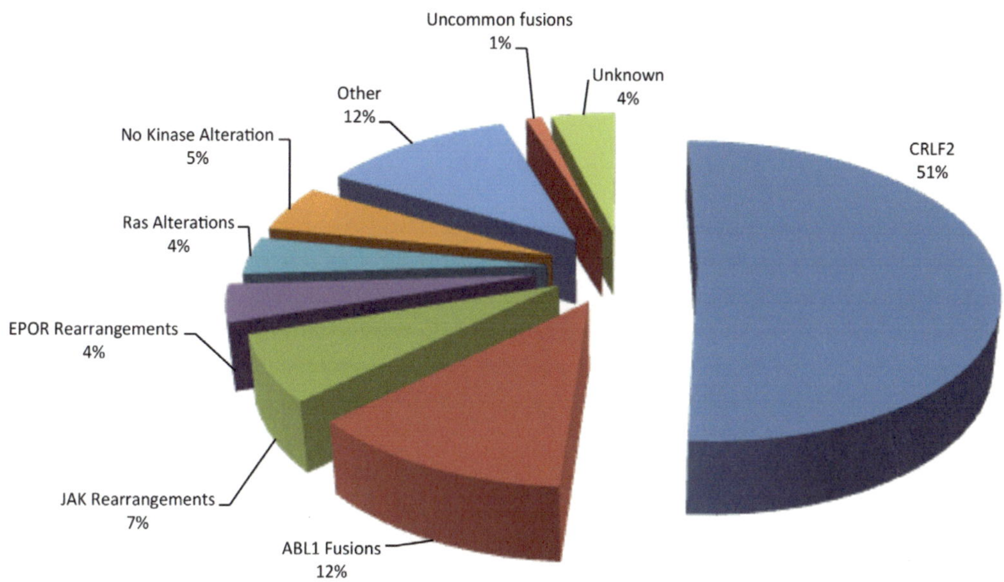

Figure 2. Ph-like ALL subtypes

The *NUP214* gene encodes a nuclear pore complex protein that is involved in nucleocytoplasmic transport. *NUP214-ABL1* is the second most prevalent fusion gene involving *ABL1*. It has been reported only in T cell ALL with a frequency of approximately 5%. So far, 60 cases of this fusion have been reported in the literature involving both childhood and adult cases of T-ALL [63, 64]. In one study by Graux et al., extrachromosomal (episomal) amplification of *ABL1* within the *NUP214-ABL1* transcript was observed in 5 out of 90 cases of T-ALL. Episomes are extrachromosomal DNA that are not visible by conventional cytogenetics [65]. The above mentioned study utilized FISH and microarray-based comparative genomic hybridization techniques to map the episomes and confirm the *ABL1* amplification. Roberts et al. have demonstrated that leukemias with ABL class fusions are sensitive in vitro to the ABL class inhibitors Imatinib and Dasatinib [58].

9.3. Genetic alterations in Ph-like ALL that include EPOR and JAKs

A number of *JAK* mutations have been identified in Ph-like B-ALL, specifically mutations in the *JAK1* pseudokinase domain, as well as the *JAK2* pseudokinase and kinase domain, and in *JAK3* [66]. However, the most common are those occurring in the *JAK2* pseudokinase domain – R683G [67]. Activating mutations in JAK kinases (*JAK1, JAK2*, and *JAK3*) have been reported in approximately 10% of Ph-like pediatric ALL. The JAK mutations were associated with alterations in *IKZF1* and *CDKN2A/CDKN2B*, and with poor outcomes [58, 67]. Approximately 50% of CRLF2 B-ALL patients show *JAK* mutations [66, 68, 69] while rearrangement or translocations involving the *JAK2* gene are characteristic of ~7% of Ph-like ALL [58].

Erythropoietin (EPO) is a hematopoietic growth factor for the erythroid lineage and regulates the production of red blood cells. The binding of EPO to its receptor EPOR leads to downstream activation of JAK2-STAT5, PI3 kinase, and MAP kinase pathways [70]. Rearrangements that involve EPOR have been found in ~4% of Ph-like ALL [58].

9.4. Ras pathway genetic alterations in Ph-like ALL

Ras pathway mutations have been described in pediatric ALL cases. In a report from the Children's Oncology Group by Zhang et al., among 23 childhood B-ALL cases with a Ph-like gene expression profile, 9% had Ras pathway mutations. However, the proportion of Ras pathway mutated cases increased to 62% among ALL with focal *ERG* deletion [71]. Among Ph-like B-ALL cases, 4% are known to have Ras pathway genetic alterations. A majority of these involve missense mutations in *KRAS* and *NRAS* [58].

9.5. IKZF1 alterations in Ph-like ALL

Aberrations in the *IKZF1* gene have been observed in 80% of pediatric B-ALL cases that harbor the *BCR-ABL* rearrangement [72] and a similar pattern is seen in Ph-like ALL. Patients with *IKZF1* deletions have increased risk for relapse and poor treatment outcomes, making *IKZF1* an independent predictor for treatment outcomes [73–75]. More recently, alterations of the *IKZF1* gene have been associated with other genetic defects including *JAK* mutations and *CRLF2* rearrangements. Mullighan et al. demonstrated that 70% of *JAK* mutated cases harbored *IKZF1* alterations [67]. Dorge et al. also performed a study which showed a higher number of Ikaros deletions in patients that have *P2RY8-CRLF2* rearrangement compared to those that are negative for the rearrangement [73]. Further, in another study of 29 pediatric B-ALL cases that showed high CRLF2 expression accompanied by *CRLF2* rearrangement, ~70% of the patients had *JAK* mutations and 80% of cases had deletions or mutations in *IKZF1* [66]. These findings provide evidence that *CRLF2* rearrangements are significantly associated with alterations in *IKZF1*, as well as *JAK* mutations. Moreover, in patients harboring *CRLF2* rearrangements, *JAK* mutations and *IKZF1* deletions/mutations have a poor survival outcome, suggesting that these three lesions cooperate to worsen prognosis and treatment outcome of high-risk B-ALL. Therefore, they can serve as therapeutic targets, as well as prognostic tools that can be used effectively in risk-stratification and treatment strategies to improve treatment outcomes in CRLF2 and other high-risk B-ALL patients.

9.6. Rearrangement of CRLF2 in Ph-like ALL

Overexpression of CRLF2 is responsible for more cases of Ph-like ALL than any other genetic alteration [58]. The *CRLF2* gene is located in the pseudoautosomal region 1 (PAR1) of Xp/Yp. Three types of *CRLF2* gene alterations can result in overexpression of the CRLF2 protein on the surface of the leukemic cells. One involves the juxtaposition of Xp/Yp into the immunoglobulin heavy chain locus at 14q32 resulting in *IgH-CRLF2* rearrangement. The other involves a focal deletion of PAR1 that juxtaposes the regulatory elements of the purinergic receptor gene *P2RY8* to *CRLF2* resulting in a chimeric fusion gene *P2RY8-CRLF2*. Thirdly, a less common missense mutation in exon 6 of *CRLF2*, F232C, results in constitutive CRLF2 dimerization [66, 76]. CRLF2 overexpression is present only in B-ALL cases without rearrangements in *ETV6 (TEL), KMT2A (MLL), TCF3*, and *BCR-ABL*. It is also worth noting that more than half of Down syndrome associated ALL overexpress CRLF2 resulting in poor outcomes in these patients [69]. CRLF2 is overexpressed in approximately 8% of childhood and adult ALL and comprises ~50% of Ph-like ALL [58].

10. Biology of CRLF2 B-ALL – The most common form of Ph-like ALL

10.1. CRLF2–TSLP cytokine receptor component in CRLF2 B-ALL

CRLF2 is a type I cytokine receptor that, along with the IL7 receptor alpha (IL-7Rα), forms a heterodimeric receptor complex for the cytokine TSLP (thymic stromal lymphopoietin). In normal B-cell progenitors the expression of CRLF2 is undetectable by flow cytometry, although TSLP cytokine acts on these cells to induce proliferation [77]. In contrast, the high levels of CRLF2 on CRLF2 B-ALL cells can easily be detected by flow cytometry [68]. In CRLF2 B-ALL cells, TSLP has been shown to increase the phosphorylation of STAT5, AKT, and S6, indicating increased JAK-STAT and AKT/mTOR signaling [78]. Studies of TSLP effects in a range of cell types indicates that it can also indicate cell survival signals through the activation of several biological pathways including ERK, MAPK, PI3K/AKT/mTORC1, and NFκB, at least in some cell types [79]. The physiological significance of the signaling induced by TSLP in CRLF2 B-ALL cells remains to be determined [78].

10.2. Role of JAK mutations in CRLF2 B-ALL

Overexpression of *CRLF2* is believed to cooperate with other genetic lesions leading to leukemogenesis and chemoresistance. In most patients, overexpression of CRLF2 and *CRLF2* gene rearrangements has been associated with deletions and/or mutations of the *IKZF1* gene. Mutations in *JAK1* or *JAK2* are present in half of all cases of CRLF2-overexpressing B-ALL and can result in constitutive activation of this pathway [66, 68, 69].

To understand the contributions of CRLF2 and JAK2 to leukemogenesis, several groups have conducted studies using *CRLF2* and *JAK* mutants. Results from cellular models that utilized murine Ba/F3 cells transduced with combinations of patient-derived mutant *JAK1* or *JAK2*, and *CRLF2* achieved cytokine-independent growth in cells that contained both *CRLF2* and *JAK2* mutants. This cytokine independent growth did not occur in cells that were transduced with wildtype CRLF2 alone or JAK2 mutants alone. Co-immunoprecipitation studies demonstrated that human CRLF2 and phosphorylated mutant JAK2 interact physically [76, 80]. These research findings provide evidence that supports the hypothesis that CRLF2 and JAK2 can cooperate to produce leukemogenesis. Indeed, Hertzberg et al. showed that almost all patients with *JAK* mutations harbor *CRLF2* gene rearrangements[80] This is in keeping with CRLF2 serving as a scaffold to facilitate signaling of mutant *JAK2* [81]. However, ~50% of CRLF2 B-ALL patients show no *JAK* mutations, suggesting that another factor might be inducing JAK activation. This is certainly consistent with the role of endogenous TSLP-induced CRLF2-mediated JAK phosphorylation in CRLF2 B-ALL. TSLP has been shown to increase both JAK-STAT and AKT/mTOR phosphorylation in human CRLF2 B-ALL cells – including those with activating *JAK* mutations [78].

10.3. Inherited background variability and susceptibility to CRLF2 B-ALL

Aside from these acquired genetic variations that contribute to leukemogenesis, other studies using Genome Wide Association techniques are employed to determine whether inherited (germline) genetic variations increase susceptibility to the development of high-risk Ph-like ALL. In a major study, 75 Ph-like ALL patients were compared to 6,661 non-ALL controls and two Single Nucleotide Polymorphisms (SNPs) within the *GATA3* gene achieved genome-wide significance (rs3824662 and rs3781093). The results showed that both SNPs were over-represented in Ph-like ALL and were associated with higher risk of relapse [82]. More importantly, the *GATA3* SNP (rs3824662) was associated with *CRLF2* rearrangement, *JAK* mutations, and *IKZF1* deletions [82]. *GATA3* is one of the six-membered *GATA* transcription factor family that is involved in the reprogramming of somatic cells to pluripotency[83]. More specifically, *GATA3* is critical for T cell development [84] and genetic alterations in *GATA3* have been observed in T-ALL patients [85] and in other hematopoietic disorders such as AML and Hodgkin Lymphoma [86, 87]. Taken together, these studies provide evidence that in addition to acquired genetic alterations such as *CRLF2*, inherited genetic variations such as *GATA3* SNPs may also contribute to increased susceptibility to developing CRLF2 B-ALL and increased risk of relapse. Thus, germline and somatic genetic alterations may play an important role in leukemogenesis.

10.4. CRLF2 B-ALL and health disparities

CRLF2 B-ALL is five times more prevalent in patients of Hispanic/Latino origin and after initial treatment they experience a higher rate of relapse. This high prevalence of CRLF2 B-ALL in Hispanics is further supported by studies that have been conducted in regions where there is a high proportion of Hispanics. For example, the highest incidence of childhood ALL is in Hispanics compared to other ethnic groups in California [88]. In a study of pediatric B-ALL patients, 18 of 51 (35.3%) Hispanic/Latino patients harbored *CRLF2* rearrangements compared to 11 of 154 (7.1%) patients of other ethnicities [66]. Harvey et al. further demonstrated that in addition to *JAK* mutations and *IKZF1* deletions, *CRLF2* rearrangement was also significantly associated with Hispanic/Latino ethnicity [66]. It has been established that populations originating from different ancestries can be distinguished by genetic polymorphisms that are unique to their ancestors [89]. Therefore, the current approach to studying the mechanisms that contribute to the racial disparities relating to incidence and outcome of ALL is to evaluate ancestry-related genetic alterations in conjunction with external factors such as the environment and socioeconomic status [90, 91]. Recent studies to identify ALL susceptibility genes in the Hispanic population demonstrated that *ARID5B* and *GATA3* SNPs are more frequent in Hispanics compared to other ethnicities [82, 92]. These SNPs have been associated with higher ALL incidence (ALL susceptibility), increased frequency of relapse, and poorer outcome [82, 92]. A possible explanation for the increased frequency of these SNPs in Hispanics is their shared genetic ancestry with Native Americans that also exhibit increased frequency of the SNPs [92]. While ancestry-related studies can provide a basis for disease, there is still a need for studies that will identify the biological factors that contribute to the health disparity. Thus, there is a need for the development of preclinical animal models that can be used to evaluate Hispanic patient samples, thereby allowing us to effectively study CRLF2 B-ALL in context of racial disparities.

10.5. Challenges of preclinical models of CRLF2 B-ALL

Current strategies to treat Ph-like ALL and more specifically CRLF2 B-ALL include: 1) stratification of patients using prognostic and clinical factors (age, gender, race, white blood cell count, CNS involvement, testicular involvement, steroid pretreatment and MRD, cell morphology, immunotyping and genetic alterations); and 2) administer treatment regimen based on risk group. Since 91% of the Ph-like ALL subset of patients (including CRLF2 B-ALL) is characterized by activated kinase signaling, tyrosine kinase inhibitors are currently recommended as part of the treatment regimen for these patients [58]. Recent studies were aimed at evaluating the effects of tyrosine kinase inhibitors, more specially JAK inhibitors and PI3K/mTOR inhibitors on CRLF2 B-ALL cells in vitro and in vivo [78, 93, 94]. Results from these studies have shown that *CRLF2* rearranged B-ALL cells are sensitive to these inhibitors in vitro and in vivo. While JAK inhibitors and all other tyrosine kinase inhibitors have shown some promise, they have not been effective in all Ph-like B-ALL and not all CRLF2 B-ALL harbor JAK mutations. Since TSLP has been shown to increase activation of the JAK-STAT, PI3K/AKT/mTOR signaling pathways, it is important to conduct studies of disease mechanisms and evaluate therapeutic candidates in context of TSLP and other cytokines that are often present in the cancer microenvironment. Though some in vitro studies were performed in the presence of TSLP [78], in vivo studies in context of TSLP stimulation are lacking. Therefore systematic evaluation of the contributions of TSLP to CRLF2 B-ALL leukemogenesis and the assessment of therapies to treat these patients are required to gain a better understanding of the etiology and treatment outcome of the disease.

Human-mouse xenograft models are ideal in vivo models for studying disease mechanisms and for evaluating therapies for leukemia, particularly in context of inherited genetic variability. NOD/SCID mice have been shown to be receptive to the engraftment of human leukemia cells [95]. The development of additional mouse strains, such as the NOD/Scid/IL- 2Rγ null (NSG) strain have significantly increased the ability of human ALL cells to engraft [96]. These animal models are effective because mouse cytokines act on the human leukemia cells by providing the necessary growth signals required to facilitate proliferation and maintenance of leukemia cells [97]. However, while most mouse cytokines can activate receptors on human cells, some mouse cytokines are species-specific, e.g., IL-3, GM-CSF, and TSLP [97]. This poses a challenge in effectively recapitulating the systemic or BM microenvironment present in patients. It is important to conduct studies as far as possible with the full complement of cytokines present under physiological conditions in order to truly identify disease mechanisms and evaluate therapies.

10.6. Novel pre-clinical xenograft models that provide human cytokines

The lack of cross species cytokine activity has been partially addressed for studies of myeloid leukemia by the recent development of so-called "cytokine mice" [98]. These immune-deficient mice express human IL-3, SCF, and GMCSF, three cytokines that play important roles in the production of myeloid lineage cells and show no or poor cross species activity. Xenografts from cytokine mice showed enhanced AML engraftment [98]. Alternative strategies have been used to produce mice that express human IL-15 and FLT3 and other cytokines, which have resulted in enhanced production of functional human natural killer cells, dendritic cells, monocytes/macrophages, and erythrocytes [97]. However, human TSLP has not been included as part of the complement of cytokines used in these studies.

Current xenografts that evaluate therapeutic candidates for CRLF2 B-ALL do not include human TSLP [94], which is required to provide the human CRLF2-mediated signals that were demonstrated by previous groups in vitro [78]. There is a need to develop new preclinical animal models that include TSLP and other species-specific cytokines in order to accurately evaluate disease mechanisms. A model that includes TSLP and allows for modulating the levels of TSLP will be of great value to the study of CRLF2 B-ALL. The rationale for this is that CRLF2, the receptor for the endogenous ligand TSLP, is overexpressed on CRLF2 B-ALL cells and has contributed to increased pathway signaling in these cells. Additionally, the role of TSLP in the initiation and maintenance of CRLF2 B-ALL is unknown. Current studies in our laboratories are aimed at developing a human TSLP+ xenograft model that provides human TSLP to activate CRLF2-mediated signals in human CRLF2 B-ALL cells transplanted into xenograft mice. This model will be used to study disease mechanisms and identify therapies to effectively treat CRLF2 B-ALL.

11. Conclusion

In summary, great strides have been made in effectively treating pediatric leukemia. Risk stratification based on clinical features combined with intensified therapies has contributed to this outcome. Increasingly, more precise molecular phenotyping available from whole genome analyses make it possible to identify and study specific subtypes of high risk leukemias. Mechanistic studies that identify druggable targets in aberrant pathways are likely to fuel rapid advances in the future. This progress will depend on the development of relevant preclinical models for studying disease mechanisms and for evaluating candidate therapies.

Author details

Chandrika Gowda[1], Olivia L. Francis[2], Yali Ding[1], Parveen Shiraz[3], Kimberly J. Payne[2,3*] and Sinisa Dovat[1]

*Address all correspondence to: kpayne@llu.edu

1 Department of Pediatrics, Pennsylvania State University College of Medicine, Hershey, PA, USA

2 Department of Pathology and Human Anatomy, Loma Linda University, School of Medicine, Loma Linda, CA, USA

3 Department of Medicine, Loma Linda University, School of Medicine, Loma Linda, CA, USA

References

[1] Schultz KR, Pullen DJ, Sather HN, Shuster JJ, Devidas M, Borowitz MJ, et al. Risk- and response-based classification of childhood B-precursor acute lymphoblastic leukemia: A combined analysis of prognostic markers from the Pediatric Oncology Group (POG) and Children's Cancer Group (CCG). Blood. 2007;109(3):926-35.

[2] Smith M, Arthur D, Camitta B, Carroll AJ, Crist W, Gaynon P, et al. Uniform approach to risk classification and treatment assignment for children with acute lymphoblastic leukemia. J Clin Oncol. 1996;14(1):18-24.

[3] Carroll WL, Bhojwani D, Min DJ, Raetz E, Relling M, Davies S, et al. Pediatric acute lymphoblastic leukemia. Hematology Am Soc Hematol Educ Program. 2003:102-31.

[4] Pui CH, Robison LL, Look AT. Acute lymphoblastic leukaemia. Lancet. 2008;371(9617):1030-43.

[5] Ross ME, Zhou X, Song G, Shurtleff SA, Girtman K, Williams WK, et al. Classification of pediatric acute lymphoblastic leukemia by gene expression profiling. Blood. 2003;102(8):2951-9.

[6] Mullighan CG. The molecular genetic makeup of acute lymphoblastic leukemia. Hematology Am Soc Hematol Educ Program. 2012;2012:389-96.

[7] Mullighan CG. Molecular genetics of B-precursor acute lymphoblastic leukemia. J Clin Invest. 2012;122(10):3407-15.

[8] Braoudaki M, Tzortzatou-Stathopoulou F. Clinical cytogenetics in pediatric acute leukemia: An update. Clin Lymphoma Myeloma Leuk. 2012;12(4):230-7.

[9] Bhojwani D, Howard SC, Pui CH. High-risk childhood acute lymphoblastic leukemia. Clin Lymphoma Myeloma. 2009;9 Suppl 3:S222-30.

[10] Pui CH, Evans WE. Treatment of acute lymphoblastic leukemia. N Engl J Med. 2006;354(2):166-78.

[11] Pui CH, Gaynon PS, Boyett JM, Chessells JM, Baruchel A, Kamps W, et al. Outcome of treatment in childhood acute lymphoblastic leukaemia with rearrangements of the 11q23 chromosomal region. Lancet. 2002;359(9321):1909-15.

[12] Krivtsov AV, Armstrong SA. MLL translocations, histone modifications and leukaemia stem-cell development. Nat Rev Cancer. 2007;7(11):823-33.

[13] Mullighan CG, Downing JR. Genome-wide profiling of genetic alterations in acute lymphoblastic leukemia: Recent insights and future directions. Leukemia. 2009;23(7): 1209-18.

[14] de Boer J, Walf-Vorderwulbecke V, Williams O. In focus: MLL-rearranged leukemia. Leukemia. 2013;27(6):1224-8.

[15] Pieters R, Schrappe M, De Lorenzo P, Hann I, De Rossi G, Felice M, et al. A treatment protocol for infants younger than 1 year with acute lymphoblastic leukaemia (Interfant-99): An observational study and a multicentre randomised trial. Lancet. 2007;370(9583):240-50.

[16] Armstrong SA, Staunton JE, Silverman LB, Pieters R, de Boer ML, Minden MD, et al. MLL translocations specify a distinct gene expression profile that distinguishes a unique leukemia. Nat Genet. 2002;30(1):41-7.

[17] Karabacak BH, Erbey F, Bayram I, Yilmaz S, Acipayam C, Kilinc Y, et al. Fms-like tyrosine kinase 3 mutations in childhood acute leukemias and their association with prognosis. Asian Pacific journal of cancer prevention: APJCP. 2010;11(4):923-7.

[18] Stirewalt DL, Radich JP. The role of FLT3 in haematopoietic malignancies. Nature Reviews Cancer. 2003;3(9):650-U1.

[19] Armstrong SA, Mabon ME, Silverman LB, Li A, Gribben JG, Fox EA, et al. FLT3 mutations in childhood acute lymphoblastic leukemia. Blood. 2004;103(9):3544-6.

[20] Taketani T, Taki T, Sugita K, Furuichi Y, Ishii E, Hanada R, et al. FLT3 mutations in the activation loop of tyrosine kinase domain are frequently found in infant ALL with MLL rearrangements and pediatric ALL with hyperdiploidy. Blood. 2004;103(3):1085-8.

[21] Wellmann S, Moderegger E, Zelmer A, Bettkober M, von Stackelberg A, Henze G, et al. FLT3 mutations in childhood acute lymphoblastic leukemia at first relapse. Leukemia. 2005;19(3):467-8.

[22] Stam RW, den Boer ML, Schneider P, Nollau P, Horstmann M, Beverloo HB, et al. Targeting FLT3 in primary MLL-gene-rearranged infant acute lymphoblastic leukemia. Blood. 2005;106(7):2484-90.

[23] Bernt KM, Hunger SP. Current concepts in pediatric Philadelphia chromosome-positive acute lymphoblastic leukemia. Frontiers in oncology. 2014;4:54.

[24] Uckun FM, Nachman JB, Sather HN, Sensel MG, Kraft P, Steinherz PG, et al. Clinical significance of Philadelphia chromosome positive pediatric acute lymphoblastic leukemia in the context of contemporary intensive therapies: A report from the Children's Cancer Group. Cancer. 1998;83(9):2030-9.

[25] Schultz KR, Bowman WP, Aledo A, Slayton WB, Sather H, Devidas M, et al. Improved early event-free survival with imatinib in Philadelphia chromosome-positive acute lymphoblastic leukemia: A children's oncology group study. J Clin Oncol. 2009;27(31):5175-81.

[26] Shah NP, Kantarjian HM, Kim DW, Rea D, Dorlhiac-Llacer PE, Milone JH, et al. Intermittent target inhibition with dasatinib 100 mg once daily preserves efficacy and improves tolerability in imatinib-resistant and intolerant chronic-phase chronic myeloid leukemia. J Clin Oncol. 2008;26(19):3204-12.

[27] Ottmann OG, Pfeifer H. Management of Philadelphia chromosome-positive acute lymphoblastic leukemia (Ph+ ALL). Hematology Am Soc Hematol Educ Program. 2009:371-81.

[28] de Labarthe A, Rousselot P, Huguet-Rigal F, Delabesse E, Witz F, Maury S, et al. Imatinib combined with induction or consolidation chemotherapy in patients with de novo Philadelphia chromosome-positive acute lymphoblastic leukemia: Results of the GRAAPH-2003 study. Blood. 2007;109(4):1408-13.

[29] Yanada M, Takeuchi J, Sugiura I, Akiyama H, Usui N, Yagasaki F, et al. High complete remission rate and promising outcome by combination of imatinib and chemotherapy for newly diagnosed BCR-ABL-positive acute lymphoblastic leukemia: A phase II study by the Japan Adult Leukemia Study Group. J Clin Oncol. 2006;24(3): 460-6.

[30] Mullighan CG, Su X, Zhang J, Radtke I, Phillips LA, Miller CB, et al. Deletion of IKZF1 and prognosis in acute lymphoblastic leukemia. N Engl J Med. 2009;360(5): 470-80.

[31] Kastner P, Dupuis A, Gaub MP, Herbrecht R, Lutz P, Chan S. Function of Ikaros as a tumor suppressor in B cell acute lymphoblastic leukemia. Am J Blood Res. 2013;3(1): 1-13.

[32] Payne KJ, Dovat S. Ikaros and tumor suppression in acute lymphoblastic leukemia. Crit Rev Oncog. 2011;16(1-2):3-12.

[33] Collins-Underwood JR, Mullighan CG. Genetic alterations targeting lymphoid development in acute lymphoblastic leukemia. Curr Top Dev Biol. 2011;94:171-96.

[34] Gurel Z, Ronni T, Ho S, Kuchar J, Payne KJ, Turk CW, et al. Recruitment of Ikaros to pericentromeric heterochromatin is regulated by phosphorylation. Journal of Biological Chemistry. 2008;283(13):8291-300.

[35] Marcais A, Jeannet R, Hernandez L, Soulier J, Sigaux F, Chan S, et al. Genetic inactivation of Ikaros is a rare event in human T-ALL. Leukemia research. 2010;34(4):426-9.

[36] Dovat S, Payne KJ. Tumor suppression in T cell leukemia—the role of Ikaros. Leukemia Research. 2010;34(4):416-7.

[37] Ronni T, Payne KJ, Ho S, Bradley MN, Dorsam G, Dovat S. Human Ikaros function in activated T cells is regulated by coordinated expression of its largest isoforms. Journal of Biological Chemistry. 2007;282(4):2538-47.

[38] Popescu M, Gurel Z, Ronni T, Song CH, Hung KY, Payne KJ, et al. Ikaros Stability and Pericentromeric Localization Are Regulated by Protein Phosphatase 1. Journal of Biological Chemistry. 2009;284(20):13869-80.

[39] Wang HJ, Song CH, Gurel Z, Song N, Ma JS, Ouyang HS, et al. Protein Phosphatase 1 (PP1) and Casein Kinase II (CK2) Regulate Ikaros-Mediated Repression of TdT in Thymocytes and T-Cell Leukemia. Pediatric Blood & Cancer. 2014;61(12):2230-5.

[40] Dovat S, Song CH, Payne KJ, Li ZJ. Ikaros, CK2 kinase, and the road to leukemia. Molecular and Cellular Biochemistry. 2011;356(1-2):201-7.

[41] Nachman JB, Heerema NA, Sather H, Camitta B, Forestier E, Harrison CJ, et al. Outcome of treatment in children with hypodiploid acute lymphoblastic leukemia. Blood. 2007;110(4):1112-5.

[42] Holmfeldt L, Wei L, Diaz-Flores E, Walsh M, Zhang J, Ding L, et al. The genomic landscape of hypodiploid acute lymphoblastic leukemia. Nat Genet. 2013;45(3): 242-52.

[43] Zhuang Y, Soriano P, Weintraub H. The helix-loop-helix gene E2A is required for B cell formation. Cell. 1994;79(5):875-84.

[44] Kamps MP, Murre C, Sun XH, Baltimore D. A new homeobox gene contributes the DNA binding domain of the t(1;19) translocation protein in pre-B ALL. Cell. 1990;60(4):547-55.

[45] Monica K, Galili N, Nourse J, Saltman D, Cleary ML. PBX2 and PBX3, new homeobox genes with extensive homology to the human proto-oncogene PBX1. Mol Cell Biol. 1991;11(12):6149-57.

[46] Kilstrup-Nielsen C, Alessio M, Zappavigna V. PBX1 nuclear export is regulated independently of PBX-MEINOX interaction by PKA phosphorylation of the PBC-B domain. EMBO J. 2003;22(1):89-99.

[47] Andersen MK, Autio K, Barbany G, Borgstrom G, Cavelier L, Golovleva I, et al. Paediatric B-cell precursor acute lymphoblastic leukaemia with t(1;19)(q23;p13): Clinical and cytogenetic characteristics of 47 cases from the Nordic countries treated according to NOPHO protocols. Br J Haematol. 2011;155(2):235-43.

[48] Felice MS, Gallego MS, Alonso CN, Alfaro EM, Guitter MR, Bernasconi AR, et al. Prognostic impact of t(1;19)/ TCF3-PBX1 in childhood acute lymphoblastic leukemia in the context of Berlin-Frankfurt-Munster-based protocols. Leuk Lymphoma. 2011;52(7):1215-21.

[49] Kamps MP, Look AT, Baltimore D. The human t(1;19) translocation in pre-B ALL produces multiple nuclear E2A-Pbx1 fusion proteins with differing transforming potentials. Genes Dev. 1991;5(3):358-68.

[50] Thorsteinsdottir U, Krosl J, Kroon E, Haman A, Hoang T, Sauvageau G. The oncoprotein E2A-Pbx1a collaborates with Hoxa9 to acutely transform primary bone marrow cells. Mol Cell Biol. 1999;19(9):6355-66.

[51] Diakos C, Xiao Y, Zheng S, Kager L, Dworzak M, Wiemels JL. Direct and indirect targets of the E2A-PBX1 leukemia-specific fusion protein. PLoS One. 2014;9(2):e87602.

[52] McWhirter JR, Neuteboom ST, Wancewicz EV, Monia BP, Downing JR, Murre C. Oncogenic homeodomain transcription factor E2A-Pbx1 activates a novel WNT gene in pre-B acute lymphoblastoid leukemia. Proc Natl Acad Sci U S A. 1999;96(20):11464-9.

[53] Fu X, McGrath S, Pasillas M, Nakazawa S, Kamps MP. EB-1, a tyrosine kinase signal transduction gene, is transcriptionally activated in the t(1;19) subset of pre-B ALL, which express oncoprotein E2a-Pbx1. Oncogene. 1999;18(35):4920-9.

[54] Crist WM, Carroll AJ, Shuster JJ, Behm FG, Whitehead M, Vietti TJ, et al. Poor prognosis of children with pre-B acute lymphoblastic leukemia is associated with the t(1;19)(q23;p13): A Pediatric Oncology Group study. Blood. 1990;76(1):117-22.

[55] Piccaluga PP, Malagola M, Rondoni M, Ottaviani E, Testoni N, Laterza C, et al. Poor outcome of adult acute lymphoblastic leukemia patients carrying the (1;19)(q23;p13) translocation. Leuk Lymphoma. 2006;47(3):469-72.

[56] Jeha S, Pei D, Raimondi SC, Onciu M, Campana D, Cheng C, et al. Increased risk for CNS relapse in pre-B cell leukemia with the t(1;19)/TCF3-PBX1. Leukemia. 2009;23(8):1406-9.

[57] Den Boer ML, van Slegtenhorst M, De Menezes RX, Cheok MH, Buijs-Gladdines JGCAM, Peters STCJM, et al. A subtype of childhood acute lymphoblastic leukaemia with poor treatment outcome: A genome-wide classification study. Lancet Oncol. 2009;10(2):125-34.

[58] Roberts KG, Li Y, Payne-Turner D, Harvey RC, Yang YL, Pei D, et al. Targetable kinase-activating lesions in Ph-like acute lymphoblastic leukemia. N Engl J Med. 2014;371(11):1005-15.

[59] Zuna J, Zaliova M, Muzikova K, Meyer C, Lizcova L, Zemanova Z, et al. Acute Leukemias with ETV6/ABL1 (TEL/ABL) Fusion: Poor Prognosis and Prenatal Origin. Gene Chromosome Canc. 2010;49(10):873-84.

[60] Mustjoki S, Hernesniemi S, Rauhala A, Kahkonen M, Almqvist A, Lundan T, et al. A novel dasatinib-sensitive RCSD1-ABL1 fusion transcript in chemotherapy-refractory adult pre-B lymphoblastic leukemia with t(1;9)(q24;q34). Haematologica. 2009;94(10): 1469-71.

[61] Hidalgo-Curtis C, Chase A, Drachenberg M, Roberts MW, Finkelstein JZ, Mould S, et al. The t(1;9)(p34;q34) and t(8;12)(p11;q15) fuse pre-mRNA processing proteins SFPQ (PSF) and CPSF6 to ABL and FGFR1. Genes Chromosomes Cancer. 2008;47(5):379-85.

[62] Soler G, Radford-Weiss I, Ben-Abdelali R, Mahlaoui N, Ponceau JF, Macintyre EA, et al. Fusion of ZMIZ1 to ABL1 in a B-cell acute lymphoblastic leukaemia with a t(9;10) (q34;q22.3) translocation. Leukemia. 2008;22(6):1278-80.

[63] De Braekeleer E, Douet-Guilbert N, Rowe D, Bown N, Morel F, Berthou C, et al. ABL1 fusion genes in hematological malignancies: A review. Eur J Haematol. 2011;86(5):361-71.

[64] Burmeister T, Gokbuget N, Reinhardt R, Rieder H, Hoelzer D, Schwartz S. NUP214-ABL1 in adult T-ALL: The GMALL study group experience. Blood. 2006;108(10): 3556-9.

[65] Graux C, Cools J, Melotte C, Quentmeier H, Ferrando A, Levine R, et al. Fusion of NUP214 to ABL1 on amplified episomes in T-cell acute lymphoblastic leukemia. Nat Genet. 2004;36(10):1084-9.

[66] Harvey RC, Mullighan CG, Chen IM, Wharton W, Mikhail FM, Carroll AJ, et al. Rearrangement of CRLF2 is associated with mutation of JAK kinases, alteration of IKZF1, Hispanic/Latino ethnicity, and a poor outcome in pediatric B-progenitor acute lymphoblastic leukemia. Blood. 2010;115(26):5312-21.

[67] Mullighan CG, Zhang J, Harvey RC, Collins-Underwood JR, Schulman BA, Phillips LA, et al. JAK mutations in high-risk childhood acute lymphoblastic leukemia. Proc Natl Acad Sci U S A. 2009;106(23):9414-8.

[68] Russell LJ, Capasso M, Vater I, Akasaka T, Bernard OA, Calasanz MJ, et al. Deregulated expression of cytokine receptor gene, CRLF2, is involved in lymphoid transformation in B-cell precursor acute lymphoblastic leukemia. Blood. 2009;114(13): 2688-98.

[69] Mullighan CG, Collins-Underwood JR, Phillips LA, Loudin MG, Liu W, Zhang J, et al. Rearrangement of CRLF2 in B-progenitor- and Down syndrome-associated acute lymphoblastic leukemia. Nat Genet. 2009;41(11):1243-6.

[70] Hardee ME, Arcasoy MO, Blackwell KL, Kirkpatrick JP, Dewhirst MW. Erythropoietin biology in cancer. Clin Cancer Res. 2006;12(2):332-9.

[71] Zhang J, Mullighan CG, Harvey RC, Wu G, Chen X, Edmonson M, et al. Key pathways are frequently mutated in high-risk childhood acute lymphoblastic leukemia: A report from the Children's Oncology Group. Blood. 2011;118(11):3080-7.

[72] Mullighan CG, Miller CB, Radtke I, Phillips LA, Dalton J, Ma J, et al. BCR-ABL1 lymphoblastic leukaemia is characterized by the deletion of Ikaros. Nature. 2008;453(7191):110-4.

[73] Dorge P, Meissner B, Zimmermann M, Moricke A, Schrauder A, Bouquin JP, et al. IKZF1 deletion is an independent predictor of outcome in pediatric acute lymphoblastic leukemia treated according to the ALL-BFM 2000 protocol. Haematologica. 2013;98(3):428-32.

[74] Yang YL, Hung CC, Chen JS, Lin KH, Jou ST, Hsiao CC, et al. IKZF1 deletions predict a poor prognosis in children with B-cell progenitor acute lymphoblastic leukemia: A multicenter analysis in Taiwan. Cancer Sci. 2011;102(10):1874-81.

[75] Kuiper RP, Waanders E, van der Velden VH, van Reijmersdal SV, Venkatachalam R, Scheijen B, et al. IKZF1 deletions predict relapse in uniformly treated pediatric precursor B-ALL. Leukemia. 2010;24(7):1258-64.

[76] Yoda A, Yoda Y, Chiaretti S, Bar-Natan M, Mani K, Rodig SJ, et al. Functional screening identifies CRLF2 in precursor B-cell acute lymphoblastic leukemia. Proc Natl Acad Sci U S A. 2010;107(1):252-7.

[77] Scheeren FA, van Lent AU, Nagasawa M, Weijer K, Spits H, Legrand N, et al. Thymic stromal lymphopoietin induces early human B-cell proliferation and differentiation. Eur J Immunol. 2010.

[78] Tasian SK, Doral MY, Borowitz MJ, Wood BL, Chen IM, Harvey RC, et al. Aberrant STAT5 and PI3K/mTOR pathway signaling occurs in human CRLF2-rearranged B-precursor acute lymphoblastic leukemia. Blood. 2012;120(4):833-42.

[79] Zhong J, Sharma J, Raju R, Palapetta SM, Prasad TS, Huang TC, et al. TSLP signaling pathway map: A platform for analysis of TSLP-mediated signaling. Database (Oxford). 2014;2014:bau007.

[80] Hertzberg L, Vendramini E, Ganmore I, Cazzaniga G, Schmitz M, Chalker J, et al. Down syndrome acute lymphoblastic leukemia, a highly heterogeneous disease in which aberrant expression of CRLF2 is associated with mutated JAK2: A report from the International BFM Study Group. Blood. 2010;115(5):1006-17.

[81] Lu X, Huang LJ, Lodish HF. Dimerization by a cytokine receptor is necessary for constitutive activation of JAK2V617F. J Biol Chem. 2008;283(9):5258-66.

[82] Perez-Andreu V, Roberts KG, Harvey RC, Yang W, Cheng C, Pei D, et al. Inherited GATA3 variants are associated with Ph-like childhood acute lymphoblastic leukemia and risk of relapse. Nat Genet. 2013;45(12):1494-8.

[83] Shu J, Zhang K, Zhang M, Yao A, Shao S, Du F, et al. GATA family members as inducers for cellular reprogramming to pluripotency. Cell Res. 2015;25(2):169-80.

[84] Wei G, Abraham BJ, Yagi R, Jothi R, Cui K, Sharma S, et al. Genome-wide analyses of transcription factor GATA3-mediated gene regulation in distinct T cell types. Immunity. 2011;35(2):299-311.

[85] Zhang J, Ding L, Holmfeldt L, Wu G, Heatley SL, Payne-Turner D, et al. The genetic basis of early T-cell precursor acute lymphoblastic leukaemia. Nature. 2012;481(7380):157-63.

[86] Hahn CN, Chong CE, Carmichael CL, Wilkins EJ, Brautigan PJ, Li XC, et al. Heritable GATA2 mutations associated with familial myelodysplastic syndrome and acute myeloid leukemia. Nat Genet. 2011;43(10):1012-7.

[87] Enciso-Mora V, Broderick P, Ma Y, Jarrett RF, Hjalgrim H, Hemminki K, et al. A genome-wide association study of Hodgkin's lymphoma identifies new susceptibility loci at 2p16.1 (REL), 8q24.21, and 10p14 (GATA3). Nat Genet. 2010;42(12):1126.

[88] Chokkalingam AP, Hsu LI, Metayer C, Hansen HM, Month SR, Barcellos LF, et al. Genetic variants in ARID5B and CEBPE are childhood ALL susceptibility loci in Hispanics. Cancer Causes Control. 2013;24(10):1789-95.

[89] Li JZ, Absher DM, Tang H, Southwick AM, Casto AM, Ramachandran S, et al. Worldwide human relationships inferred from genome-wide patterns of variation. Science. 2008;319(5866):1100-4.

[90] Bhatia S. Influence of race and socioeconomic status on outcome of children treated for childhood acute lymphoblastic leukemia. Curr Opin Pediatr. 2004;16(1):9-14.

[91] Buffler PA, Kwan ML, Reynolds P, Urayama KY. Environmental and genetic risk factors for childhood leukemia: Appraising the evidence. Cancer Invest. 2005;23(1): 60-75.

[92] Xu H, Cheng C, Devidas M, Pei D, Fan Y, Yang W, et al. ARID5B genetic polymorphisms contribute to racial disparities in the incidence and treatment outcome of childhood acute lymphoblastic leukemia. J Clin Oncol. 2012;30(7):751-7.

[93] Wong J, Welschinger R, Hewson J, Bradstock KF, Bendall LJ. Efficacy of dual PI-3K and mTOR inhibitors in vitro and in vivo in acute lymphoblastic leukemia. Oncotarget. 2014;5(21):10460-72.

[94] Maude SL, Tasian SK, Vincent T, Hall JW, Sheen C, Roberts KG, et al. Targeting JAK1/2 and mTOR in murine xenograft models of Ph-like acute lymphoblastic leukemia. Blood. 2012;120(17):3510-8.

[95] Liem NL, Papa RA, Milross CG, Schmid MA, Tajbakhsh M, Choi S, et al. Characterization of childhood acute lymphoblastic leukemia xenograft models for the preclinical evaluation of new therapies. Blood. 2004;103(10):3905-14.

[96] Agliano A, Martin-Padura I, Mancuso P, Marighetti P, Rabascio C, Pruneri G, et al. Human acute leukemia cells injected in NOD/LtSz-scid/IL-2Rgamma null mice generate a faster and more efficient disease compared to other NOD/scid-related strains. Int J Cancer. 2008;123(9):2222-7.

[97] Chen Q, Khoury M, Chen J. Expression of human cytokines dramatically improves reconstitution of specific human-blood lineage cells in humanized mice. Proc Natl Acad Sci U S A. 2009;106(51):21783-8.

[98] Wunderlich M, Chou FS, Link KA, Mizukawa B, Perry RL, Carroll M, et al. AML xenograft efficiency is significantly improved in NOD/SCID-IL2RG mice constitutively expressing human SCF, GM-CSF and IL-3. Leukemia. 2010;24(10):1785-8.

Chapter 2

Early T-cell Precursor Acute Lymphoblastic Leukemia – A Characteristic Neoplasm Presenting the Phenotype of Common Hematopoietic Progenitors for both Myeloid and Lymphoid Lineages

Hiroko Tsunemine and Takayuki Takahashi

Additional information is available at the end of the chapter

http://dx.doi.org/10.5772/60901

Abstract

Introduction: Early T-cell precursor acute lymphoblastic leukemia (ETP-ALL) is a subtype of T-ALL and its clinical entity was established in recent years based on characteristic immunophenotyping and gene expression profiles. The cellular origin of ETP-ALL is supposed to be from common hematopoietic progenitors both for lymphoid and myeloid lineages because this leukemia phenotypically exhibits lymphoid, myeloid, and stem cell features. ETP-ALL comprises 5–15% of all T-ALL and is associated with a poor prognosis. The purpose of this chapter is to clarify the etiology, clinical picture, and therapeutic strategy of ETP-ALL showing two cases of this leukemia in our institution.

Cellular origin of ETP-ALL: The normal early T-cell precursors (ETPs) are considered to be a subset of early thymocytes which are originated from the bone marrow and subsequently reside in the thymus, retaining multilineage differentiation potential as the common lymphoid-myeloid hematopoietic progenitors. ETP-ALL is supposed to be a neoplastic counterpart of ETPs.

Immunophenotype and diagnosis of ETP-ALL: ETP-ALL is characterized by the lack of expression of T-lineage cell surface antigens (CD1a and CD8, weak or no expression of CD5) and expression of myeloid and hematopoietic stem cell markers such as CD13, CD33, CD34, and CD117. These characteristic immunophenotypic profiles have provided a scoring system or a criterion for the diagnosis of ETP-ALL, which distinguishes ETP-ALL from classical T-ALL.

Clinical pictures: Clinical features are not substantially different between ETP-ALL and classical T-ALL, although ETP-ALL is associated with a higher rate of relapse and induction failure and a significantly worse overall survival. Two cases of ETP-ALL in our institution, which exhibited unique clinical pictures, that is, marked intestinal involvement and lymphoma-like systemic lymphadenopathy, respectively, will be discussed later in this chapter.

Gene profiles: Whole-genome sequencing studies on ETP-ALL have demonstrated several recurrent mutations involving genes coding cytokines, RAS signaling mediators (NRAS, KRAS, FLT3, IL7R, JAK3, LAK1, SH2B3, and BRAF), epigenetic controllers (EZH2, EED, SUZ12, SETD2, EP300 and DNMT3A), and hematopoietic transcriptional regulators (GATA3, ETV6, RUNX1, IKZF1, and EP300). These mutational spectrums are similar to those of acute myeloid leukemia.

Therapeutic strategies: These gene profiles suggest that treatment of ETP-ALL may benefit from a new chemotherapeutic approach, which is directed to the myeloid or stem cell natures of this leukemia, such as high-dose cytarabine, or epigenetic or molecular targeting therapy. Allogeneic stem cell transplantation (allo-SCT) may be a promising option for the treatment of ETP-ALL.

Conclusion: More precise and extensive cellular and molecular investigations are required to establish definite cellular origin and genetic or epigenetic nature of ETP-ALL. Accumulation of ETP-ALL cases and larger clinical trials will establish an effective therapeutic strategy for this high risk leukemia.

Keywords: Early T-cell precursor acute lymphoblastic leukemia

---

1. Introduction

T-cell acute lymphoblastic leukemia (T-ALL) is a clonal malignant disorder of immature T-cells that accounts for 10–15% of childhood and 25% of adult ALL patients [1]. Despite the relatively high morbidity and mortality of T-ALL when compared to B-cell ALL, the prognosis of T-ALL has dramatically improved following the advancement of chemotherapy, and its long-term survival has become as high as 85% in both pediatric and adult T-ALL patients [2, 3]. However, a refractory subset of pediatric T-ALL associated with a poor prognosis has remained. In 2009, a study performed at St. Jude Children's Research Hospital identified a distinct subtype of pediatric T-ALL, which was designated as early T-cell precursor ALL (ETP-ALL) [4]. This new subtype of T-ALL was defined according to the characteristic gene expression profile and immunophenotypes of the leukemic cells and was found to be associated with a high rate of remission induction failure or relapse when the patients were treated with conventional chemotherapy [4].

The purpose of this chapter is to clarify the recent advances in the biology, genetics, clinical characteristics, and therapeutic strategy of ETP-ALL and discuss two cases experienced at our institution.

http://dx.doi.org/10.5772/60901

2. Cellular origin of ETP-ALL

Normal early T-cell precursors (ETPs) are a subset of thymocytes, which have newly immigrated from the bone marrow to the thymus, and they retain multilineage differentiation potential, suggesting their direct derivation from hematopoietic stem cells [5-7]. The initial stage of thymocyte development is characterized by the generation of cells that lack the expression of CD4 or CD8 antigen. Along with the differentiation of these double negative cells, a minimum of four distinct differentiation stages have been identified according to the differential expressions of CD44 and CD25, that is, DN1, DN2, DN3, and DN4 stages. The potential for myeloid, dendritic, and natural killer cell differentiation is retained at both the DN1 and early DN2 stages [6]. The ability to confer multilineage differentiation is lost at the DN3 stage, and provably, at the latter half of DN2 progression [8]. Therefore, it may be reasonable that the tumor-initiating cells in ETP-ALL could originate from DN1 and/or DN2 thymocytes (Figure 1). However, in recent years, a mouse model of T-ALL using a Sleeping-Beauty-based transposon system suggested that ETP-ALL may be derived from more mature T-cells [9]. Thus, the exact cellular origin of ETP-ALL remains to be elucidated.

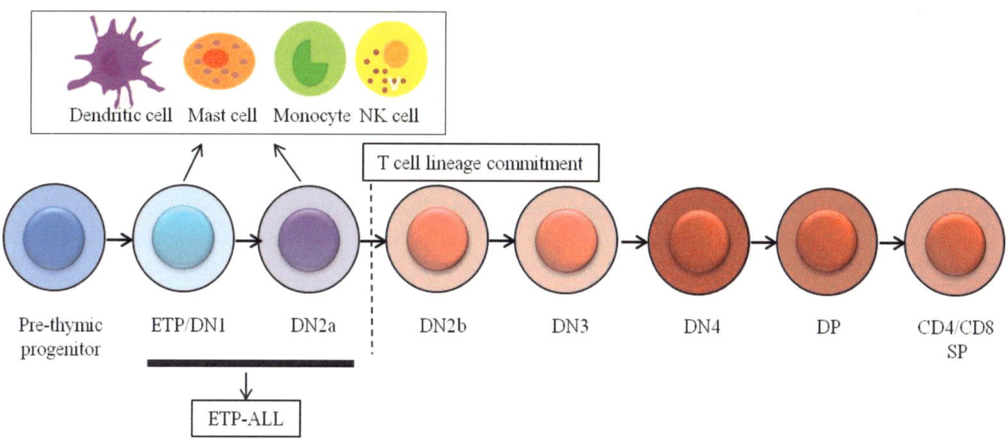

Figure 1. Early T-cell development and supposed cellular origin of ETP-ALL.

3. Immunophenotyping and diagnosis of ETP-ALL

Immunophenotyping of ETP-ALL cells is characterized by the lack of CD1a and CD8 expressions, weak CD5 expression (< 75% positive blasts), and the expression of one or more of the following myeloid or stem cell antigens on at least 25% of the leukemic cells: CD117, CD34, HLA-DR, CD13, CD33, CD11b, and/or CD65 [4]. Subsequently, a study proposed a scoring system based on the expression of commonly available eleven markers: CD5, CD8, CD13, CD33, CD34, HLA-DR, CD2, smCD3, CD4, CD10, and CD56 (Figure 2A) [10]. The specificity and sensitivity of this scoring system were 100% and 94%, respectively, when applied to the patients in the St. Jude cohort (Figure 2B) [10]. Recently, another study attempted to make a more simple diagnosis of ETP-ALL using the expression of CD5 and concluded that CD5-negative T-ALL could be diagnosed as ETP-ALL because CD5 negativity was associated with positive myeloid/stem cell antigens but not CD1a and CD8 expressions (Figure 3) [11]. Currently, precise immunophenotyping is the most important tool to make a diagnosis of ETP-ALL, and this analysis enables us to distinguish ETP-ALL from classical T-ALL.

(A) Scoring system based on 11 marker expression

Score	-2	-1	+1	+2
CD5	≥75%			<75%
CD8	≥5%			<5%
CD13			≥25%	≥75%
CD33			≥25%	≥75%
CD34			≥25%	≥75%
HLA-DR			≥25%	≥75%
CD2		≥75%	<20%	
CD3		≥75%	<20%	
CD4		≥75%	<20%	
CD10		≥75%	<20%	
CD56			≥20%	

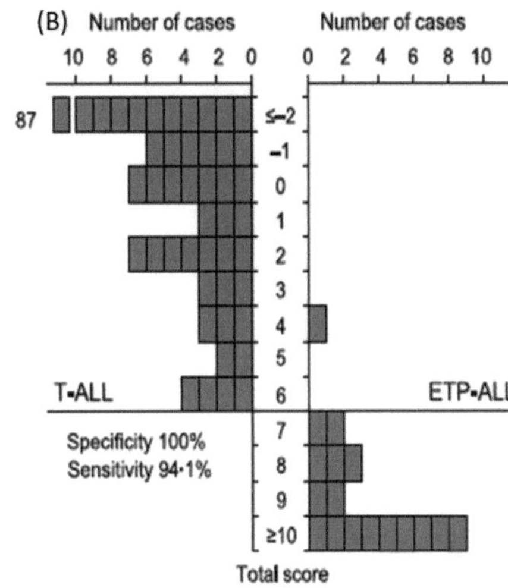

Figure 2. A scoring system for immunophenotypical diagnosis of ETP-ALL. A: Scoring system based on the expression of 11 markers., B: Distribution of total score of 11-marker expression in ETP-ALL patients (right) and T-ALL (left) of the St Jude cohort. (Extract of Ref.10).

4. Clinical characteristics

Following the early reports from the St. Jude Children's Research Hospital and the Associazione Italiana Ematologica Oncologica Pediatrica (AIEOP), comparative studies on the clinical characteristics between ETP-ALL and classical T-ALL were performed in six institutions: the Tokyo Children's Cancer Study Group [10], the Shanghai Children's Medical Center [12], the German Multicenter Study Group for adult ALL [13], Colombia University Medical Center [14], All India Institute of Medical Sciences [11], and the Medical Research Council UK-ALL 2003 trial [15] (Table 1). According to the results of these clinical studies, ETP-ALL was observed to comprise 5.5–16% of all T-ALL cases. The clinical characteristics were similar between ETP-ALL and classical T-ALL with regard to gender, hemoglobin concentration, and central nervous system involvement. However, ETP-ALL patients presented with a lower white blood cell (WBC) count [11, 12, 15], lower frequency of the mediastinal mass [13, 14], and higher age (10 years or older) [4, 11] at presentation when compared to those with classical T-ALL. Regarding the cytogenetic profile, Coustan-Smith et al. reported that ETP-ALL had

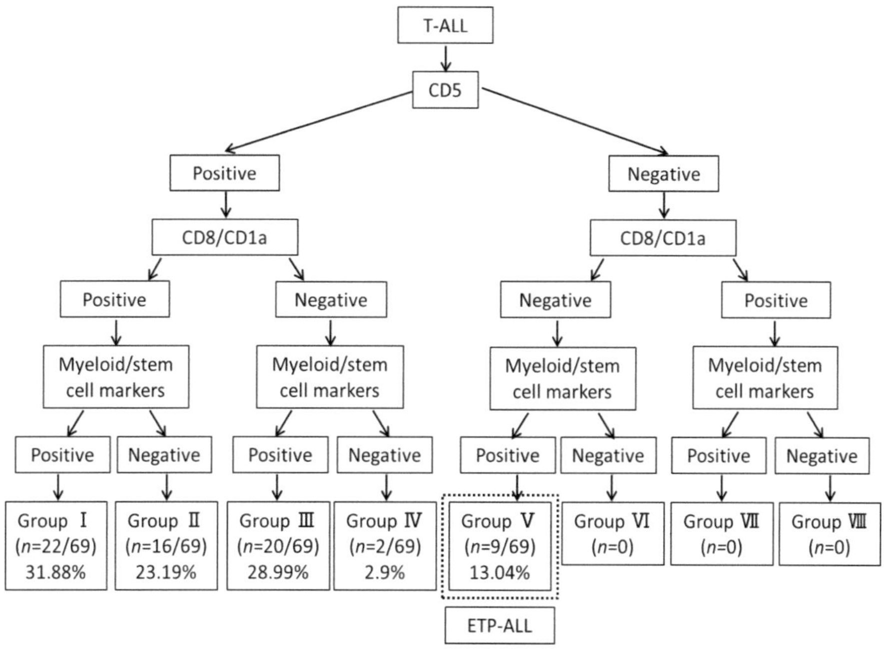

Figure 3. A flowchart for the diagnosis of ETP-ALL based on CD5 expression (Extract of Ref.11).

more 13q- and DNA copy number abnormalities than those in classical T-ALL [4]. Conversely, Allen et al. reported that the majority of patients with ETP-ALL exhibited a normal karyotype without recurrent cytogenetic abnormalities [14]. The monoclonal rearrangement of T-cell receptor genes was observed in 71% of the ETP-ALL cases, showing no significant difference between the two T-ALL subgroups [14].

	St. Jude cohort		TCCSG L99-15 study		AIMS cohort		SCMC study		GMALL study		Columbia university		UKALL 2003	
	Coustan-Smith E, et al. [4]		Inukai T, et al. [10]		Chopra A, et al. [11]		Ma M, et al. [12]		Neuman M, et al.[13]		Allen A, et al. [14]		Patrick K, et al. [15]	
	ETP-ALL	T-ALL	ETP-ALL	T-ALL	ETP-ALL	T-ALL	ETP-ALL	T-ALL	ETP-ALL	T-ALL	ETP-ALL	T-ALL	ETP-ALL	T-ALL
Number of patients	17	122	5	86	9	60	12	62	57	121	7	41	35	187
Age (years old)	≥10		≥10		median		N.R.		≥36		>10		>10	
	13 (76.5%)	49 (40.2%)	3 (60%)	39 (45.3%)	22	9.9			30 (52.6%)	53 (43.8%)	5 (72%)	24 (58%)	18 (51%)	83 (44%)
Gender							N.R.							
Male	14	92	2	67	53	8			47	84	6	28	22	138
Female	3	30	3	19	7	1			10	37	1	13	13	49
WBC ($\times 10^9$/L)	≥100		≥100		median				>30		>50		≥50	
	3 (17.6%)	58 (47.5%)	1 (20%)	42 (48.8%)	7.5	117.5	16.8± 18.1	125.8± 107	19 (37.3%)	41 (36.6%)	1 (14.3%)	16 (39%)	16 (46%)	139 (74%)
Mediastinal mass	2 (11.8%)	39 (32.0%)	3 (60%)	51 (59.3%)	22.20%	2.75%	N.R.		14 (27.5%)	52 (46.8%)	1 (14.3%)	25 (61%)	1 (3%)	13 (7%)
CNS involvement	4 (23.5%)	49 (40.2%)	0 (0%)	3 (3.5%)	N.R.		N.R.		4 (8.7%)	4 (3.8%)	N.R.		N.R.	
Abnormal karyotype	14 (82.4%)	N.R.	N.R.		N.R.		N.R.		N.R.		3 (42.9%)	10 (24.4%)	N.R.	
Treatment outcome	10-year of RF or relapse		Remission failure		CR rate		CR rate		CR rate		Relapse hazard risk		Relapse rate	
	72%	10%	0%	4.7%	33.3%	49.3%	75%	90.30%	42 (79.2%)	93 (82.3%)	4.08	1	18.6%	9.6%
Event free survival	10-year EFS		4-year EFS		60-days EFS		5-year EFS		9-year remission rate		N.R.		5-year EFS	
	22%	69%	40.00%	70.90%	37.6%	80.8%	11.1± 10.1%	57.6± 5.6%	46%	57%			76.6%	84.6%
Overall survival	10-year OS		N.R.		60-days OS		5-year OS		10-year OS		N.R.		5-year OS	
	19%	84%			96.6%	77.5%	3.3± 11.0%	64.7± 6.3%	35%	38%			82.4%	90.9%

RF,remission failure; N.R.,not reported; CR, complete remission

Table 1. Comparative studies on the clinical characteristics between ETP-ALL and classical T-ALL.

As for the prognosis, ETP-ALL is associated with a higher rate of relapse and induction failure. ETP-ALL is additionally associated with a significantly worse overall survival with a 10-year event free survival (EFS) and overall survival (OS) rates of 22% and 19%, respectively, as compared with 69% EFS and 84% OS for all other subtypes of T-ALL, respectively, in the St. Jude cohort [4]. Similar results were obtained in the cohorts of four other institutions [4, 10-12]. More recently, however, two clinical studies showed no significant differences in the EFS and OS rates between the patients with ETP-ALL and classical T-ALL [14, 15]. Although the reason for this discrepancy is unclear, differences in the therapeutic protocol and patient cohort may have influenced the results of these clinical studies. However, an increased risk of relapse in the patients with ETP-ALL [4, 10-12, 15], especially children [4, 14], was a common result in all these previous studies. Thus, larger prospective studies are needed to determine the real prognosis of this T-ALL subtype.

5. Gene profiles

The expression levels of oncogenic transcription factor genes were examined to establish genetic profiles of ETP-ALL in the St Jude Children's Research Hospital and AIEOP studies. Pediatric ETP-ALL had a higher expression of oncogenic transcription factors: *LMO1*, *LMO2*, *LYL1*, and *ERG* [4, 16]. *LMO1* and *LMO2* are binding partners with hematopoietic basic helix-loop-helix transcription factors, such as *SCL/TAL1* or *LYL1*. These proteins interact together to form a transcription factor complex, and they are hypothesized to act through a common mechanism which leads to oncogenesis of T-ALL [17]. McCormack et al. demonstrated that *LYL1* is critical for the oncogenic function of *LMO2*, including the upregulation of a stem cell-like gene signature, aberrant self-renewal of thymocytes, and subsequent generation of T-cell leukemia in *LMO2*-transgenic mice. Moreover, *LMO2* and *LYL1* are co-expressed in leukemic cells from the patients with ETP-ALL, and *LYL1* is indispensable for the growth of ETP-ALL cell lines [18]. Whole-genome sequencing studies showed that ETP-ALL had a high frequency of activating mutations in the genes involved in cytokine receptor and RAS signaling (e.g., *NRAS*, *KRAS*, *FLT3*, *IL-7R*, *JAK3*, *LAK1*, *SH2B3*, and *BRAF*) and inactivating mutations in the genes encoding key transcription factors involved in hematopoietic development (e.g., *GATA3*, *ETV6*, *RUNX1*, *IKZF1*, and *EP300*) and involved in epigenetic gene control (e.g., *EZH2*, *EED*, *SUZ12*, *SETD2*, and *EP300* genes) [16]. The gene mutations which affect cytokine receptor regulation and/or RAS signaling pathway are observed in two-thirds of ETP-ALL cases but only in 19% of non-ETP T-ALL cases [16]. These mutational gene spectrums in ETP-ALL are similar to those in acute myeloid leukemia (AML), but not in T- or B-lineage ALLs. Furthermore, the global transcriptional profile of ETP-ALL is similar to that of normal hematopoietic stem cells, AML stem cells, and murine ETP. The activating mutations in the interleukin-7 receptor (IL-7R) gene were reported to be sufficient to generate ETP-ALL in mice, and this murine ETP-ALL model showed the blockage of thymocyte differentiation at the DN2 stage, at which the developmental potentials for both myeloid and T-cell lineages coexists [19]. These findings suggesting ETP-ALL is a neoplasm at the stage of less mature hematopoietic progenitor or stem cells may account for the capacity of ETP-ALL to exert myeloid differentiation.

Gene expression profiling was also investigated in adult ETP-ALL patients. Whole-exome sequencing in adult ETP-ALL cells demonstrated a distinct mutation spectrum from that of pediatric ETP-ALL, particularly in affecting genes involved in epigenetic regulation with higher frequencies of *DNMT3A* and *FAT3* mutations [20]. *DNMT3A*, one of the genes for DNA-methyl-transferase, is a frequent mutational target in AML [21], whereas *FAT3* mutations have been frequently reported in ovarian carcinomas but not AML [22]. The incidence of *DNMT3A* mutations showed a clear age relationship [20]. Adult ETP-ALL patients also had mutations in the genes known to be involved in leukemogenesis, including *ETV6*, *NOTCH1*, *JAK1*, and *NF1*. In addition, more than 60% of the adult patients with ETP-ALL harbored at least a single genetic lesion in *DNMT3A*, *FLT3*, or *NOTCH1* [20]. Furthermore, adult ETP-ALL showed higher expression levels of *BAALC*, *IGFBP7*, *WT-1*, and *MN1* than those in classical T-ALL [4, 13, 18]. As described above, the high expression of *BAALC* and *ERG* were predictive for unfavorable outcomes in adult T-ALL [23, 24]. *IGFBP7* is a stem cell-associated gene, which is functionally highly related to *BAALC* and overexpressed in early T-ALL [25]. The *WT-1* gene is commonly overexpressed in AML [26], and its overexpression is associated with a poor prognosis in thymic T-ALL patients [27]. The overexpression of the *MN1* gene is additionally associated with a shorter survival in the patients with AML without karyotypic abnormalities [28, 29]. The *FLT3* mutations which are frequently observed in AML were found in 37.5% of the adult ETP-ALL but only in 1–3% of the classical T-ALL patients (37.5%) [13], although these *FLT3* mutations in ETP-ALL more frequently generated tyrosine kinase domain (TDK) abnormalities rather than internal tandem duplication (ITD) mutations, which are frequently observed in AML. In relation to the above-mentioned observations, mice that received a transplant of FLT3-ITD-transduced bone marrow cells developed myeloproliferative diseases, while those that received a transplant of FLT3-TDK-transduced bone marrow cells developed lymphoid disorders [30]. Collectively, it may be reasonable to separate ETP-ALL from classical T-ALL due to the distinct genetic profiles between ETP-ALL and other T-ALL subtypes, and the characteristic gene profile of ETP-ALL may provide new therapeutic strategies for this leukemia.

6. Therapeutic strategies

Coustan-Smith et al. previously reported that the patients with ETP-ALL showed a poor initial response to standard intensive chemotherapies and unfavorable outcomes [4]. Subsequently, six clinical studies showed that ETP-ALL was associated with a very high risk for relapse, whereas two additional studies showed no significant differences in both the EFS and OS rates between the patients with ETP-ALL and classical T-ALL [14, 15]. In the TLLSGL99-15 study, three of four relapsed ETP-ALL patients were successfully treated with allogenic hematopoietic stem cell transplantation (allo-SCT), indicating that allo-SCT could be an effective therapeutic option for ETP-ALL [10]. Prior to this report, the Berlin-Frankfurt-Munster group showed that allo-SCT was superior to chemotherapy alone for high-risk childhood T-ALL [31]. The UKALL 2003 study, which showed better outcomes of ETP-ALL, suggested the beneficial effects of a more intensive chemotherapeutic regimen and the employment of dexamethasone and pegylated asparaginase [15]. High-dose cytarabine combined with epigenetic treatment may be a promising option for ETP-ALL according to the results of whole-genome sequencing, which showed that the mutational spectrum of ETP-ALL was similar to that of AML and that the transcriptional profile was similar to that of normal hematopoietic stem cells and granulocyte-macrophage progenitor cells [4], although these hypotheses need to be proven in future investigations. Additionally, other potential targets have been suggested according to the genetic alterations in the transcription factors. Stat4 phosphorylation was observed in *IL-7R* mutant-induced ETP-ALL cell lines, and consequently, ruxolitinib which is a selective JAK1 and JAK2 inhibitor, was shown to inhibit the proliferation of cells from the ETP-ALL cell lines and prolong the survival of mice xeno-transplanted with the *IL-7R* mutated ETP-ALL cells [19]. Tyrosine kinase inhibitors may be effective when *FLT3* mutations harboring ETP-ALL are molecularly targeted [13]. The antiapoptotic B-cell lymphoma-2 (BCL-2) protein is another attractive molecular target. BCL-2 is highly expressed in ETP-ALL and gradually decreases its expression along with the differentiation toward mature T-cells. ABT-199, an orally bioavailable BCL-2 specific inhibitor, was demonstrated to induce apoptosis of ETP-ALL cells from patients with this subtype of leukemia and dramatically reduced the tumor burden in the bone marrow, spleen, and peripheral blood in mice transplanted with ETP-ALL patient-derived xenografts [32, 33]. In addition, a WT-1 peptide cancer vaccine may be a therapeutic option for relapsed patients or those with minimal residual disease in *WT-1*-overexpressed ETP-ALL, because this approach has demonstrated objective clinical responses in other hematological neoplasms and solid tumors [34].

7. Case study

For a better understanding of ETP-ALL, we herein present two cases of ETP-ALL in our institution, which exhibited unique clinical pictures.

Case 1: A 24-year-old man developed epigastralgia and low-grade fever four months before the admission to our hospital. On gastrofiberscopy performed in a hospital, multiple non-ulcerative mucosal nodules were observed. A biopsy specimen from the nodule histologically showed diffuse infiltration of small lymphocytes, which were positive for CD3, CD7, CD8, and CD56 but negative for TIA-1, Epstein-Barr virus-encoded small RNAs-in situ hybridization (EBER-ISH), and a suspected pathological diagnosis was lymphomatoid gastroenteropathy. Three months later, the patient was admitted to our hospital due to the exacerbation of abdominal distress. On this admission, he presented with multiple ulcerative nodules in the gastric mucosa (Figure 4), marked wall thickening of the small intestine, hepatosplenomegaly (Figure 5) and multiple nodular lesions in the bilateral lungs. A histological examination of the biopsied gastric mucosal nodule showed dense infiltration with small immature lymphocytes (Figure 6). The WBC count elevated to 3.83×10^9/L with 55% immature lymphocytes (Figure 7). Flow cytometry indicated that these cells were positive for cyCD3, CD7, CD8, CD13, and CD56 (partially), but negative for CD2, smCD3, CD34, TdT, B-cell antigens, and cytoplasmic myeloperoxidase (MPO). A multiplex PCR analysis for TCRγ chain and immunoglobulin heavy chain genes yielded negative results regarding the monoclonal gene rearrangements. A cytogenetic examination of the bone marrow cells, including abundant leukemic cells, gave a normal karyotype of 46, XY. He was subsequently diagnosed with ETP-ALL according to these immunophenotypes of abnormal lymphocytes, which fulfilled the criteria of the TCCSG L99-15 study scoring system but not the St. Jude Criteria due to the CD8 positivity. Although the leukemia was resistant to CHOP (cyclophosphamide, adriamycin, vincristine, and prednisolone) and SMILE (dexamethasone, methotrexate, ifosfamide, L-asparaginase, and etoposide) [35] regimens, a complete remission (CR) was obtained with the MEC regimen (mitoxantrone, etoposide, and cytarabine) followed by nelarabine. He underwent unrelated allogeneic bone marrow transplantation and is currently maintaining CR. Importantly, a marked intestinal involvement at presentation has not been reported in ETP-ALL.

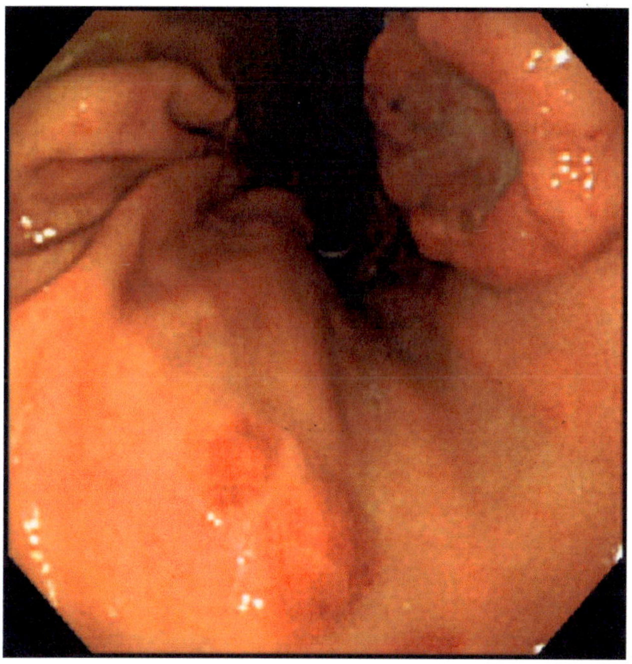

Figure 4. Gastrofiberscopy of Case 1 on admission to our hospital. Multiple ulcerative nodules were visible on the gastric mucosa.

Case 2: An 83-year-old female who presented with generalized lymphadenopathy was referred to our hospital. She was tentatively diagnosed with peripheral T-cell lymphoma-unspecified according to the findings from a biopsy specimen from a cervical lymph node, which histologically showed diffuse infiltration of CD3-positive lymphocytes and a proliferation of Langerhans cells without dysplastic features. The lymphadenopathy disappeared after CHOP chemotherapy; however, blast cells (Figure 8A) appeared in the peripheral blood and rapidly increased in number without recurrence of the lymphadenopathy after the fourth round of CHOP chemotherapy. The blast cells expressed cyCD3, CD7, CD56, CD33, and CD34, but not CD2, smCD3, CD4, and CD8. PCR of the TCRγ chain gene

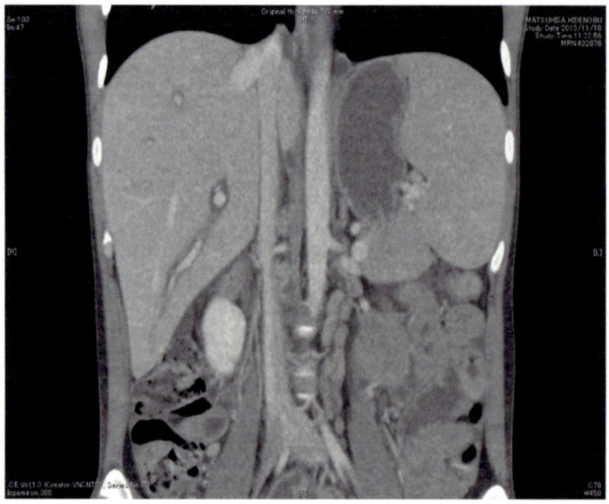

Figure 5. Contrast CT scanning of the abdomen (coronal image) in Case 1. Marked hepatosplenomegaly and wall thickening of the small intestine (arrows) were observed.

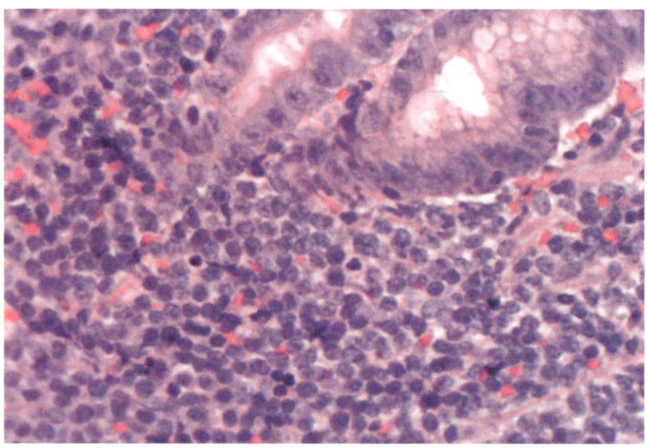

Figure 6. Histology of the biopsied gastric mucosal nodule in Case 1. Diffuse and dense infiltration of immature lymphocytes is shown (H-E staining, 100×).

demonstrated a monoclonally rearranged faint band. These blast cells were negative for MPO staining; however, some of the cells were weakly positive for both α-naphthyl butyrate (Figure 8B) and naphthol AS-D chloroacetate esterase staining (Figure 8C), suggesting their ability to differentiate toward monocytes and granulocytes. A chromosomal analysis revealed an abnormal karyotype of 46, XX, t(12;20)(q13;q11.2) in seven of the 20 bone marrow cells analyzed. A final diagnosis of ETP-ALL was made according to these immunophenotypes, which fulfilled both the TCCSG L99-15 study scoring system and St. Jude criteria. Her leukemia was resistant to any chemotherapeutic protocols for lymphoma, ALL, and AML, and she ultimately died due to disease progression.

http://dx.doi.org/10.5772/60901

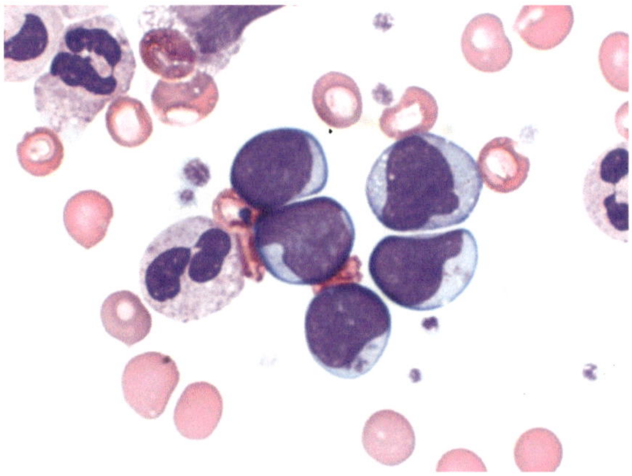

Figure 7. Abnormal lymphocytes in the peripheral blood in Case 1 (Wright-Giemsa staining, 1,000×).

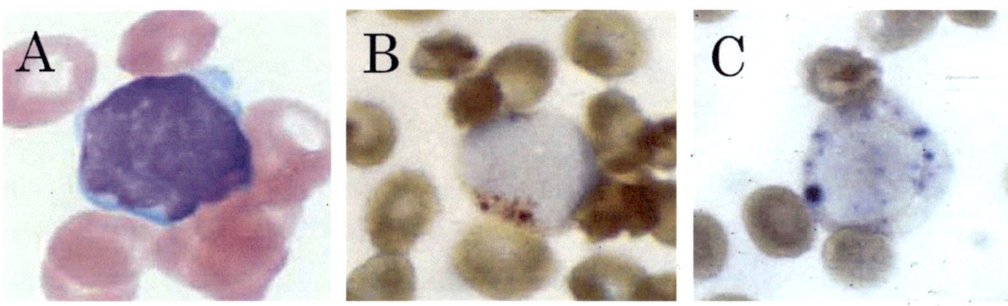

Figure 8. Abnormal lymphocytes in the peripheral blood in Case 2. A: Wright-Giemsa staining, 1,000×); B: a-naphthyl butyrate esterase staining; C: naphthol AS-D chloroacetate esterase staining. Esterase staining was performed using a kit for double esterase staining (Muto Pure Chemicals, Tokyo, Japan).

In both cases, it was difficult to make a precise diagnosis with a histopathological strategy, and the immunophenotypic analysis was crucially important to determine the final diagnosis. Both cases are very interesting in terms of the phenotypic presentation reflecting an oncogenic development at the level of granulocyte-macrophage-T-cell progenitors in early normal hematopoiesis. In addition, morphologically, leukemic cells in these two cases had a slightly condensed chromatin network of the nucleus when compared with that of classical ALL blasts and these nuclei were irregular in shape.

8. Conclusion

More precise and extensive cellular and molecular investigations are required to establish the definite cellular origin and genetic or epigenetic nature of ETP-ALL. An accumulation of ETP-ALL cases and larger clinical trials will establish effective therapeutic strategies for this high-risk leukemia.

Author details

Hiroko Tsunemine and Takayuki Takahashi*

*Address all correspondence to: takahashi.takayuki@shinkohp.or.jp

Department of Hematology, Shinko Hospital, Kobe, Japan

The authors declare that there are no conflicts of interest with any individuals or companies.

References

[1] Pui CH, Evans WE. Treatment of acute lymphoblastic leukemia. N Engl J Med. 2006;354:166-78.

[2] Hoelzer D, Gokbuget N, Digel W, Faak T, Kneba M, Reutzel R, et al. Outcome of adult patients with T-lymphoblastic lymphoma treated according to protocols for acute lymphoblastic leukemia. Blood. 2002;99:4379-85.

[3] LeClerc JM, Billett AL, Gelber RD, Dalton V, Tarbell N, Lipton JM, et al. Treatment of childhood acute lymphoblastic leukemia: results of Dana-Farber ALL Consortium Protocol 87-01. J Clin Oncol. 2002;20:237-46.

[4] Coustan-Smith E, Mullighan CG, Onciu M, Behm FG, Raimondi SC, Pei D, et al. Early T-cell precursor leukaemia: a subtype of very high-risk acute lymphoblastic leukaemia. Lancet Oncol. 2009;10:147-56.

[5] Rothenberg EV, Moore JE, Yui MA. Launching the T-cell-lineage developmental programme. Nat Rev Immunol. 2008;8:9-21.

[6] Bell JJ, Bhandoola A. The earliest thymic progenitors for T cells possess myeloid lineage potential. Nature. 2008;452:764-7.

[7] Wada H, Masuda K, Satoh R, Kakugawa K, Ikawa T, Katsura Y, et al. Adult T-cell progenitors retain myeloid potential. Nature. 2008;452:768-72.

[8] Yui MA, Feng N, Rothenberg EV. Fine-scale staging of T cell lineage commitment in adult mouse thymus. J Immunol. 2010;185:284-93.

[9] Berquam-Vrieze KE, Nannapaneni K, Brett BT, Holmfeldt L, Ma J, Zagorodna O, et al. Cell of origin strongly influences genetic selection in a mouse model of T-ALL. Blood. 2011;118:4646-56.

[10] Inukai T, Kiyokawa N, Campana D, Coustan-Smith E, Kikuchi A, Kobayashi M, et al. Clinical significance of early T-cell precursor acute lymphoblastic leukaemia: results of the Tokyo Children's Cancer Study Group Study L99-15. Br J Haematol. 2012;156:358-65.

[11] Chopra A, Bakhshi S, Pramanik SK, Pandey RM, Singh S, Gajendra S, et al. Immunophenotypic analysis of T-acute lymphoblastic leukemia. A CD5-based ETP-ALL perspective of non-ETP T-ALL. Eur J Haematol. 2014;92:211-8.

[12] Ma M, Wang X, Tang J, Xue H, Chen J, Pan C, et al. Early T-cell precursor leukemia: a subtype of high risk childhood acute lymphoblastic leukemia. Front Med. 2012;6:416-20.

[13] Neumann M, Heesch S, Gokbuget N, Schwartz S, Schlee C, Benlasfer O, et al. Clinical and molecular characterization of early T-cell precursor leukemia: a high-risk subgroup in adult T-ALL with a high frequency of FLT3 mutations. Blood Cancer J. 2012;2:e55.

[14] Allen A, Sireci A, Colovai A, Pinkney K, Sulis M, Bhagat G, et al. Early T-cell precursor leukemia/lymphoma in adults and children. Leuk Res. 2013;37:1027-34.

[15] Patrick K, Wade R, Goulden N, Mitchell C, Moorman AV, Rowntree C, et al. Outcome for children and young people with early T-cell precursor acute lymphoblastic leukaemia treated on a contemporary protocol, UKALL 2003. Br J Haematol. 2014;166:421-4.

[16] Zhang J, Ding L, Holmfeldt L, Wu G, Heatley SL, Payne-Turner D, et al. The genetic basis of early T-cell precursor acute lymphoblastic leukaemia. Nature. 2012;481:157-63.

[17] Aifantis I, Raetz E, Buonamici S. Molecular pathogenesis of T-cell leukaemia and lymphoma. Nat Rev Immunol. 2008;8:380-90.

[18] McCormack MP, Shields BJ, Jackson JT, Nasa C, Shi W, Slater NJ, et al. Requirement for Lyl1 in a model of Lmo2-driven early T-cell precursor ALL. Blood. 2013;122:2093-103.

[19] Treanor LM, Zhou S, Janke L, Churchman ML, Ma Z, Lu T, et al. Interleukin-7 receptor mutants initiate early T cell precursor leukemia in murine thymocyte progenitors with multipotent potential. J Exp Med. 2014;211:701-13.

[20] Neumann M, Heesch S, Schlee C, Schwartz S, Gokbuget N, Hoelzer D, et al. Whole-exome sequencing in adult ETP-ALL reveals a high rate of DNMT3A mutations. Blood. 2013;121:4749-52.

[21] Ley TJ, Ding L, Walter MJ, McLellan MD, Lamprecht T, Larson DE, et al. DNMT3A mutations in acute myeloid leukemia. N Engl J Med. 2010;363:2424-33.

[22] Integrated genomic analyses of ovarian carcinoma. Nature. 2011;474:609-15.

[23] Baldus CD, Burmeister T, Martus P, Schwartz S, Gokbuget N, Bloomfield CD, et al. High expression of the ETS transcription factor ERG predicts adverse outcome in acute T-lymphoblastic leukemia in adults. J Clin Oncol. 2006;24:4714-20.

[24] Baldus CD, Martus P, Burmeister T, Schwartz S, Gokbuget N, Bloomfield CD, et al. Low ERG and BAALC expression identifies a new subgroup of adult acute T-lymphoblastic leukemia with a highly favorable outcome. J Clin Oncol. 2007;25:3739-45.

[25] Heesch S, Schlee C, Neumann M, Stroux A, Kuhnl A, Schwartz S, et al. BAALC-associated gene expression profiles define IGFBP7 as a novel molecular marker in acute leukemia. Leukemia. 2010;24:1429-36.

[26] Menssen HD, Renkl HJ, Rodeck U, Maurer J, Notter M, Schwartz S, et al. Presence of Wilms' tumor gene (wt1) transcripts and the WT1 nuclear protein in the majority of human acute leukemias. Leukemia. 1995;9:1060-7.

[27] Heesch S, Goekbuget N, Stroux A, Tanchez JO, Schlee C, Burmeister T, et al. Prognostic implications of mutations and expression of the Wilms tumor 1 (WT1) gene in adult acute T-lymphoblastic leukemia. Haematologica. 2010;95:942-9.

[28] Heuser M, Beutel G, Krauter J, Dohner K, von Neuhoff N, Schlegelberger B, et al. High meningioma 1 (MN1) expression as a predictor for poor outcome in acute myeloid leukemia with normal cytogenetics. Blood. 2006;108:3898-905.

[29] Grosveld GC. MN1, a novel player in human AML. Blood Cells Mol Dis. 2007;39:336-9.

[30] Hosoya T, Kuroha T, Moriguchi T, Cummings D, Maillard I, Lim KC, et al. GATA-3 is required for early T lineage progenitor development. J Exp Med. 2009;206:2987-3000.

[31] Schrauder A, Reiter A, Gadner H, Niethammer D, Klingebiel T, Kremens B, et al. Superiority of allogeneic hematopoietic stem-cell transplantation compared with chemotherapy alone in high-risk childhood T-cell acute lymphoblastic leukemia: results from ALL-BFM 90 and 95. J Clin Oncol. 2006;24:5742-9.

[32] Chonghaile TN, Roderick JE, Glenfield C, Ryan J, Sallan SE, Silverman LB, et al. Maturation stage of T-cell acute lymphoblastic leukemia determines BCL-2 versus BCL-XL dependence and sensitivity to ABT-199. Cancer Discov. 2014;4:1074-87.

[33] Peirs S, Matthijssens F, Goossens S, Van de Walle I, Ruggero K, de Bock CE, et al. ABT-199 mediated inhibition of BCL-2 as a novel therapeutic strategy in T-cell acute lymphoblastic leukemia. Blood. 2014;124:3738-47.

[34] Van Driessche A, Berneman ZN, Van Tendeloo VF. Active specific immunotherapy targeting the Wilms' tumor protein 1 (WT1) for patients with hematological malignancies and solid tumors: lessons from early clinical trials. Oncologist. 2012;17:250-9.

[35] Yamaguchi M, Kwong KL, Kim WS, Maeda Y, Hashimoto C, Suh C, et al. Phase II study of SMILE chemotherapy for newly diagnosed stage IV, relapsed or refractory extranodal natural killer (NK)/T-cell lymphoma, nasal type: the NK-Cell Tumor Study Group Study. J Clin Oncol. 2011;29:4410-16.

Chapter 3

Leukemia and Retroviral Disease

Lorena Loarca, Neil Sullivan, Vanessa Pirrone and Brian Wigdahl

Additional information is available at the end of the chapter

http://dx.doi.org/10.5772/61254

Abstract

Two human retroviruses, identified as the human T-cell leukemia virus type 1 (HTLV-1) and human immunodeficiency virus type 1 (HIV-1), have been shown to affect millions of people worldwide. In the context of coinfection, the impact of their interactions with respect to HTLV-1-induced adult T-cell leukemia and neurologic disease as well as HIV-1 disease progression has been an understudied area of investigation. HTLV-1/HIV-1 coinfections occur frequently, particularly in large metropolitan areas of the Americas, Africa, Europe, and Japan. The retroviruses HTLV-1 and HIV-1 share some similarities with regard to their genetic structure, general mechanisms of replication, modes of transmission, and cellular tropism; however, there are also significant differences in the details of these properties as well, and they also differ significantly with respect to the etiology of their pathogenic and disease outcomes. Both viruses impair the host immune system with HIV-1 demonstrated to cause the hallmark lethal disease known as the acquired immune deficiency syndrome (AIDS), while HTLV-1 infection has been shown to cause several different forms of T-cell leukemia. In addition, both viruses have also been shown to cause a spectrum of neurologic disorders with HIV-1 shown to cause an array of neurologic syndromes referred to as HIV-1-associated neurologic disorders or HAND, while HTLV-1 has been shown to be the etiologic agent of HTLV-1-associated myelopathy/tropical spastic paraparesis or HAM/TSP. The natural history of the coinfection, however, is different from that observed in monoinfections. Several studies have demonstrated utilizing a number of in vitro models of HTLV-1/HIV-1 coinfection that the two viruses interact in a manner that results in enhanced expression of both viral genomes. Nevertheless, there remains unresolved controversy regarding the overall impact of each virus on progression of disease caused by both viruses during the course of coinfection. Although combination antiretroviral therapy has been shown to work very effectively with respect to maintaining HIV-1 viral loads in the undetectable range, these therapeutic strategies exhibit no benefit for HTLV-1-infected individuals, unless administered immediately after exposure. Furthermore, the treatment options for HTLV-1/HIV-1-coinfected patients are very limited. In recent years, allogeneic stem cell transplantation (alloSCT) has been used for the treatment of leukemia. In this regard, the case of a leukemic patient positive for HIV-1 who was cured of their HIV-1 infection while treated with alloSCT for acute myeloid leukemia has also been examined with regard to impact on HIV-1 disease.

Keywords: HIV-1, HTLV-1, coinfection, ATL/ATLL, HAM/TSP

1. Introduction

HTLV-1/HIV-1 coinfection is very common among drug users, particularly in metropolitan areas [1, 2]. It is estimated that in endemic areas, 10% of HIV-1-infected patients are coinfected with HTLV-1 [3]. The frequency of HTLV-1 and HIV-1 coinfections is on the rise, especially in Africa and South America [4]. Both HTLV-1 and HIV-1 are retroviruses capable of integrating their proviral DNA genome into the host cell chromosome, thereby establishing a latent infection, both of which share quiescent $CD4^+$ T cells as their primary target. However, the life cycle, pathogenesis, and clinical syndromes of these two viruses after infection are very different within this cellular compartment [5, 6]. In the absence of therapeutic intervention, there is a striking difference in the prevalence of disease caused by the two viruses with overt clinical disease far less common after HTLV-1 infection, perhaps because HTLV-1 has existed within the human population for far longer than HIV-1 and therefore may be more highly adapted to its human host. This could explain why HTLV-1 has been shown to cause T-cell transformation and clonal expansion of immortalized cells, whereas HIV-1 induces $CD4^+$ T-cell death [7]. Since the first cases of HIV-1 were reported early in the 1980s, there has been much progress with respect to investigating the viral replication cycle, mechanisms of pathogenesis, as well as the diagnosis and treatment of HIV-1 infection. There are now more than 30 antiretroviral drugs available for the management of HIV-1 infection, with them, their modes of inhibition and novel drug discovery techniques have been reviewed previously [8]. A number of drug combinations have been shown to be quite effective with regard to reducing HIV-1 titers to undetectable levels with subsequent maintenance of this well-controlled state for many years if not decades, yet they do not cure individuals because the drugs are effective against actively replicating virus and not the latent, integrated provirus. In the absence of treatment and subsequent to the development of drug resistance, particularly in the precombination antiretroviral therapy (cART) era, HIV-1 has been shown to induce severe immunosuppression leading to AIDS with the ultimate development of opportunistic infections and cancers. In the case of HTLV-1 infection, most patients remain asymptomatic for many years before the onset of disease. In contrast to HIV-1, only a small percentage of untreated HTLV-1 carriers develop clinically apparent disease [9, 10]. HTLV-1 may cause neurologic problems, skin and inflammatory disorders, leukemia, and leukemia/lymphoma [9, 10]. The treatments available for HTLV-1-related complications are limited, and the antiretrovirals used to treat HIV-1 infection are not efficacious unless taken early after first contact with the virus [6] when viral replication is responsible for expansion in the number of infected cells as compared to expansion of infected cells by cell division with the associated integrated HTLV-1 provirus expanding within the transformed cell population in the absence of infectious HTLV-1 production [5]. The clinical implications and the molecular interactions between HTLV-1 and HIV-1 remain understudied. The management of patients coinfected with HTLV-1/HIV-1 is clearly a challenge. Although it is well known that both HTLV-1 and HIV-1 may cause progressive diseases within the central nervous system, the focus here will center on the interaction of these two retroviruses within the immune system and more specifically examine the impact of HIV-1 infection on the leukemogenic process induced by HTLV-1 in coinfected individuals as well as the impact of HTLV-1 infection on HIV-1 disease. A summary of the epidemiology of the two viruses within the human population is shown in Table 1.

	HIV-1	**HTLV-1**
Prevalence	35 million people	20 million people
Transmission	· Sexual transmission · Parenteral transmission (blood transfusions, organ transplantation, and via infected sharp objects) · Mother to child (breast-feeding and during delivery)	· Sexual transmission · Parenteral transmission (blood transfusions, organ transplantation, and via infected sharp objects) · Mother to child (breast-feeding and during delivery)
Endemic areas	Africa, Eastern Europe, South Asia, and China	Caribbean region, Central Africa, and South Japan

Table 1. Epidemiological comparison of HTLV-1 and HIV-1 infection and disease

2. Introduction to Human T-cell Leukemia Virus type 1 (HTLV-1)

HTLV-1 is a single-stranded positive-sense RNA, a type C retrovirus, and the etiologic agent of adult T-cell leukemia (ATL) or adult T-cell leukemia/lymphoma (ATLL) and a progressive neuroinflammatory disease known as HTLV-1-associated myelopathy/tropical spastic paraparesis (HAM/TSP), with some similarities to multiple sclerosis due to the progressive destruction/loss of myelination [11] (also reviewed in [68]). It was the first human retrovirus discovered [10, 12] and isolated in the United States in the late 1970s, with parallel discoveries by investigators in Japan [13–15]. In this regard, in the United States, HTLV-1 particles were detected in fresh peripheral blood lymphocytes and in the T-cell lymphoblastoid cell lines, HUT 102 and CTLC-3, derived from a 28-year-old African American man suffering from cutaneous T-cell lymphoma [13]. At nearly the same time, the Japanese investigators isolated HTLV-1 from a series of cell lines derived from cases of adult T-cell leukemia [13, 15]. Over the years, HTLV-1 has been shown to be associated with the human population for a much longer period of time than the HIV-1 with HTLV-1 being detected in remains of a 1,500 Chilean mummy [16], while HIV-1 sequences have been detected in humans only as far back as the 1920s, many decades before its discovery in the mid-1980s. Based on extensive studies performed over the past three to four decades concerning clinical parameters, epidemiology, molecular biology and virology, immunology, cancer biology, neurobiology, and immune- and neuropathogenesis of HTLV-1 infection, the virus appears to be much more adapted to the human population with greater than 95% of the infected individuals harboring the virus asymptomatically with only small percentages of individuals presenting with symptomatic disease in the form of leukemia or neurologic disease [9, 17]. This epidemiologic pattern is quite different than the widespread highly lethal disease of the immune and nervous systems caused by the HIV-1 in the absence of highly active antiretroviral therapy (HAART) [18] (also reviewed in [19]).

2.1. HTLV-1 genetic architecture and viral replication

The HTLV-1 genome comprises four main genetic components that include gag, pol, env, and pX sequences (Figure 1). The gag, pol, and env genes encode the structural proteins and enzymatic proteins, with a 5 and 3 long terminal repeat (LTR) at each end of the genome, typical of all viruses in the Retroviridae family. Gag proteins have been designated the group-specific antigens, which encode the inner virion structural components such as matrix, capsid, and nucleocapsid. The pro and pol genes encode the protease, integrase, and viral RNA-dependent DNA polymerase or reverse transcriptase, respectively, and the env gene that encodes the viral surface and transmembrane envelope proteins [63]. What makes HTLV-1 unique compared to other retroviruses is the pX region. This region encodes multiple accessory and regulatory proteins that give HTLV-1 its unique phenotype, one of which is the multifunction oncoprotein Tax. Tax has been shown to alter the course of gene expression at a number of points during the course of viral infection and in this regard has been shown to regulate viral replication, modulate cellular gene expression, induce inflammation, and block apoptosis to pinpoint just a few, with many of its functions being identified by Tax mutagenesis [20]. More importantly, this protein is known for its ability to transform T lymphocytes into cancerous leukemic cells, as described in the following sections. HTLV-1 infection of susceptible cells via transmission involving transfer of virus from an infected cell to an uninfected cell occurs very efficiently as a result of specific cell–cell interactions and less efficiently from cell-free viral particle-driven transmission [21–23]. The replication cycle of HTLV-1 begins with the interaction between the viral Env glycoproteins and the specific cellular receptor proteins. At least three cellular receptors have been found to facilitate viral attachment and entry into the cell, and these include the glucose transporter 1 (GLUT1) [24, 25], neuropilin-1 (NRP-1) [26–28], and heparan sulfate proteoglycans (HSPG) [29–31]. During the membrane fusion process and after entry of the viral capsid into the cytoplasm, the viral genomic RNA is reverse transcribed into DNA, by the viral particle-associated reverse transcriptase. During the process of reverse transcription, the newly synthesized proviral DNA is transported to the nuclear membrane. After the translocation of the proviral DNA into the nucleus, it is subsequently integrated into the host cell chromosomal material, which is catalyzed by the activity of the viral-encoded, particle-associated integrase. Following integration, the transcription of viral RNAs and the translation of viral proteins are carried out by host machinery with the subsequent assembly of viral particles and release of infectious virions into the extracellular environment.

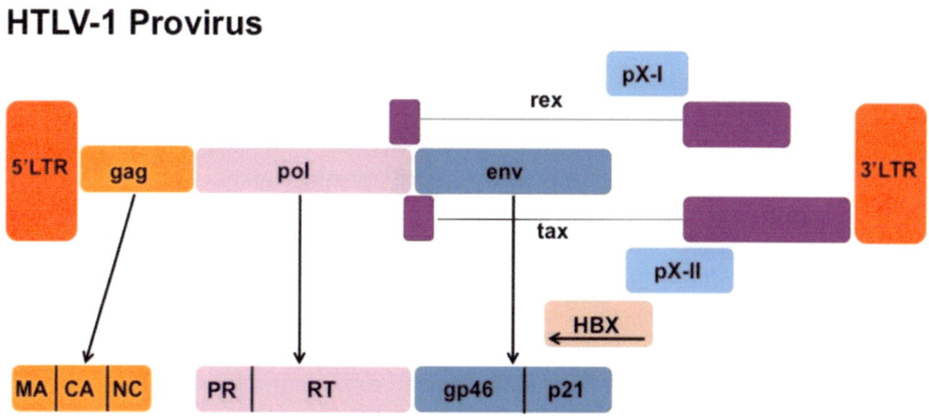

Figure 1. HTLV-1 genomic architecture. A schematic representation of the proviral genome organization, open reading frames, and viral products of HTLV-1. The organization of the ~9-kb genome is depicted along with the genes and their transcriptional splicing.

2.2. HTLV-1 infectivity, transmission, and pathogenesis

Although the tropism of HTLV-1 may not represent a direct representation of cells that can be infected *in vivo*, studies performed *in vitro* are often performed to get an approximation regarding the cell types that may be targeted by a virus during the course of *in vivo* infection. If proven susceptible and productive for viral replication, these cell types may then be used for virus propagation or studies concerning viral pathogenesis. In this regard, during *in vitro* propagation of HTLV-1, a wide variety of non-T-cell types have been shown to be susceptible to viral infection, including human primary endothelial cells [32], monocytes [33], microglial cells [33], B cells [34], mammary epithelial cells [35], and dendritic cells (DCs) [36], although the relative level of viral production between the different cell types was shown to differ greatly. In parallel with these observations, HTLV-1 infection *in vivo has* been shown to occur primarily in $CD4^+$ T-cell subsets and to a lesser extent in $CD8^+$ T cells in both asymptomatic and symptomatic HTLV-1-infected patients [37]. Furthermore, Koyanagi and colleagues [37] demonstrated HTLV-1 tropism for $CD8^+$ T cells, monocytes, and B cells in the majority of the asymptomatic HTLV-1-positive individuals studied, as well as in patients with HTLV-1-related ATL or HAM/TSP. Other groups have also confirmed these observations and have reported that HTLV-1 also infects macrophages [37], DCs [38], synovial fluid cells [39], and astrocytes [40] among others when the target cells are examined *in vivo*. Perhaps of great importance in the pathogenesis of HTLV-1-associated neurologic disease is the penetration of the virus into the bone marrow compartment with increasing numbers of HTLV-1 DNA^+/RNA^-progenitor cells detected in patients suffering from HAM/TSP as compared to patients with ATL [41], thus further demonstrating another layer of complexity with respect to target cell identification that likely involves latency, immune invasion, and adaptation to the host.

HTLV-1 has been shown to be transmitted primarily via three routes: (i) mother-to-child transmission [42], (ii) sexual intercourse [43], and (iii) parenteral transmission. The vertical transmission of HTLV-1 from mother to child occurs via the transfer of maternally infected lymphocytes to the fetus or newborn through the placenta [44], during delivery [45, 46], or by breastfeeding [47]. Sexual transmission is a common route of HTLV-1 transmission. Sexual transmission of HTLV-1 occurs more efficiently from male to female than from female to male. This might be due in part to the higher numbers of HTLV-1-infected lymphocytes found in semen than in vaginal secretions [48]. The parenteral transmission of HTLV-1 includes blood or cellular blood products transferred during the transfusion process [49], organ transplantation [50], and possibly percutaneous exposure of the virus via sharing of contaminated objects such as razor blades and needles, particularly among drug users and healthcare workers [48]. Parenteral transmission represents a large proportion of infected individuals. Regardless of how the virus is acquired, the infected cells produce numerous progeny virion. Particularly in the case of T lymphocytes, they too are activated and clonally proliferate, further driving the expansion and number of cells harboring provirus DNA.

2.3. Cancers and other diseases associated with HTLV-1 infection

Currently, there are approximately 20 million individuals living with HTLV-1 worldwide [7]. In highly endemic regions such as the Caribbean Basin, Central Africa, and southern Japan, more than 1% of the population is infected with HTLV-1 (reviewed in [51] and [52]). Approximately 95% of the individuals infected with HTLV-1 remain as asymptomatic carriers throughout their lives [9, 17]. As previously indicated, HTLV-1 is the etiological agent for causing two distinct disease phenotypes, ATL and HAM/TSP, the first involving a $CD4^+$ T-cell malignancy and the second involving a progressive neurological disease. Interestingly, the specific response of the immune system to the virus seems to influence which clinical manifestation presents and likely includes other factors such as route of transmission, host genetics, and perhaps aspects of viral genetics.

Less than 5% of the HTLV-1-infected individuals develop ATL after a long period of latency, which in some cases can be greater than 50 years [53]. ATL is more prevalent in men than in women with a median onset age of 55 years. ATL can present as four overlapping clinical manifestations that are broken down into smoldering, chronic, acute, and lymphoma [54, 55]. Approximately 5% of the patients with ATL have been shown to develop the smoldering type of disease presenting with a number of minor symptoms with leukemic cells infiltrating the skin causing surface lesions leading to a breach in the epithelial layer of the skin [56]. It has been estimated that 20% of the HTLV-1-positive patients will develop a chronic form of the disease. These patients experience similar manifestations as individuals with smoldering ATL, but they also develop abnormalities in their viscera, leading to impairment of spleen, liver, and lymphatic functions as well as a slight increase in the levels of leukemic cells [54].

In the acute phase of ATL, the disease progresses quickly, and patients exhibit generalized swelling of the lymph nodes, elevated calcium and lactate dehydrogenase levels, impairment of liver and spleen function, skin lesions, bone wounds, and release of cytokines by malignant cells. All of these abnormalities cause patients to experience fever, cough, malaise, dehydration, lethargy, shortness of breath, and inflammation of the lymph nodes. About 55% of patients with ATL experience the acute form of the disease. Furthermore, around 20% of the

ATL cases are of the lymphoma type, and they experience inflammation of the lymph nodes, with no evidence of leukemic cells in the periphery, and general suppression of their immune system function as summarized in Figure 2. The survival rate associated with ATL from the time of first disease manifestations is approximately 24.3, 10.2, and 6.2 months for the chronic, lymphoma, and acute types, respectively [55]. The actual process of transforming T lymphocytes and developing ATL is dependent on the HTLV-1 oncoprotein Tax in part as well as a number of other factors indicated above.

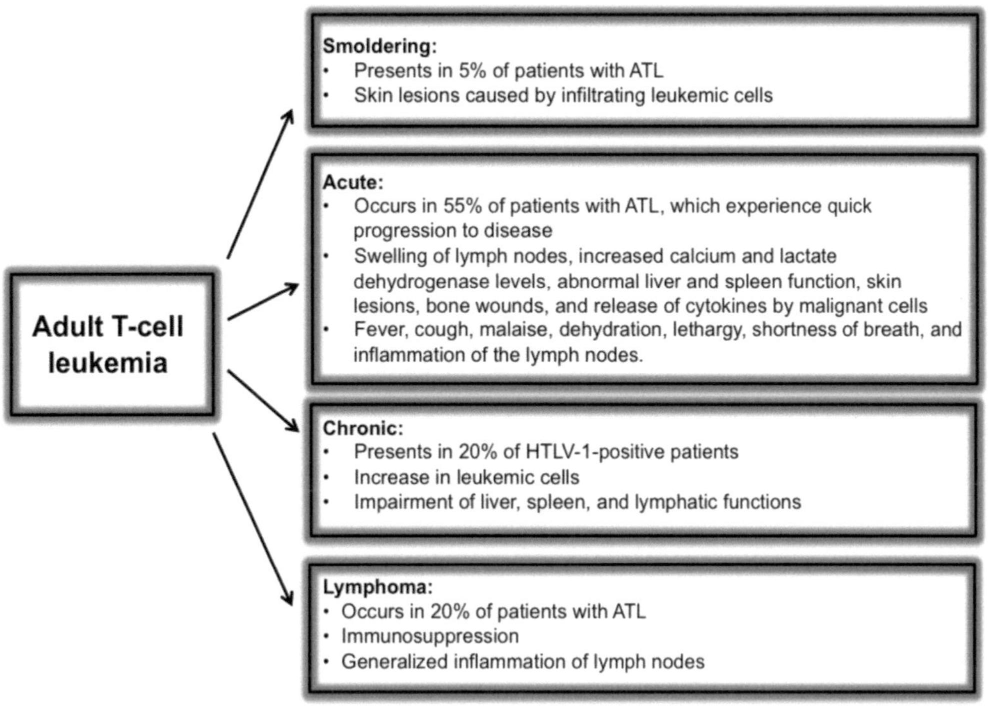

Figure 2. Summary of pathogenic forms of HTLV-1-induced leukemia. A summary of disease outcomes and symptomatology during the course of HTLV-1-induced leukemia.

Like most other RNA viruses, due to the constraints of genome size, as compared to larger DNA viruses, the proteins they encode usually have multiple functions. The multifunction oncoprotein Tax is a 353 amino acid phosphoprotein that is a transcriptional activator of the LTR, and the protein is primarily responsible for transformation of T lymphocytes. It has been shown that selected domains of Tax are responsible for interacting with the host transcription factors NF-κB, ATF/CREB, Sp1, Ets-1, and many others in conjunction with their cognate binding sites. This leads to enhanced chromatin remodeling, transactivation of the LTR, activation of host genes, and enhanced viral gene expression. More importantly in the process of cellular transformation is its chronic activation of signaling pathways (JAK/STAT), expression of cytokines and their receptors (IL-2, IL-2Rα), and interaction with cellular tumor suppressors (p53) and cell cycle kinases and regulators (p15, p16, and p21), to name a few, all of which increase the probability of uncontrolled cell division and transformation exhaustively reviewed [10, 57, 58]. As of now, it is not fully understood how and why Tax, which is a strong inducer of transformation, only induces ATL in 5% of infected individuals. This could be, in part, the immune system efficiently removing infected cells and/or combating Tax with specific host restriction factors. Additionally, Tax has been shown to be secreted from infected cells and have bystander effects, such as pro-inflammatory cytokines and the infiltration of Tax-specific $CD8^+$ T cells into the CNS, thus playing a part in HAM/TSP [59–64].

HTLV-1 infection also causes HAM/TSP, a neuroinflammatory disorder that mostly affects the spinal cord and brain due to chronic proinflammatory cytokines, the destruction of myelin, and the cells that secrete it, oligodendrocytes [64–66]. It was first thought that there might be a hormonal component regulating HAM/TSP, as it occurs more frequently and progresses more rapidly in women than in men, particularly if the first signs of disease occur before menopause [67]. The onset of HAM/TSP usually happens after 20–30 years of latency [4], and the average age in which patients experience the first signs of disease is about 43 years of age [68]. The early phase of HAM/TSP is presented with a profound inflammatory response resulting in lower back pain, weakness in the lower limbs, and impairment of urinary and sexual functions. Eventually, a chronic degenerative disorder develops characterized by the progressive loss of myelin in the thoracic and lumbar regions of the spinal cord [67]. Damage to the central nervous system (CNS) also occurs in patients with HAM/TSP, likely mediated by particular cells of the immune system such as $CD4^+$ T cells, $CD8^+$ T cells, DCs, and cells of the monocyte–macrophage lineage. For instance, it has been proposed (28) that at least three mechanisms participate in the process of myelin degradation that occurs in HAM/TSP: (i) direct injury caused by $CD8^+$ T cells, (ii) damage mediated by an uncontrolled cytokine storm, and (iii) an autoimmune response. Previous studies have shown that infiltrating activated Tax-specific $CD8^+$ cytotoxic T lymphocytes (CTLs) in the peripheral blood and cerebrospinal fluid (CSF) induced lysis of HTLV-1-infected cells triggering a pro-inflammatory cytokine storm. There is evidence that HTLV-1 has been found in the CNS. The release of pro-inflammatory factors such as TNF-α and IFN-γ secreted by activated $CD8^+$ CTLs injures the CNS. Further damage may occur as a result of the molecular mimicry between the Tax protein and the neuronal antigen heterogeneous ribonuclear protein-A1 (hnRNP-A1), which may cause an autoimmune response [69].

Both HTLV-1 and HIV-1 have been shown to penetrate the bone marrow to varying degrees during the course of monoinfection, and it is assumed to be the case during the course of coinfection with both viruses but less information is available in this regard. Clearly, the relative penetration of the two viruses into the bone marrow compartment during the course of coinfection may have dramatic effects on HTLV-1- and HIV-1-induced pathogenesis and disease caused by either viruses, and these pathogenic processes will also be a subject of this review. These interactions may periodically alter the balance between immune control and HTLV-1 infection, and the periodic imbalance has also been associated with the etiology of other inflammatory diseases such as arthropathy, pulmonary alveolitis, uveitis, dermatitis, Sjögren's syndrome, Behçet's disease, thyroid disease, prostatitis, cystitis, hepatitis, polymyositis, arthritis, and a sarcoidosis-like disorder [67].

3. Introduction to HIV-1 infection, pathogenesis, and disease

In 1981, the first cases of AIDS were reported in the United States. At the beginning of the epidemic, AIDS was first identified in homosexual men and drug users. However, the epidemic rapidly spread to the general population primarily by heterosexual intercourse [70]. In 1983, a retrovirus was isolated at the Pasteur Institute in France from a lymph node biopsy from a homosexual man with lymphadenopathy presenting with AIDS-like symptoms [71]. Almost in parallel at the National Cancer Institute in Bethesda, United States, the same virus was identified from samples of patients suffering from AIDS [72]. In 1986, the virus was named the human immunodeficiency virus (HIV) and demonstrated to be the causative agent of AIDS [73].

There are two types of HIV, HIV type 1 (HIV-1) and HIV type 2 (HIV-2), which are genetically and morphologically related viruses that share similarities in their mechanisms of replication and transmission. However, HIV-1 and HIV-2 differ in clinical disease progression and geographical distribution. HIV-1 leads to overt disease much faster than HIV-2, with worldwide distribution, whereas HIV-2 infections are more prevalent in West Africa [74]. HIV-1 is divided into four genetically different groups: M (main), O (outlier), N (non-M, non-O), and P. The group M, which accounts for 98% of the HIV-1 cases worldwide, is further classified into nine subtypes, with subtype B being the most prevalent within North America [75].

3.1. HIV-1 genetic architecture, entry, and viral replication

HIV-1 is also a type C retrovirus that belongs to the genus lentivirus. On a genomic level, HIV-1 is similar to HTLV-1 in a number of aspects. They both contain 5 and 3 LTR and gag, pol, and env genes. However, HIV-1 lacks the pX region and encodes for other accessory proteins that have some overlapping function with those of HTLV-1. HIV-1 proviral DNA encodes for the accessory proteins Tat, Vpu, Nef, Vif, Rev, and Vpr (Figure 3) [6, 76]. Tat is similar in function to Tax in the sense it can transactivate the LTR but does not function in cell transformation. Similarly, both Rev and Rex function to export unspliced and singly spliced RNAs from the nucleus. While HIV-1 shares sequence similarity at the genome level, it has been shown to utilize a different receptor for entry.

The HIV-1 envelope glycoprotein gp120 is the trimeric spike on the surface of the virion that has been shown to mediate attachment to the host target cells by engaging the CD4 receptor embedded in the plasma membrane. Subsequent structural changes mediate the exposure and interaction of the V3 region of gp120 to the chemokine coreceptors, either CXCR4 or CCR5 (although others have also been identified to facilitate this process as well), depending on V3 sequence and charge, and mediate fusion of the viral plasma membrane with the host cell membrane. Once the particle has been internalized, the capsid and associated viral enzymes and RNA remain associated in the cytoplasm in a capsid-like structure, where the viral reverse transcriptase continues to be transcribed from viral RNA to DNA (a process that is likely initiated as the viral particle interfaces with the cell surface proteins involved in viral entry). As the reverse transcription process continues to completion, the capsid structure transitions to a preintegration complex (PIC) containing the reverse transcriptase, integrase, capsid, and

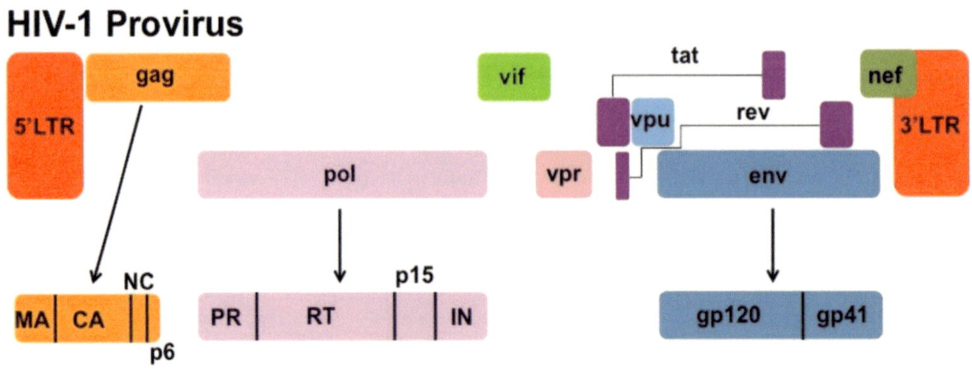

Figure 3. HIV-1 genomic architecture. A schematic representation of the proviral genome organization open reading frame and viral products of HIV-1. The organization of the ~10-kb genome is depicted along with the genes and their transcriptional splicing.

Vpr, and this structure has been shown to be transferred to the nuclear membrane. After entry into the nucleus, the proviral DNA genome is integrated into the host cell chromosome, with recent studies characterizing integration site preference and how it changes with disease progression [77–79]. Once integrated, the proviral DNA becomes part of the cellular chromatin environment and subjected to host machinery involved in the processes of transcription and translation. In conjunction with a number of cellular transcription factors and the viral transactivator proteins Tat and Vpr, transactivation directed by the LTR-driven contained within the integrated provirus is initiated and used as a template for the transcription of viral genomic RNAs and viral mRNAs with the subsequent translation of these viral mRNA into structural, enzymatic, and accessory proteins. From there, the viral polyproteins an proteins are recruited and aggregate primarily in the vicinity of the plasma membrane, resulting in the formation and release of mature infectious virions as previously reviewed [80, 81].

3.2. HIV-1 infectivity, transmission, and pathogenesis

As a result of studies performed in cell lines and primary human cells cultured *in vitro*, transplanted human cells maintained *in vivo* in engineered animals, and primary cells examined in an *ex vivo* experimental environment, HIV-1 has been shown to most efficiently infect activated CD4$^+$ T cells [82], although these cells do not need to be activated in order for infection to occur [83]. Both HIV and HTLV-1 share CD4$^+$ T cells as their cell target, which was further demonstrated by complementation viral envelopes for each other [84]. In addition to the CD4$^+$ T-cell compartment, a number of other human cellular compartments are infected by HIV-1, including cells of the monocyte–macrophage lineage, some subsets of dendritic cells, microglial cells and astrocytes within the brain, hematopoietic progenitor cells, and endothelial cells lining the blood-brain barrier [85, 86].

Studies performed *in vitro* have shown that all HIV-1 isolates infect activated peripheral blood mononuclear cells (PBMCs). Some isolates are able to infect CD4$^+$ T-cell lines, T-cell leukemia cell lines, and monocyte-derived macrophages (MDMs). The target cell population and coreceptor utilization seems to change during disease progression, and the once clear distinction between CXCR4-utilizing or X4 versus the CCR5-utilizing or R5 viruses as compared to the designations referred to as T-tropic and M-tropic now seems to be also guided by the relative utilization of different levels of the CD4 receptor present on T cells and cells of the monocyte–macrophage lineage [87]. During the acute phase of infection and to a lesser extent at later times during the course of disease, primarily due to cART combating replication competent virus, HIV-1 infects $CD4^+$ T-cell populations, with the resting memory $CD4^+$ T cells establishing a latent HIV-1 reservoir. The majority of activated and infected $CD4^+$ T cells will be eliminated, and during this T-cell depletion phase, a portion of the activated $CD4^+$ T cells will undergo a reprogramming of transcription and translation to allow them to survive and differentiate into a resting memory cell phenotype. This resting memory $CD4^+$ T-cell can contribute to the latent reservoir because it was infected and then differentiated into a resting memory cell or as the cell was differentiated into a memory cell it became infected; regardless of the mode of infection, the HIV-1 provirus survives, along with a substantial number of defective proviral genotypes [78, 79]. Because memory $CD4^+$ T cells live for many years, with a predicted half-life of 44 months [79, 88], these cells maintain one of the critical latent reservoirs of HIV-1 and a complicating factor in the pursuit to identify an effective means to cure the HIV-1-infected individual by a new generation of treatment strategies. However, there are very likely a number of additional cellular reservoirs that facilitate the persistence of HIV-1 during prolonged cART. For example, cells of the monocyte–macrophage lineage in the peripheral blood and other lymphoid tissues, resident macrophages of the central nervous system, astrocytes, DCs, follicular dendritic cells (FDCs), hematopoietic progenitor cells (HPCs) in the bone marrow, and specialized epithelial cells within the kidney likely play a role in maintaining HIV-1 during clinical latency prior to the start of any form of therapy despite ongoing immune surveillance and after the start of cART [85]. Each of these cell types present a unique challenge with respect to a cure based on the IR rate of cell turnover, the relative proviral genome transcriptional competency, the innate capacity of the virus to move out of the reservoir, the continued production of infected cells from infected precursors, and the poor drug penetrating ability into these physiological niches, with resting memory $CD4^+$ T cells and cells within the brain and bone marrow being prime examples.

It has been suggested that HIV-1 can be transmitted via free virus or HIV-1-infected cells present in infected blood and body fluids that enter the blood stream of an uninfected individual. The three routes of HIV-1 transmission are (i) via sexual intercourse, (ii) from mother to child, and (iii) parenteral transmission [76]. Sexual transmission is the most common mode of HIV-1 transmission and accounts for the 80% of infections in adults [89] and includes vaginal, anal, and oral unprotected sex between an infected individual and his or her uninfected partner. The risk of HIV-1 transmission is higher between homosexual men as compared to the risk during heterosexual intercourse and individuals whom engage in high risk behaviors [90]; however, this trend can be steadily reduced by prophylactic antiviral use and educating the public. Parenteral transmission of HIV-1 is usually associated with the transfusion of contaminated blood, transplant of infected organs, and sharing of infected sharps, needles, or syringes [76]. Mother-to-child HIV-1 transmission occurs during pregnancy, delivery, or breastfeeding. The presence of higher levels of HIV-1 RNA in blood/body fluids of the infected host has been associated with greater probabilities of transmission [91].

3.3. Diseases caused by HIV-1

According to the World Health Organization (WHO), by the end of 2013, there were 35 million people living with HIV worldwide, and 1.5 million people died as a consequence of AIDS-associated diseases [92]. The course of HIV-1 infection consists of three phases of disease: primary or acute, asymptomatic/chronic, and AIDS. After 2 weeks of initial exposure to HIV-1, approximately 50–70% of the infected patients experience nonspecific symptoms that do not last for more than 4 weeks. These symptoms include increase in body temperature, sore throat, cephalea, joint and muscle pain, general discomfort, and weight loss. Around 70% of patients will develop a rash on trunk and face [6]. This is followed by a long-term period (in many individuals, this highly variable period has been thought to be longer than 10 years but may be altered by many host and comorbidity factors) of asymptomatic chronic infection [93]. This phase is marked by a loss of $CD4^+$ T cells at an annual rate of 30 to 60 cells/mm^3 [6]. HIV-1 titers in the peripheral blood, and antibodies to HIV-1 become readily detectable [76]. Most patients do not present major symptoms; however, some experience tiredness and swollen lymph nodes. Less than 1% of patients in this phase develop AIDS within a period of 1–2 years. The more advanced disease symptoms begin when the $CD4^+$ T-cell levels drop below 500 cell/mm^3. During this stage, HIV-1-infected patients become immunocompromised, developing opportunistic infections such as oral candidiasis, pneumococcal infections, tuberculosis, and infections caused by the herpes simplex and varicella zoster viruses. When the CD4 counts decrease below 200 cells/mm^3, they are clinically diagnosed as having progressed to AIDS. Here HIV-1-infected patients are at high risk of serious diseases like systemic fungal infections, toxoplasma encephalitis, and cryptococcal meningitis, reactivation of other latent viruses such as cytomegalovirus (CMV), and other opportunistic infections, [94], which is primarily due to the decrease in T-cell count. AIDS patients are also susceptible to developing AIDS- and non-AIDS-defining cancers. Kaposi sarcoma (KS) induced by human herpes virus 8 and non-Hodgkin's lymphoma are two examples of AIDS-defining cancers. Importantly, the incidence of AIDS-defining cancers and opportunistic infections in HIV-1-infected patients has dropped since the introduction in 1996 of the highly active antiretroviral therapy (HAART) for the treatment of HIV-1 in North America, Europe, and Australia [95]. In contrast, the frequency of non-AIDS-defining cancers such as cervical and anal cancer caused by human papilloma virus, liver cancer, Hodgkin's lymphoma, lung cancer, and prostate cancer has increased among the HIV-1-infected population [95].

4. Impact of HIV-1 on HTLV-1 disease progression

The effect that HIV-1 has on the progression of HTLV-1 infection remains controversial, as there are very few studies that have directly examined the process interaction. However, it is likely that the periods of immunosuppression observed during the course of HIV-1 disease include the first 3–6 months of the primary infection, a time when the $CD4^+$ T-cell compartment is acutely targeted by HIV-1, the period involving the transition from asymptomatic clinical latency to symptomatic disease prior to therapeutic intervention, and last during the final progressive decrease in the $CD4^+$ T-cell count prior to the availability of therapy or after the development of drug resistance without the availability of alternative therapies, which may very likely alter the course of primary HTLV-1 infection, the development and control of ATL, or the etiology and progression of HAM/TSP. Although HIV-1 has not been shown to infect bone marrow stem cells, it has been shown to infect more differentiated progenitor cells. In addition, HTLV-1 has also been shown by Jacobson and coworkers [96] to penetrate the bone marrow compartment with the detection of HTLV-1 DNA in the absence or presence of detectable transcription. Given these observations, it is possible that HIV-1 infection of similar cell populations in the bone marrow may impact HTLV-1 gene expression programming and alter the functional course of these cell populations with respect to the development and control of ATL and HAM/TSP.

4.1. Incidence of HAM/TSP among HTLV-1/HIV-1-coinfected patients

Much knowledge of viral coinfection and HAM/TSP has come from longitudinal and cross-sectional studies of patient cohorts. While much still needs to be understood on a molecular biologic and immunologic level, these human studies are invaluable with respect to identifying correlations that allow one to develop experimental designs to explore mechanistic avenues to determine the role of virus–virus interactions. Based on these studies, it was determined that less than 2% of the individuals were infected with HTLV-1 develop HAM/TSP [97, 98]. Previous studies have suggested that HIV-1 increases the risk of HAM/TSP in HTLV-1/HIV-1-coinfected individuals. For example, the incidence of HAM/TSP is 9.7% among HTLV-1/HIV-1-coinfected individuals in a cohort of patients from New Orleans, Louisiana. These patients did not present with AIDS, and their $CD4^+$ T-cell levels were normal or slightly elevated [99]. The occurrence of myelopathy in HTLV-1/HIV-1-coinfected individuals was estimated in a case-control study in Rio de Janeiro, Brazil. The results indicated that 73% of the coinfected patients and 16% of the patients infected with only HIV-1 developed myelopathy [100]. Another group reported that the prevalence of HAM/TSP among HTLV-1/HIV-1-coinfected patients in Brazil was 8% [101]. Schutte and coworkers [102] observed in a cohort of patients in Pretoria, South Africa, that HTLV-1/HIV-1-coinfected individuals were prone to developing HAM/TSP at an earlier age than when infected with HTLV-1. Furthermore, the period of time in which the coinfected patients remained asymptomatic was shorter than the monoinfected patients (less than 3 years) [102]. Furthermore, Casseb and colleagues [101] demonstrated that the levels of HTLV-1 proviral DNA load in coinfected patients with HAM/TSP were five times higher than in asymptomatic coinfected individuals. HTLV-1 proviral DNA levels in PBMCs varied during the course of HTLV-1 infection [103]. High proviral DNA levels [104] along with the replication or migration of HTLV-1-infected lymphocytes to the CNS have been associated with the development of HAM/TSP [103]. Indeed, Bassi et al. [105] proposed the use of HTLV-1 proviral DNA loads as a diagnostic tool for the early detection of HAM/TSP. In this regard, other studies have established the lower limits of detection of HTLV-1 proviral DNA, and these efforts facilitated studies to distinguish between asymptomatic HTLV-1-infected patients and HAM/TSP patients. With regard to coinfection, studies have reported that HIV-1 infection increased the HTLV-1 proviral DNA levels in HTLV-1-infected patients. Yet, Césaire and colleagues [106] found no difference between the levels of HTLV-1 proviral DNA in the coinfected patients compared to those infected with only HTLV-1. Even without understanding the molecular mechanism of how one retrovirus influences pathology and disease, what is obvious is the strong association of HAM/TSP and HTLV-1/HIV-1 coinfection (Table 2).

Viral protein	Effect on HIV-1 infection	Effect on HTLV-1 infection
Tat	Transactivator protein that enhances viral transcription; can be secreted and cause apoptosis in uninfected bystander cells	Some studies have suggested that there is minimal effect by Tat on HTLV-1 infection; other studies have suggested that HIV-1 Rev is the protein that potentially enhances gene expression; some studies have shown that HIV-1 does not affect proviral load in PBMCs; there has been a link between coinfection and increased risk to develop HAM/TSP and ATL
Tax	Has been shown to be overexpressed in HTLV-1/HIV-1 coinfection; promotes nuclear transport of the reverse transcribed HIV-1 DNA; stimulates HIV-1 via activation of NF-κB (both alone and synergistically with Tat); has been shown to interact with CCR5, a major coreceptor of HIV-1, although a role in disease progression is controversial	Transactivator protein that enhances viral transcription; largely implicated in the oncogenic potential of HTLV-1; can be secreted from infected cells resulting in bystander effects such as upregulation of cytokines and chemokines, and infiltration of Tax specific $CD8^+$ T cells, which can influence HAM/TSP

Table 2. Points of intersection between HTLV-1 and HIV-1

The levels of $CD4^+$ T-cell counts and HTLV-1 disease progression in HTLV-1/HIV-1 coinfection were evaluated in a study conducted in Brazil by Casseb and coworkers. One hundred and fifty HTLV-1-infected patients were enrolled in the study; 27 of them were coinfected with HIV-1, and 15 of the coinfected patients had already reported an AIDS-defining event. $CD4^+$ T-cell counts were higher in coinfected individuals with AIDS than in HIV-1-monoinfected patients (median = 189 cells/mm^3 and 89 cells/mm^3, respectively; $p = 0.036$). Moreover, five of the coinfected subjects who had AIDS and three of the coinfected patients without AIDS showed signs of HAM/TSP. Three of the eight patients with signs of HAM/TSP also developed an opportunistic infection. Importantly, the incidence of HAM/TSP in coinfected patients with AIDS was 20 times higher than those infected with only HTLV-1 infection. These results supported previous observations that HTLV-1/HIV-1 coinfection was associated with a higher probability of a more severe HTLV-1 infection along with an increase in the levels of $CD4^+$ T cells [3]. These results have suggested the possibility that HTLV-1 may inhibit HIV-1 replication with a subsequent increase in $CD4^+$ T-cell counts, thereby enhancing HTLV-1 disease progression. Based on these observations, current research has centered on a more in-depth molecular analysis with respect to how HTLV-1 and HIV-1 impact each other during the course of dual infection.

http://dx.doi.org/10.5772/61254

5. Impact of HTLV-1 on HIV-1 disease progression

The influence of HTLV-1 infection on the development of AIDS in HIV-1-coinfected patients is not well understood. Several studies have indicated that HTLV-1 infection promotes HIV-1 replication, accelerating the development of AIDS, while other reports have shown that HTLV-1 actually inhibits HIV-1 infection [4]. The conflicting results reported are likely due in part to the diverse antiretroviral regimens used to treat HTLV-1/HIV-1-coinfected patients [104]. In addition, the timing with respect to the introduction of the second virus (HTLV-1 or HIV-1) may have great impact on HIV-1 replication and disease.

Prior to the HAART era, Bartholomew and colleagues [107] reported the results of a study conducted in Trinidad with 40 HIV-1-positive homosexual men, 6 of them coinfected with HTLV-1. The coinfected individuals were severely immunocompromised compared to the HIV-1-monoinfected patients. Irrespective of sex and $CD4^+$ T-cell counts, a retrospective case-control study performed in Bahia, Brazil, showed that people living with HTLV-1/HIV-1 coinfection exhibited a shorter lifespan than HIV-1-monoinfected patients. The mean survival time for controls was 2,430 days, whereas for HTLV-1/HIV-1-coinfected patients, it was 1,849 days, with a $p = 0.02$ when comparing the two groups [108]. The reduced survival was also observed in children [109].

Scapellato and colleagues [110] reported that in HTLV-1/HIV-1-coinfected patients naive to treatment, $CD4^+$ T-cell counts were higher in the coinfected patients than in HIV-1-monoinfected patients at the time of an AIDS-defining illness. A case-control study to characterize the phenotype of $CD4^+$ T cells during HTLV-1/HIV-1 coinfection was conducted with 701 HAART-naïve, HIV-1-positive African adults. Within this patient cohort, 29 patients were found to be coinfected with HTLV-1. Each coinfected patient was matched by age and sex with two HIV-1-monoinfected individuals. The study also included unmatched healthy controls. $CD4^+$ T-cell levels, markers of $CD4^+$ T-cell activation, and HIV viral load were the parameters used to assess HIV-1 disease progression. The results showed that coinfected patients exhibited higher levels of $CD4^+$ T cells (median = 525 cells/mm^3 and 274 cell/mm^3, respectively; $p < 0.05$) with higher levels of expression of the activation markers CD25 and CD45RO and lower expression levels of CD45RA and CD62L (markers of naïve T cells) in coinfected individuals as compared to monoinfected individuals. Furthermore, coinfected patients exhibited an increase in HIV-1 proviral DNA load as compared to monoinfected subjects. Despite the normal or higher levels of $CD4^+$ T cells, coinfected patients still progressed to AIDS [111]. These observations imply that HTLV-1 infection enhances HIV-1 progression via loss of naïve $CD4^+$ T cells, with an overall increase in total $CD4^+$ T cells and an increase in HIV-1 viral load, key features with respect to the development of AIDS. The lymphocytosis observed in coinfected patients might have been caused by the Tax oncoprotein encoded by HTLV-1. Tax inhibits the cellular mechanisms involved in DNA repair and induces cell transformation and immortalization [111, 112].

The impact of HTLV-1 on the immune response during coinfection with HIV-1 was evaluated using quiescent PBMCs from HTLV-1/HIV-1-coinfected patients as well as from HIV-1 and HTLV-1-monoinfected individuals. The Th1 cytokine pathway appeared to be overstimulated during HTLV-1/HIV-1 coinfection, as PBMCs from coinfected patients produced increased levels of IL-2 and IFN-γ compared to PBMCs from HIV-1 and HTLV-1-monoinfected individuals. These results implied that overproduction of Th1 cytokines during the course of HTLV-1/HIV-1 coinfection could be augmenting the overall negative impairment of the immune system induced by HIV-1 [113], which normally influences a Th2 response during chronic infection. Curiously, the correction to a Th1 response does not seem to correct for the shortened lifespan and a possible increase in progression to AIDS. It should be noted that there was obviously patient-to-patient variability, differences in phenotype depending on viral genotypes, and the length of time involving mono or dual infection.

6. Molecular interactions between HTLV-1 and HIV-1

To this point, we have discussed the impact that HIV-1 has on HTLV-1 disease progression, particularly on the occurrence of HAM/TSP, as well as the effect of HTLV-1 on HIV-1 infection. Clearly, HTLV-1/HIV-1 coinfection alters the course of disease caused by either virus along as assessed by proviral DNA loads, $CD4^+$ T-cell death and proliferation assessments, and overall immunologic assessment, pathogenesis, and disease indicates that the presence of both viruses negatively impacts human health as compared to the presence of either virus alone. Based on these observations, investigators have also explored the molecular interactions between HTLV-1 and HIV-1 that could be influencing the development of HTLV-1 disease or HIV/AIDS during HTLV-1/HIV-1 coinfection. *In vitro* experiments involving superinfection with the HIV-1 molecular clone HIV-1_{IIIB} on two HTLV-1-transformed cell lines, MT2 (an HTLV-1-producer cell line) and 81-66/45 cell line (an HTLV-1 nonproducer cell line), have demonstrated that HIV-1 infection activates HTLV-1 and increases the levels of HTLV-1 proviral DNA in both HTLV-1-transformed cell lines [114]. Additional studies performed by Zsabó and colleagues [115] have shown that *in vitro* HTLV-1/HIV-1 coinfection of macrophages by both viruses results in increased replication of both viruses. The presence of the HTLV-1 Tax protein promoted nuclear transport of the newly reverse transcribed HIV-1 DNA, whereas the mechanism by which HIV-1 infection enhanced HTLV-1 gene expression did not appear to involve the HIV-1 Tat protein.

In a tripartite coculture assay using Jurkat T cells transfected with an HTLV-1LTR-driven reporter construct designated Jurkat/HTLV-1-Luc with a chronically infected HTLV-1 cell line, HTLV-1-MT2, that has also been infected with HIV-1_{IIIB} via cell-to-cell transfer of virus from HIV-1_{IIIB}-infected H9 cells, Sun and coworkers demonstrated that HIV-1 infection induced an 80-fold increase in LTR-dependent HTLV-1 gene expression. It was also demonstrated that the increase in transcriptional activation of HTLV-1 genes occurred in a mechanism that was dependent on the HTLV-1 Tax protein, the HIV-1 gp120/gp41 complex, and CD40. These results suggested that HIV-1 infection promoted the development of syncytium among the cell lines examined in these studies, thereby acting as a channel for HTLV-1 Tax to translocate from the HTLV-1-infected MT2 cells to the HTLV-1-LTR-Jurkat cells, thereby providing an explanation as to how coinfection with HIV-1 and HTLV-1 may transactivate the LTR of latent provirus in neighboring cells [116]. Using an *in vitro* model of HTLV-1/HIV-1 coinfection, Roy and colleagues confirmed that HIV-1 virus alone or the accessory protein Tat can enhance HTLV-1 gene expression. Culturing the NO-HTLV-1 cell line, an HTLV-1-infected cell line established by exposure of the cells to an HTLV-1 clinical isolate, in the presence of cell-free HIV-1 virion alone (HIV-1_{IIIB}), doubled the amount of HTLV-1 gene expression [117–119]. Additionally, the NO-HTLV-1 cells were exposed to recombinant HIV-1 Tat protein alone, subsequently resulting in an increase in the expression of HTLV-1 matrix protein expression (p. 19). Furthermore, the majority of HTLV-1-infected cells colocalized with HIV-1 virions, indicating HLTV-1 gene expression and transactivation, was dependent and correlated with the presence of HIV-1 virion or Tat [2].

With respect to the interactions between HTLV-1 and HIV-1 that affect HIV-1 expression, Leung and coworkers [120] first reported that the HTLV-1 Tat protein stimulates HIV-1 via activation of NF-κB. Later, studies by Böhnlein and colleagues [121] confirmed that in vitro HTLV-1/HIV-1 coinfection assays indicated that HTLV-1 enhanced HIV-1 expression utilizing a mechanism dependent on HTLV-1 Tax. These experiments revealed that HTLV-1 Tax protein stimulates T cells and promotes transcriptional activation of the HIV-1LTR via interaction with the cellular protein HIVEN86A. Additional studies indicated that HTLV-1 Tax also works synergistically with HIV-1 Tat to increase HIV-1 via stimulation of NF-κB [122]. Culturing HTLV-1-producing MT2 cells with HIV-1 isolates from quiescent $CD4^+$ T cells from HIV-1-infected patients treated with HAART upregulated HIV-1 expression. HTLV-1 Tax or the Env glycoprotein alone was sufficient to induce HIV-1 replication [123].

7. Treatments for HIV-1 and HTLV-1 infections

The current approach to effectively treat HIV-1-infected patients involves the use of a combination of antiretroviral drugs that inhibit a number of steps within the HIV-1 replication cycle, including the reverse transcription process, integration, and proteolytic processing of structural polyproteins, thereby reducing the production of mature infectious HIV-1 virions that involves the HIV-1-encoded protease [124]. By 2011, the FDA had approved 26 antiretrovirals for the treatment of HIV-1 [6] with now more than 30 agents approved for use in humans to treat HIV-1 infection [8]. The rationale of using highly active antiretroviral therapy (HAART) or also referred as combination antiretroviral therapy (cART) in HIV-1-infected individuals has been to minimize the development of drug-resistant virus while effectively reducing the viral load to undetectable levels for prolonged periods of time, in essence, the establishment of a manageable chronic disease. As mentioned previously, although cART reduced actively replicating virus, it does not remove active or defective integrated and latent provirus. To affectively "cure" and HIV-infected individual, every copy of proviral DNA must be removed. Recently, much attention has been focused on purging and excising the latent reservoir by the shock and kill method (HDAC inhibitors) and gene-editing enzymes (zinc-finger nucleases, TALENS and CRISPR/Cas9) [125–128], as previously reviewed [129, 130]. The shock and kill strategy has involved reactivating latent virus reservoirs from resting memory $CD4^+$ T cells with this process leading to a contraction in the size of the reservoir post activation in combination with cART therapy that leads to the destruction of the activated cell and the prevention of infection of uninfected T cells. Additional therapeutic strategies have recently focused on the use of gene-editing systems involving protein-based enzymes that have been designed to seek out specific HIV-1 proviral DNA sequences and induce double-stranded DNA breaks that can induce nucleotide deletions and removal of whole gene segments [126, 130]. Many of these techniques are in basic discovery phases for the treatment of infected cells with the goal of eliminating integrated provirus. These technologies hold great promise to eliminate integrated retroviral genetic information thereby curing the infected cell.

In the case of HTLV-1 infection, reverse transcriptase inhibitors stop HTLV-1 replication *in vivo* but can only prevent infection if they are taken immediately after first contact with the virus [131, 132]. The current therapeutic options for HTLV-1 infection consist of a number of chemotherapeutic agents for lymphoma and the combination of zidovudine and interferon-α (IFN-α) for the management of acute, smoldering, and chronic ATL. The clinical management of ATL continues to be challenging because it has been shown to be a highly lethal type of cancer resistant to many of the currently available anticancer drugs (Figure 4) [124]. In 1996, Borg and colleagues [133] successfully treated and caused cancer rejection in an Afro-Caribbean female with ATL using a combination of chemotherapeutic agents (cyclophosphamide, doxorubicin, and etoposide) and allogeneic bone marrow stem cell transplantation (alloSCT). In the case of people older than 50 years, alloSCT treatment is given with low doses of chemotherapeutic drugs. Retrospective studies indicate that 30–40% of ATL patients who have undergone alloSCT treatment become long-term survivors [134]. The use of the humanized defucosylated antiCCR4 antibody in patients with ATL has also had promising results [135, 136] with HAM/TSP [137]. Concurrently, the treatment for HAM/TSP and its secondary effects involves the use of spasmolytic drugs, prednisone, danazol [138], valproic acid [139], prosultiamine [140], IFN-α [141–143], IFN-β-1a [144–146], or vitamin B1 [147].

The management of HTLV-1/HIV-1 coinfection can be challenging due to the lack of efficacy of antiretroviral therapy with respect to the inhibition of HTLV-1 replication as well as the disparate effects one therapy or compound may have on the other virus. One of the drugs commonly used for HTLV-1 infection is IFN-α. However, the clinical benefits of IFN-α for HIV-1-infected patients are controversial. *In vitro*, IFN-α downregulates HIV-1 replication in macrophages and T cells and halts the formation of mature HTLV-1 virions. Importantly, IFN-α treatment induces caspase-3-mediated apoptosis of HTLV-1/HIV-1_{IIIB}-coinfected MT-4 cells, but not HTLV-1-monoinfected MT-4 cells. Interestingly, IFN-α treatment did not affect HTLV-1 infectivity but markedly reduced HIV-1 replication, with an approximately 1000-fold decrease in HIV-1 p24 antigen expression [124]. These immediate differential affects on therapy of these two viruses also project a possible role of coinfection in influencing ATL and HAM/TSP prominence and therapeutic strategy for treatment.

The incidence of ATL in HTLV-1/HIV-1-coinfected individuals has not been widely reported yet. Shibata and colleagues reported a case involving a 43-year-old African American male with ATL that was positive for both HTLV-1 and HIV-1. The patient underwent three phases of treatment achieving at least 12 months of remission. The first stage consisted of daunorubicin, prednisone, and vincristine. Then the patient was placed on *cis*-platinum, etoposide, cytosine arabidoside, and dexamethasone. During the third phase, the patient was treated with

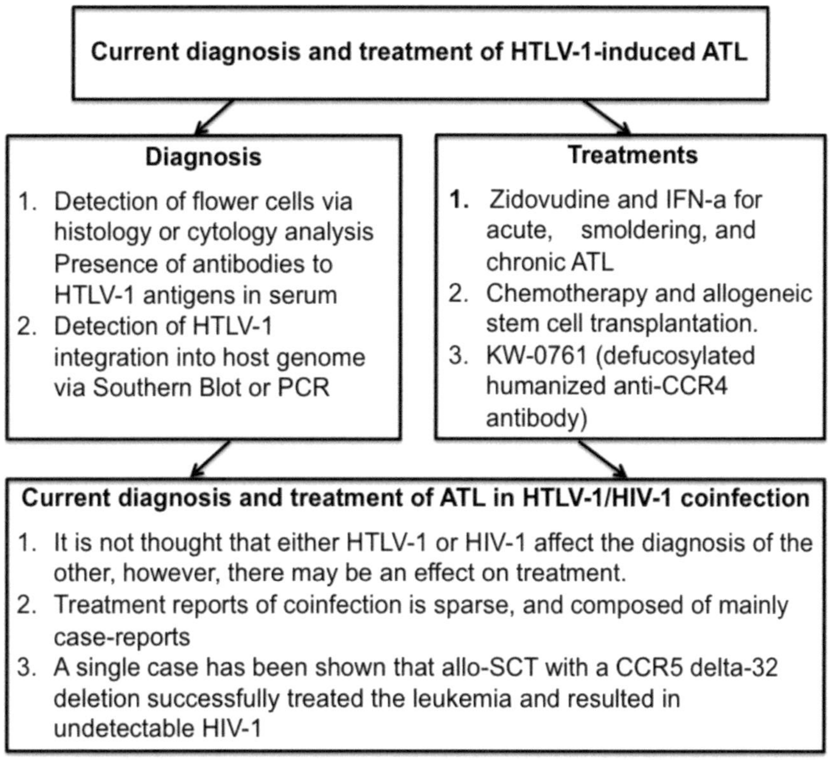

Figure 4. Current diagnosis and treatment of HTLV-1-induced ATL. Summary of criteria used to diagnose previously identifiable forms of ATL and a brief overview of currently available treatments are shown.

zidovudine. PCR analysis of PBMCs detected HTLV-1 in 1/1,000 cells and HIV-1 in a similar fraction [148].

Furthermore, Hütter and colleagues used alloSCT to treat a 40-year-old white male who suffered from acute myeloid leukemia and was also HIV-1-positive. The patient received the transplant from an HLA-matched donor who was homozygous for the CCR5 delta32 deletion. Importantly, a homozygous 32-bp deletion in the CCR5 allele has been shown to confer long-term resistance to HIV-1 infection with CCR5-utilizing viruses but not CXCR4-utilizing viruses. The patient was infected with HIV-1 more than 10 years earlier and had received cART for the previous 4 years. At the time of his leukemia, he was asymptomatic with respect to HIV disease. Initially, the patient was treated with chemotherapy, after which time he suffered from a rebound in his HIV-1 viral load and a relapse in his leukemia. At this time, he received the alloSCT, which successfully treated the leukemia. In addition, the patient stopped taking the cART and his HIV-1 viral loads were undetectable. After 20 months of follow-up, this patient was free of both the HIV-1 infection and the leukemia [149]. While these *in vitro* and *in vivo* studies and clinical trials have revealed a great deal of information about co- and monoinfection of HTLV-1/HIV-1-infected individuals, much more research is needed to help manage these lifelong chronic infections.

8. Summary and concluding remarks

We have discussed a number of diseases caused by infection with two common human retroviruses, HTLV-1 and HIV-1, alone or within the context of coinfection. As previously shown by epidemiological studies, coinfection with these two viral pathogens occurs frequently among illicit drug users, and its incidence is on the rise particularly in regions around the world where both viruses are endemic. Although HTLV-1 and HIV-1 are both retroviruses and as such share a number of genomic structural features, similar events within the replication cycle, and common modes of transmission, the overall pathogenic outcomes and the associated diseases they cause are very different except, for the most part, they all occur within the context of the immune and nervous systems with other end organs also involved. Additional information relevant to epidemiology, virology, immunology, immune- and neuropathogenesis, diagnosis, molecular mechanisms of disease, treatment, and clinical management are also discussed within the context of mono- and coinfection with these two important human retroviruses. Despite large bodies of information available concerning the molecular pathogenesis and disease resulting from monoinfections, there is much less information concerning the molecular interactions between HTLV-1 and HIV-1 replication machinery as well as the implications each virus has on disease progression resulting from the pathogenic outcomes when both viruses are replication in the same cells or neighboring cells within the same tissue compartment. Clearly, studies of HTLV-1/HIV-1 coinfection have been complicated by the fact that most of these studies have been conducted after the initiation of cART for suppression of HIV-1 infection (although many of the coinfection studies have been performed in countries where delivery of optimal cART has been difficult). With regard to the molecular interactions between the two viruses, even though both viruses target $CD4^+$ T cells, HIV-1 infection usually results in lytic replication in activated T-cell populations, whereas HTLV-1 infection usually results in more limited replication and gene expression and ultimately induces clonal expansion of selected $CD4^+$ T-cell populations. Interestingly, the bone marrow compartment is penetrated by both HTLV-1 and HIV-1 during the course of disease; the penetration of this compartment appears to seed each virus into different cellular compartments [41, 85, 150]. With respect to HIV-1, the stem cell population within this compartment appears to be spared of viral infection with virus only seeded into more committed or differentiated progenitor cell compartments. The binding of HIV-1 particles to stem cells has been shown to alter their functional properties despite the absence of detectable levels of viral entry into stem cells. However, following HTLV-1 infection, there appears to be differential gene expression within cellular compartments within the bone marrow with much greater numbers of DNA^+RNA^+ progenitor cells in individuals suffering from HAM/TSP as compared to individuals with ATL where there are far fewer DNA^+RNA^+ progenitor cells [61, 64]. The significance of these molecular interactions within the context of bone marrow cell populations remains unresolved during the course of monoinfections and remains to be examined in HTLV-1/HIV-1 coinfections. The interaction of both viruses with the bone marrow compartment during the course of mono- and coinfection within the same or different bone marrow-infected cell populations will likely play an important role in the pathogenesis of diseases caused by both viruses. Clearly, studies with a greater number of larger coinfection cohorts will be required to approach defining molecular mechanisms, diagnosis, treatment, prevention, and overall clinical management of diseases caused by HTLV-1/HIV-1 coinfection. It would also seem important to obtain a better understanding concerning the relationship between the timing of HIV-1 infection relative to the course of HTLV-1-induced disease. Interestingly and perhaps relevant to thinking about this problem is the epidemiologic data suggesting that individuals that suffer from ATL as compared to HAM/TSP are more likely to have been infected by mucosal membrane exposure early in life often as a result of vertical transmission of HTLV-1 as compared to a blood stream exposure of the virus as a result of IV transmission associated with illicit drug abuse [151]. Clearly, the immunosuppression that occurs as a result of primary HIV-1 infection and later during the course of disease with individuals that first seek medical attention for symptoms consistent with HIV-1 disease prior to the start of cART may have great impact on the initial phases of HTLV-1 disease depending on the size and functionality of the T-cell compartment during the primary HTLV-1 infection. If these predictable periods of immunosuppression occur at critical phases of already ongoing HTLV-1-induced disease, the impact of HIV-1 on the course of HTLV-1 disease could be significant whether the individual is headed toward neuroinflammatory or leukemic disease. Clearly, these interactions will pose significant challenges with respect to the clinical management of HTLV-1-induced disease, while HTLV-1 infection could alter the course of HIV-1 disease depending on what impact the neuroinflammatory state associated with the development of HAM/TSP may have on HIV-1 infection of the $CD4^+$ T-cell compartment and what impact of polyclonal or monoclonal expansion of the $CD4^+$ T-cell compartment associated with HTLV-1-induced leukemogenesis may have on productive HIV-1 infection and replication in these T-cell compartments. Finally, the discussion of an HIV-1-positive patient suffering from ATL and another case with an HIV-1-positive patient with acute myeloid leukemia with respect to the impact of bone marrow stem cell replacement therapy on controlling HTLV-1-induced cancer and impact on ongoing HIV-1 disease was examined. In both cases, HIV-1 disease was well controlled at the time of the bone marrow transplant. Interestingly, they both achieved remission of the leukemia, and the HIV-1 and HTLV-1 titers of the first case were very low after treatment, and in the second case, the HIV-1 infection has been apparently cured. This is clearly a better understanding of the molecular interactions between HTLV-1 and HIV-1 and their respective host cell targets with regard to cellular coinfection or cellular interactions altered by viral coinfection of different cellular compartments.

The clinical management of HTLV-1 and HIV-1 mono- and HTLV-1/HIV-1 coinfection will be greatly enhanced by the identification of additional druggable viral or cellular targets to enhance the effective long-term clinical management of HTLV-1- and HIV-1-induced disease outcomes stemming from monoinfections (long-term suppression of viral gene expression in either case with minimal impact of viral infection on host cell function) prior to the encounter of the second virus. A second therapeutic approach will involve curing HTLV-1- and HIV-1-infected patients by elimination of susceptible target cell populations by targeted elimination of cellular receptor epitopes rendering normally susceptible cells refractile to viral infection while maintaining the normal cellular function of these host cell proteins. In parallel with these types of experimental studies, additional types of experimentation will involve the eradication of HTLV-1 and HIV-1 infections by site-specific excision of integrated HTLV-1 and HIV-1 proviral DNA with minimal off target impact on host cell function. Clearly, this is exciting technology with great promise to completely eliminate latent or persistent viral infections without having to activate latent viral gene expression to kill latently infected cells [125–130, 152]. The goal of eliminating both defective and completely functional HIV-1 and HTLV-1 will likely be very critical since it is entirely possible that nonactivatable defective proviruses may still be able to drive the expression of viral proteins (gp120, Tat, Vpr, and Nef) that may cause detrimental effects to neighboring or distant cells in the absence of lytic infectious virus production. Many challenges await this experimental approach, including the exact nature of existing viral reservoirs, the genetic variability of the latent virus, and the delivery of excision technologies to tissue-specific reservoirs, including memory $CD4^+$ T-cell subpopulations, specific cell populations within the monocyte–macrophage lineage, as well as cell populations within the brain and other tissues. Perhaps central to basic and translational science is the development of tomorrow's translational solutions to today's challenges leading to effective solutions to clinical problems.

Author details

Lorena Loarca[1], Neil Sullivan[2,3], Vanessa Pirrone[2,3] and Brian Wigdahl[2,3*]

*Address all correspondence to: brian.wigdahl@drexelmed.edu

1 Division of Gastroenterology and Hepatology, Mayo Clinic and Medical School, Rochester, MN, USA

2 Center for Molecular Virology and Translational Neuroscience, Institute for Molecular Medicine and Infectious Disease, Drexel University College of Medicine, Philadelphia, USA

3 Department of Microbiology and Immunology, Drexel University College of Medicine, Philadelphia, USA

References

[1] Khabbaz RF, Onorato IM, Cannon RO, Hartley TM, Roberts B, Hosein B, et al. Seroprevalence of HTLV-1 and HTLV-2 among intravenous drug users and persons in clinics for sexually transmitted diseases. N Engl J Med 1992;326:375–80.

[2] Upal R, SA Simpson, D Mondal, S Eloby-Childress, EL Winsor, and MA Beilke. Upregulation of HTLV-1 and HTLV-2 Expression by HIV-1 In Vitro. J Med Virol 2008;80:494–500.

[3] Casseb J, MP Posada-Vergara, P Montanheiro, LMI Fukumori, I Olah, J Smid, et al. T CD4+ cells count among patients co-infected with human immunodeficiency virus

type 1 (HIV-1) and human T-cell leukemia virus type 1 (HTLV-1): high prevalence of tropical spastic paraparesis/HTLV-1-associated myelopathy (TSP/HAM). Rev Inst Med Trop Sao Paulo 2007;49.

[4] Casoli C, E Pilotti, and U Bertazzoni. Molecular and cellular interactions of HIV-1/HTLV coinfection and impact on AIDS progression. AIDS Rev 2007;3:140–9.

[5] Brites C, Sampalo J, Oliveira A. HIV/human T-cell lymphotropic virus coinfection revisited: impact on AIDS progression. AIDS Rev 2009;11:8–16.

[6] Knipe DM. aPMH. Fields Virology. Wolters Kluwer Health/Lippincott Williams & Wilkins 2013;2.

[7] Barrios CS, L Castillo, CZ Giam, L Wu, and MA Beilke. Inhibition of HIV type 1 replication by human T lymphotropic virus types 1 and 2 tax proteins in vitro. AIDS Res Hum Retroviruses 2013;29:1061–7.

[8] Engelman A, Cherepanov P. The structural biology of HIV-1: mechanistic and therapeutic insights. Nat Rev Microbiol 2012;10:279–90.

[9] Proietti FA, Carneiro-Proietti AB, Catalan-Soares BC, Murphy EL. Global epidemiology of HTLV-I infection and associated diseases. Oncogene 2005;24:6058–68.

[10] Yao J, Wigdahl B. Human T cell lymphotropic virus type I genomic expression and impact on intracellular signaling pathways during neurodegenerative disease and leukemia. Front Biosci 2000;5:D138–68.

[11] Hollsberg P, Hafler DA. Seminars in medicine of the Beth Israel Hospital, Boston. Pathogenesis of diseases induced by human lymphotropic virus type I infection. N Engl J Med 1993;328:1173–82.

[12] Poiesz BJ, Ruscetti FW, Gazdar AF, Bunn PA, Minna JD, Gallo RC. Detection and isolation of type C retrovirus particles from fresh and cultured lymphocytes of a patient with cutaneous T-cell lymphoma. Proc Natl Acad Sci U S A 1980;77:7415–9.

[13] Hinuma Y, Nagata K, Hanaoka M, Nakai M, Matsumoto T, Kinoshita KI, et al. Adult T-cell leukemia: antigen in an ATL cell line and detection of antibodies to the antigen in human sera. Proc Natl Acad Sci U S A 1981;78:6476–80.

[14] Uchiyama T, J Yodoi, K Sagawa, K Takatsuki, and H Uchino. Adult T-cell leukemia: clinical and hematologic features of 16 cases. Blood 1977;50:481–92.

[15] Yoshida M, Seiki M, Yamaguchi K, Takatsuki K. Monoclonal integration of human T-cell leukemia provirus in all primary tumors of adult T-cell leukemia suggests causative role of human T-cell leukemia virus in the disease. Proc Natl Acad Sci U S A 1984;81:2534–7.

[16] Sonoda S, Li HC, Cartier L, Nunez L, Tajima K. Ancient HTLV type 1 provirus DNA of Andean mummy. AIDS Res Hum Retroviruses 2000;16:1753–6.

[17] Abrams A, Akahata Y, Jacobson S. The prevalence and significance of HTLV-I/II seroindeterminate Western blot patterns. Viruses 2011;3:1320–31.

[18] Matinella A, Lanzafame M, Bonometti MA, Gajofatto A, Concia E, Vento S, et al. Neurological complications of HIV infection in pre-HAART and HAART era: a retrospective study. J Neurol 2015.

[19] McArthur JC, Steiner J, Sacktor N, Nath A. Human immunodeficiency virus-associated neurocognitive disorders: Mind the gap. Ann Neurol 2010;67:699–714.

[20] Semmes OJ, Jeang KT. Mutational analysis of human T-cell leukemia virus type I Tax: regions necessary for function determined with 47 mutant proteins. J Virol 1992;66:7183–92.

[21] Derse D, Mikovits J, Waters D, Brining S, Ruscetti F. Examining the molecular genetics of HTLV-I with an infectious molecular clone of the virus and permissive cell culture systems. J Acquir Immune Defic Syndr Hum Retrovirol 1996;12:1–5.

[22] Koralnik IJ, Lemp JF, Jr., Gallo RC, Franchini G. In vitro infection of human macrophages by human T-cell leukemia/lymphotropic virus type I (HTLV-I). AIDS Res Hum Retroviruses 1992;8:1845–9.

[23] Seto A, Isono T, Ogawa K. Infection of inbred rabbits with cell-free HTLV-I. Leuk Res 1991;15:105–10.

[24] Jin Q, Agrawal L, VanHorn-Ali Z, Alkhatib G. Infection of CD4+ T lymphocytes by the human T cell leukemia virus type 1 is mediated by the glucose transporter GLUT-1: evidence using antibodies specific to the receptor's large extracellular domain. Virology 2006;349:184–96.

[25] Manel N, Kim FJ, Kinet S, Taylor N, Sitbon M, Battini JL. The ubiquitous glucose transporter GLUT-1 is a receptor for HTLV. Cell 2003;115:449–59.

[26] Jin Q, Alkhatib B, Cornetta K, Alkhatib G. Alternate receptor usage of neuropilin-1 and glucose transporter protein 1 by the human T cell leukemia virus type 1. Virology 2010;396:203–12.

[27] Lambert S, Bouttier M, Vassy R, Seigneuret M, Petrow-Sadowski C, Janvier S, et al. HTLV-1 uses HSPG and neuropilin-1 for entry by molecular mimicry of VEGF165. Blood 2009;113:5176–85.

[28] Ghez D, Lepelletier Y, Lambert S, Fourneau JM, Blot V, Janvier S, et al. Neuropilin-1 is involved in human T-cell lymphotropic virus type 1 entry. J Virol 2006;80:6844–54.

[29] Ghez D, Y Lepelletier, KS Jones, C Pique, and O Hermine. Current topics regarding the HTLV-1 receptor complex. Retrovirology 2010;7:99:109.

[30] Jones KS, Petrow-Sadowski C, Bertolette DC, Huang Y, Ruscetti FW. Heparan sulfate proteoglycans mediate attachment and entry of human T-cell leukemia virus type 1 virions into CD4+ T cells. J Virol 2005;79:12692–702.

[31] Pinon JD, Klasse PJ, Jassal SR, Welson S, Weber J, Brighty DW, et al. Human T-cell leukemia virus type 1 envelope glycoprotein gp46 interacts with cell surface heparan sulfate proteoglycans. J Virol 2003;77:9922–30.

[32] Ho DD, TR Rota, and MS Hirsch. Infection of human endothelial cells by human T-lymphotropic virus type I. PNAS 1984;81:7588–90.

[33] Hoffman PM, Dhib-Jalbut S, Mikovits JA, Robbins DS, Wolf AL, Bergey GK, et al. Human T-cell leukemia virus type I infection of monocytes and microglial cells in primary human cultures. Proc Natl Acad Sci U S A 1992;89:11784–8.

[34] Shohken T, JL Ambrus, DJ Volkman, DL Longo, H Mitsuya, MS Reitz, and AS Fauci. Human T cell lukemia/lymphoma virus I infection and subsequent cloning of normal human B cells. J Exp Med 1985;162:393–8.

[35] LeVasseur RJ, SO Southern, and PJ Southern. Mammary epithelial cells support and transfer productive human T-cell lymphotropic virus infections. J Hum Virol 1998;1:214–23.

[36] Jones KS, C Petrow-Sadowski, YK Huang, DC Bertolette, and FW Ruscetti. Cell-free HTLV-1 infects dendritic cells leading to transmission and transformation of CD4(+) T cells. Nat Med 2008;14:429–36.

[37] Koyanagi Y, Y Itoyama, N Nakamura, K Takamatsu, J Kira, T Iwamasa, et al. In vivo infection of human T-cell leukemia virus type I in non-T cells. Virology 1993;196:25–33.

[38] Macatonia SE, JK Cruickshank, P Rudge, and SC Knight. Dendritic cells from patients with tropical spastic paraparesis are infected with HTLV-1 and stimulate autologous lymphocyte proliferation. AIDS Res Hum Retroviruses 1992;8:1699–706.

[39] Kitajima I, K Yamamoto, K Sato, Y Nakajima, T Nakajima, I Maruyama, et al. Detection of human T cell lymphotropic virus type I proviral DNA and its gene expression in synovial cells in chronic inflammatory arthropathy. J Clin Invest 1991;88:1315–22.

[40] Lehky TJ, CH Fox, S Koenig, MC Levin, N Flerlage, S Izumo, et al. Detection of human T-lymphotropic virus type I (HTLV-I) tax RNA in the central nervous system of HTLV-I-associated myelopathy/tropical spastic paraparesis patients by in situ hybridization. Ann Neurol 1995;37:167–75.

[41] Levin MC, Krichavsky M, Fox RJ, Lehky T, Jacobson S, Fox C, et al. Extensive latent retroviral infection in bone marrow of patients with HTLV-I-associated neurologic disease. Blood 1997;89:346–8.

[42] Hino S, K Yamaguchi, S Katamine, H Sugiyama, T Amagasaki, K Kinoshita, et al. Mother-to-child transmission of human T-cell leukemia virus type-I. Jpn J Cancer Res 1985;76:474–80.

[43] Tajima K, S Tominaga, T Suchi, T Kawagoe, H Komoda, Y Hinuma, et al. Epidemiological analysis of the distribution of antibody to adult T-cell leukemia virus-associat-

ed antigen: possible horizontal transmission of adult T-cell leukemia virus. Jpn J Cancer Res 1982;73:893–901.

[44] Fujino TaYN. HTLV-I transmission from mother to child. J of Reprod Immunol 2000;47:197–206.

[45] Hori M, Y Ami, S Kushida, M Kobayashi, K Uchida, T Abe, et al. Intrauterine transmission of human T-cell leukemia virus type I in rats. J Virol 1995;69:11302–1305.

[46] Best JM. Laboratory diagnosis of intrauterine and perinatal virus infections. Clin Diagn Virol 1996;5:121–9.

[47] Hino S. Establishment of the milk-borne transmission as a key factor for the peculiar endemicity of human T-lymphotropic virus type 1 (HTLV-1): the ATL Prevention Program Nagasaki. Proc Jpn Acad Ser B Phys Biol Sci 2011;87:152–66.

[48] Paiva AaJC. Sexual transmission of human T-cell lymphotropic virus type. Rev Soc Bras Med Trop 2014;47:265–74.

[49] Manns A, RJ Wilks, EL Murphy, G Haynes, JP Figueroa, M Barnett, et al. A prospective study of transmission by transfusion of HTLV-I and risk factors associated with seroconversion. Int J Cancer 1992;51:886–91.

[50] Toro C BR, Aguilera A, Bassani S, Rodriguez C, Calderon E, et al. Infection with human T-lymphotropic virus type I in organ transplant donors and recipients in Spain. J Med Virol 2005;76:268–70.

[51] Gessain A, Cassar O. Epidemiological aspects and world distribution of HTLV-1 infection. Front Microbiol 2012;3:388.

[52] Vrielink HaWR. HTLV-I/II prevalence in different geographic locations. Transfus Med Rev 2004;18:46–57.

[53] Murphy EL, B Hanchard, JP Figueroa, WN Gibbs, WS Lofters, M Campbell, et al. Modelling the risk of adult T-cell leukemia/lymphoma in persons infected with human T-lymphotropic virus type I. Int J Cancer 1989;43:250–3.

[54] Kawano F, Yamaguchi K, Nishimura H, Tsuda H, Takatsuki K. Variation in the clinical courses of adult T-cell leukemia. Cancer 1985;55:851–6.

[55] Shimoyama M. Diagnostic criteria and classification of clinical subtypes of adult T-cell leukaemia-lymphoma. A report from the Lymphoma Study Group (1984–87). Br J Haematol 1991;79:428–37.

[56] Yamaguchi K, Nishimura H, Kohrogi H, Jono M, Miyamoto Y, Takatsuki K. A proposal for smoldering adult T-cell leukemia: a clinicopathologic study of five cases. Blood 1983;62:758–66.

[57] Currer R, Van Duyne R, Jaworski E, Guendel I, Sampey G, Das R, et al. HTLV tax: a fascinating multifunctional co-regulator of viral and cellular pathways. Front Microbiol 2012;3:406.

[58] Grassmann R, Aboud M, Jeang KT. Molecular mechanisms of cellular transformation by HTLV-1 Tax. Oncogene 2005;24:5976–85.

[59] Alefantis T, Flaig KE, Wigdahl B, Jain P. Interaction of HTLV-1 Tax protein with calreticulin: implications for Tax nuclear export and secretion. Biomed Pharmacother 2007;61:194–200.

[60] Alefantis T, Jain P, Ahuja J, Mostoller K, Wigdahl B. HTLV-1 Tax nucleocytoplasmic shuttling, interaction with the secretory pathway, extracellular signaling, and implications for neurologic disease. J Biomed Sci 2005;12:961–74.

[61] Barmak K, Harhaj E, Grant C, Alefantis T, Wigdahl B. Human T cell leukemia virus type I-induced disease: pathways to cancer and neurodegeneration. Virology 2003;308:1–12.

[62] Alefantis T, Mostoller K, Jain P, Harhaj E, Grant C, Wigdahl B. Secretion of the human T cell leukemia virus type I transactivator protein tax. J Biol Chem 2005;280:17353–62.

[63] Jain P, Mostoller K, Flaig KE, Ahuja J, Lepoutre V, Alefantis T, et al. Identification of human T cell leukemia virus type 1 tax amino acid signals and cellular factors involved in secretion of the viral oncoprotein. J Biol Chem 2007;282:34581–93.

[64] Grant C, Barmak K, Alefantis T, Yao J, Jacobson S, Wigdahl B. Human T cell leukemia virus type I and neurologic disease: events in bone marrow, peripheral blood, and central nervous system during normal immune surveillance and neuroinflammation. J Cell Physiol 2002;190:133–59.

[65] Ahuja J, Lepoutre V, Wigdahl B, Khan ZK, Jain P. Induction of pro-inflammatory cytokines by human T-cell leukemia virus type-1 Tax protein as determined by multiplexed cytokine protein array analyses of human dendritic cells. Biomed Pharmacother 2007;61:201–8.

[66] Harhaj EW, Harhaj NS, Grant C, Mostoller K, Alefantis T, Sun SC, et al. Human T cell leukemia virus type I Tax activates CD40 gene expression via the NF-kappa B pathway. Virology 2005;333:145–58.

[67] Lepoutre V, P Jain, K Quann, B Wigdahl, and ZK Khan. Role of resident CNS cell populations in HTLV-1-associated neuroinflammatory disease. Front Biosci 2009;14:1152–68.

[68] Uchiyama T. Human T cell leukemia virus type I (HTLV-I) and human diseases. Annu Rev Immunol 1997;15:15–37.

[69] Barmak K, EW Harhaj, and B Wigdahl. Mediator of central nervous system damage during the progression of human T-cell leukemia type I-associated myelopathy/tropical spastic paraparesis. J Neurovirol 2003;9:522–9.

[70] Barré-Sinoussi F, AL Ross, and JF Delfraissy. Past, present and future: 30 years of HIV research. Nat Rev 2013;11:877–83.

[71] Barré-Sinoussi F, JC Chermann, F Rey, MT Nugeyre, S Chamaret, J Gruest, et al. Isolation of a T-lymphotropic retrovirus from a patient at risk for acquired immune deficiency syndrome (AIDS). Science 1983;220:868–71.

[72] Sarngadharan MG, AL DeVico, L Bruch, J Schüpbach, and RC Gallo. HTLV-III: the etiologic agent of AIDS. Princess Takamatsu Symp 1984;15:301–8.

[73] Coffin J. A Haase, JA Levy, L Montagnier, S Oroszlan, N Teich, et al. What to call the AIDS virus? (Letter) Nature 1986;321:10.

[74] Nyamweya S, A Hegedus, A Jaye, S Rowland-Jones, KL Flanagan, and DC Macallan. Comparing HIV-1 and HIV-2 infection: lessons for viral immunopathogenesis. Rev Med Virol 2013;23:221–40.

[75] Hemelaar J, Gouws E, Ghys PD, Osmanov S, Isolation W-UNfH, Characterisation. Global trends in molecular epidemiology of HIV-1 during 2000–2007. AIDS 2011;25:679–89.

[76] Moss JA. HIV/AIDS Review. Radiol Technol 2013;84:247–70.

[77] Wagner TA, McLaughlin S, Garg K, Cheung CY, Larsen BB, Styrchak S, et al. HIV latency. Proliferation of cells with HIV integrated into cancer genes contributes to persistent infection. Science 2014;345:570–3.

[78] Maldarelli F, Wu X, Su L, Simonetti FR, Shao W, Hill S, et al. HIV latency. Specific HIV integration sites are linked to clonal expansion and persistence of infected cells. Science 2014;345:179–83.

[79] Cohn LB, Silva IT, Oliveira TY, Rosales RA, Parrish EH, Learn GH, et al. HIV-1 integration landscape during latent and active infection. Cell 2015;160:420–32.

[80] Costin JM. Cytopathic Mechanisms of HIV-1. Virol J 2007;4:100–23.

[81] Nisole S, Saib A. Early steps of retrovirus replicative cycle. Retrovirology 2004;1:9.

[82] Folks T, J Kelly, S Benn, A Kinter, J Justement, J Gold, et al. Susceptibility of normal human lymphocytes to infection with HTLV-III/LAV. J Immunol 1986;136:4049–53.

[83] Zack JA, SJ Arrigo, SR Weitsman, AS Go, A Haislip, and IS Chen. HIV-1 entry into quiescent primary lymphocytes: molecular analysis reveals a labile, latent viral structure. Cell 1990;61:213–22.

[84] Klase Z, Jeang KT. Reciprocal functional pseudotyping of HIV-1 and HTLV-1 viral genomes by the heterologous counterpart envelope proteins. Virology 2013;443:106–12.

[85] Alexaki A, Liu Y, Wigdahl B. Cellular reservoirs of HIV-1 and their role in viral persistence. Curr HIV Res 2008;6:388–400.

[86] Alexaki A, Wigdahl B. HIV-1 infection of bone marrow hematopoietic progenitor cells and their role in trafficking and viral dissemination. PLoS Pathog 2008;4:e1000215.

[87] Musich T, O'Connell O, Gonzalez-Perez MP, Derdeyn CA, Peters PJ, Clapham PR. HIV-1 non-macrophage-tropic R5 envelope glycoproteins are not more tropic for entry into primary CD4+ T-cells than envelopes highly adapted for macrophages. Retrovirology 2015;12:25.

[88] Finzi D, Blankson J, Siliciano JD, Margolick JB, Chadwick K, Pierson T, et al. Latent infection of CD4+ T cells provides a mechanism for lifelong persistence of HIV-1, even in patients on effective combination therapy. Nat Med 1999;5:512–7.

[89] U.S. Dept of Health and Human Services. HIV/AIDS Surveillance Report, 2006. Atlanta, GA: Centers for Disease Control and Prevention, U.S. Department of Health and Human Services; 2008.

[90] White PJ, Fox J, Weber J, Fidler S, Ward H. How Many HIV infections may be averted by targeting primary infection in men who have sex with men? Quantification of changes in transmission-risk behavior, using an individual-based model. J Infect Dis 2014;210 Suppl 2:S594–9.

[91] Cohen MS, and CL Gay. Treatment to prevent transmission of HIV-1. Clin Infect Dis 2010; 50(S3):S85–S95 2010;50:S85–95.

[92] WHO–HIV Department. Global summary of the AIDS epidemic, 2013. http://wwwwhoint/hiv/data/epi_core_dec2014png?ua=1 2014.

[93] World Health Organization. Interim WHO clinical staging of HIV/AIDS and HIV/AIDS case definitions for surveillance. http://www.who.int/hiv/pub/guidelines/clinicalstaging.pdf; 2005.

[94] Crowe SM, Carlin JB, Stewart KI, Lucas CR, Hoy JF. Predictive value of CD4 lymphocyte numbers for the development of opportunistic infections and malignancies in HIV-infected persons. J Acquir Immune Defic Syndr 1991;4:770–6.

[95] Oliveira Cobuccia RN, PH Lima, P Carvalho de Souza, VV Costa, MC de Mesquita Cornetta, JV Fernandes, et al. Assessing the impact of HAART on the incidence of defining and non-defining AIDS cancers among patients with HIV/AIDS: A systematic review. J Infect Public Health 2015;8:1–10.

[96] Jacobson S, Krichavsky M, Flerlage N, Levin M. Immunopathogenesis of HTLV-I associated neurologic disease: massive latent HTLV-I infection in bone marrow of HAM/TSP patients. Leukemia 1997;11 Suppl 3:73–5.

[97] Caskey MF, DJ Morgan, AF Porto, SP Giozza, AL Muniz, GO Orge, MJ Travassos, et al. Clinical manifestations associated with HTLV type i infection: a cross-sectional study. AIDS Res Hum Retroviruses 2007 Mar; 23(3): 365–371 2007;23.

[98] Manns A, Hisada M, La Grenade L. Human T-lymphotropic virus type I infection. Lancet 1999;353:1951–8.

[99] Beilke MA, S Japa, C Moeller-Hadi, and S Martin-Schild. Tropical spastic paraparesis/human T leukemia virus type 1–associated myelopathy in HIV type 1–Coinfected Patients. Clin Infect Dis 2005;41:e57–63.

[100] Harrison LH, B.Vaz, DM Taveira, TC Quinn, CJ Gibbs, SH de Souza, et al. Myelopathy among Brazilians coinfected with human T-cell lymphotropic virus type I and HIV. Neurology 1997;48:13–8.

[101] Casseb J. ACP de Oliveira, MP Vergara, P Montanheiro, F Bonasser, CM Ferreira, et al. Presence of tropical spastic paraparesis/human T-cell lymphotropic virus type 1-associated myelopathy (TSP/HAM)-like among HIV-1-infected patients. J Med Virol 2008;80:392–8.

[102] Schutte CM, T Townsend, R Van Coller, and S Olorunju. Comparison of HTLV-associated myelopathy (HAM) in HIV-positive and HIV-negative patients at a tertiary South African hospital. S Afr Med J 2013;103:43–6.

[103] Takenouchi N, Y Yamano, K Usuku, M Osame, and S Izumo. Usefulness of proviral load measurement for monitoring of disease activity in individual patients with human T-lymphotropic virus type I-associated myelopathy/tropical spastic paraparesis. J Neurovirol 2003;9:29–35.

[104] Furtado M, RG Andrade, LC Romanelli, MA Ribeiro, JG Ribas, EB Torres, et al. Monitoring the HTLV-1 proviral load in the peripheral blood of asymptomatic carriers and patients with HTLV-associated myelopathy/tropical spastic paraparesis from a Brazilian cohort: ROC curve analysis to establish the threshold for risk disease. J Med Virol 2008;80:392–8.

[105] Bassi SS, R Coutinho, V Nilla Olavarria, F Martin, B Galvão-Castro, and MF Rios Grassi. HTLV-1 proviral load as an indicative marker of HAM/TSP: a systematic review of studies of patients with HAM/TSP. Retrovirology 2014;11:36.

[106] Césaire R, A Dehée, A Lézin, N Désiré, O Bourdonné, F Dantin, et al. Quantification of HTLV type I and HIV type I DNA load in coinfected patients: HIV type 1 infection does not alter HTLV type I proviral amount in the peripheral blood compartment. AIDS Res Hum Retroviruses 2001;17:799–805.

http://dx.doi.org/10.5772/61254

[107] Bartholomew C, W Blattner, and F Cleghorn. Progression to AIDS in homosexual men co-infected with HIV and HTLV-1 in Trinidad. Lancet 1987;2:1469.

[108] Brites C, R Alencar, R Gusmão, C Pedroso, EM Netto, D Pedral-Sampaio, et al. Co-infection with HTLV-1 is associated with a shorter survival time for HIV-1-infected patients in Bahia, Brazil. AIDS 2001;15:2053–5.

[109] Pedroso C, Netto EM, Weyll N, Brites C. Coinfection by HIV-1 and human lymphotropic virus type 1 in Brazilian children is strongly associated with a shorter survival time. J Acquir Immune Defic Syndr 2011;57 Suppl 3:S208–11.

[110] Scapellato PG, E Bottaro, MT Brieschke, JL Scapellato, A Dato, AD Intile, R Davaro, GI Vidal. CD4 cell count among HIV-infected patients with an AIDS-defining disease: higher count in patients coinfected than in those not coinfected with human T-cell lymphotropic virus type I. J Acquir Immune Defic Syndr 2003;33:279–80.

[111] Gudo E, N Bhatt, D Ramalho, C Monteiro, A Tanuri, W Savino, et al. Co-infection by human immunodeficiency virus type 1 (HIV-1) and human T cell leukemia virus type 1 (HTLV-1): does immune activation lead to a faster progression to AIDS? BMC Infect Dis 2009;9:211–23.

[112] Marriott SJ, and OJ Semmes. Impact of HTLV-I Tax on cell cycle progression and the cellular DNA damage repair response. Oncogene 2005;24:5986–95.

[113] Abrahão MH, RG Lima, E Netto, and C Brites. Short communication: human lymphotropic virus type 1 coinfection modulates the synthesis of cytokines by peripheral blood mononuclear cells from HIV type 1-infected individuals. AIDS Res Hum Retroviruses 2012;28:806–8.

[114] De Rossi A, D Saggioro, ML Calabró, R Cenzato, and L Chieco-Bianchi. Reciprocal activation of human T-lymphotropic viruses in HTLV-I-transformed cells superinfected with HIV-1. J Acquir Immune Defici Syndr 1991;4:380–5.

[115] Szabó J, Z Beck, E Csomán, X Liu, I Andrikó, J Kiss, et al. Differential patterns of interaction between HIV type 1 and HTLV type I in monocyte-derived macrophages cultured in vitro: implications for in vivo coinfection with HIV type 1 and HTLV type I. AIDS Res Hum Retroviruses 1999;18:1653–66.

[116] Sun J, B Barbeau, and MJ Tremblay. HIV-1-mediated syncytium formation promotes cell-to-cell transfer of Tax protein and HTLV-I gene expression. Virus Res 2006;118:120–9.

[117] Beilke MA. Human T-cell lymphotropic virus type I-associated uveitis in an African American. Am J Ophthalmol 1995;119:104–5.

[118] Beilke MA, Greenspan DL, Impey A, Thompson J, Didier PJ. Laboratory study of HIV-1 and HTLV-I/II coinfection. J Med Virol 1994;44:132–43.

[119] Roy U, Simpson SA, Mondal D, Eloby-Childress S, Winsor EL, Beilke MA. Upregulation of HTLV-1 and HTLV-2 expression by HIV-1 in vitro. J Med Virol 2008;80:494–500.

[120] Leung K, and GJ Nabel. HTLV-1 transactivator induces interleukin-2 receptor expression through an NF-kB like factor. Nature 1988;23:776–8.

[121] Böhnlein E, M Siekevitz, DW Ballard, JW Lowenthal, L Rimsky, H Bogérd, et al. Stimulation of the human immunodeficiency virus type 1 enhancer by the human T-cell leukemia virus type I tax gene product involves the action of inducible cellular proteins. J Virol 1989;63:1578–86.

[122] Cheng H, J Tarnok, and WP Parks. Human immunodeficiency virus type 1 genome activation induced by human T-cell leukemia virus type 1 tax protein is through cooperation of NF-kB and Tat. J Virol 1998;72:6911–6.

[123] Moriuchi H, and M Moriuchi. In vitro induction of HIV-1 replication in resting CD4(+) T cells derived from individuals with undetectable plasma viremia upon stimulation with human T-cell leukemia virus type I. Virology 2000;278:514–9.

[124] Moens B, C Pannecouque, G López, M Talledo, E Gotuzzo, R Khouri, et al. Simultaneous RNA quantification of human and retroviral genomes reveals intact interferon signaling in HTLV-1-infected CD4+ T cell lines. Virol J 2012:171–85.

[125] Ebina H, Kanemura Y, Misawa N, Sakuma T, Kobayashi T, Yamamoto T, et al. A high excision potential of TALENs for integrated DNA of HIV-based lentiviral vector. PLoS One 2015;10:e0120047.

[126] Hu W, Kaminski R, Yang F, Zhang Y, Cosentino L, Li F, et al. RNA-directed gene editing specifically eradicates latent and prevents new HIV-1 infection. Proc Natl Acad Sci U S A 2014;111:11461–6.

[127] Ebina H, Misawa N, Kanemura Y, Koyanagi Y. Harnessing the CRISPR/Cas9 system to disrupt latent HIV-1 provirus. Sci Rep 2013;3:2510.

[128] Deeks SG. HIV: Shock and kill. Nature 2012;487:439–40.

[129] Manjunath N, Yi G, Dang Y, Shankar P. Newer gene editing technologies toward HIV gene therapy. Viruses 2013;5:2748–66.

[130] Dampier W, Nonnemacher MR, Sullivan NT, Jacobson JM, Wigdahl B. HIV Excision utilizing CRISPR/Cas9 technology: attacking the proviral quasispecies in reservoirs to achieve a cure. MOJ Immunol 2014;1.

[131] Macchi B, Balestrieri E, Ascolani A, Hilburn S, Martin F, Mastino A, et al. Susceptibility of primary HTLV-1 isolates from patients with HTLV-1-associated myelopathy to reverse transcriptase inhibitors. Viruses 2011;3:469–83.

[132] Ishitsuka K, Tamura K. Human T-cell leukaemia virus type I and adult T-cell leukaemia-lymphoma. Lancet Oncol 2014;15:e517–26.

[133] Borg A, JA Yin, PR Johnson, J Tosswill, M Saunders, and D Morris. Successful treatment of HTLV-1-associated acute adult T-cell leukaemia lymphoma by allogeneic bone marrow transplantation. Br J Haematol 1996;94:713–5.

[134] Okamura J, N Uike, A Utsunomiya, R Tanosaki. Allogeneic stem cell transplantation for adult T-cell leukemia/lymphoma. Int J Hematol 2007;86:118–25.

[135] Yamamoto K, Utsunomiya A, Tobinai K, Tsukasaki K, Uike N, Uozumi K, et al. Phase I study of KW-0761, a defucosylated humanized anti-CCR4 antibody, in relapsed patients with adult T-cell leukemia-lymphoma and peripheral T-cell lymphoma. J Clin Oncol 2010;28:1591–8.

[136] Ishida T, Joh T, Uike N, Yamamoto K, Utsunomiya A, Yoshida S, et al. Defucosylated anti-CCR4 monoclonal antibody (KW-0761) for relapsed adult T-cell leukemia-lymphoma: a multicenter phase II study. J Clin Oncol 2012;30:837–42.

[137] Yamauchi J, Coler-Reilly A, Sato T, Araya N, Yagishita N, Ando H, et al. Mogamulizumab, an anti-CCR4 antibody, targets human T-lymphotropic virus type 1-infected CD8+ and CD4+ T cells to treat associated myelopathy. J Infect Dis 2015;211:238–48.

[138] Boostani R, Saber H, Etemadi M. Effects of danazol on clinical improvement of patients with human T-cell lymphotropic virus type I associated myelopathy/tropical spastic paraparesis (HAM/TSP): a placebo-controlled clinical trial. Iran J Basic Med Sci 2013;16:213–6.

[139] Olindo S, Belrose G, Gillet N, Rodriguez S, Boxus M, Verlaeten O, et al. Safety of long-term treatment of HAM/TSP patients with valproic acid. Blood 2011;118:6306–9.

[140] Nakamura T, Matsuo T, Fukuda T, Yamato S, Yamaguchi K, Kinoshita I, et al. Efficacy of prosultiamine treatment in patients with human T lymphotropic virus type I-associated myelopathy/tropical spastic paraparesis: results from an open-label clinical trial. BMC Med 2013;11:182.

[141] Kinpara S, Kijiyama M, Takamori A, Hasegawa A, Sasada A, Masuda T, et al. Interferon-alpha (IFN-alpha) suppresses HTLV-1 gene expression and cell cycling, while IFN-alpha combined with zidovudine induces p53 signaling and apoptosis in HTLV-1-infected cells. Retrovirology 2013;10:52.

[142] Saito M, Nakagawa M, Kaseda S, Matsuzaki T, Jonosono M, Eiraku N, et al. Decreased human T lymphotropic virus type I (HTLV-I) provirus load and alteration in T cell phenotype after interferon-alpha therapy for HTLV-I-associated myelopathy/tropical spastic paraparesis. J Infect Dis 2004;189:29–40.

[143] Feng J, Misu T, Fujihara K, Saito H, Takahashi T, Kohnosu T, et al. Interferon-alpha significantly reduces cerebrospinal fluid CD4 cell subsets in HAM/TSP. J Neuroimmunol 2003;141:170–3.

[144] Viana GM, Silva MA, Souza VL, Lopes NB, Silva DL, Nascimento Mdo D. Interferon beta-1a treatment in HTLV-1-associated myelopathy/tropical spastic paraparesis: a case report. Rev Inst Med Trop Sao Paulo 2014;56:443–5.

[145] Costa DT, Sundberg M, Passos L, Muniz AL, Santos S. Interferon Beta-1a improves urinary symptoms, reduces proviral load, and modifies the immune response in a patient with HAM/TSP. Case Rep Neurol Med 2012;2012:958786.

[146] Oh U, Yamano Y, Mora CA, Ohayon J, Bagnato F, Butman JA, et al. Interferon-beta1a therapy in human T-lymphotropic virus type I-associated neurologic disease. Ann Neurol 2005;57:526–34.

[147] Kira J. Therapeutic benefits of an oral vitamin B1 derivative for human T lymphotropic virus type I-associated myelopathy/tropical spastic paraparesis (HAM/TSP). BMC Med 2013;11:183.

[148] Shibata D, RK Brynes, A Rabinowitz, CA Hanson, ML Slovak, TJ Spira, et al. Ann Intern Med 1989;111:871–5.

[149] Hütter GD, D Nowak, M Mossner, S Ganepola, A Müßig, K Allers, et al. Long-term control of HIV by CCR5 Delta32/Delta32 stem-cell transplantation. N Engl J Med 2009;360:692–8.

[150] Carr JM, Ramshaw HS, Li P, Burrell CJ. CD34+ cells and their derivatives contain mRNA for CD4 and human immunodeficiency virus (HIV) co-receptors and are susceptible to infection with M- and T-tropic HIV. J Gen Virol 1998;79 (Pt 1):71–5.

[151] Araujo A, Sheehy N, Takahashi H, Hall WW. Concomitant infections with human immunodeficiency virus type 1 and human T-lymphotropic virus types 1 and 2. In: Brogden K, Guthmiller J, editors. Polymicrobial Diseases. Washington DC: ASM Press; 2002. p. 75–97.

[152] Tanaka A, Takeda S, Kariya R, Matsuda K, Urano E, Okada S, et al. A novel therapeutic molecule against HTLV-1 infection targeting provirus. Leukemia 2013;27:1621–7.

Chapter 4

Gene Mutations in Acute Myeloid Leukemia — Incidence, Prognostic Influence, and Association with Other Molecular Markers

Olga Blau

Additional information is available at the end of the chapter

http://dx.doi.org/10.5772/60928

Abstract

Acute myeloid leukemia (AML) is a clonal disorder affecting pluripotent stem cells and is characterized by ineffective hematopoiesis. Most AML patients harbor cytogenetic and molecular defects that identify entities with peculiar biologic and clinical data and distinct therapeutic responses. Approximately 50%–60% of de novo AML and 80%–95% of secondary AML patients display chromosomal aberrations. Structural chromosomal rearrangements are the most common cytogenetic abnormalities in de novo AML, with an incidence of 40%. Last years, large collaborative studies have demonstrated the importance of cytogenetic aberrations for the prognosis of AML patients.

The large group of patients with cytogenetically normal (CN) AML refers to the intermediate risk category. It is known that this group of patients is very heterogeneous with respect to prognosis. The recent large-scale sequencing of AML genomes is now providing opportunities for patient stratification and personalized approaches to treatments that are based on individual mutation profiles. Genes recurrently mutated in AML belong to distinct functional groups or pathways. A few recurring gene mutations with prognostic relevance in AML have been identified and have become incorporated into current prognostication models. For patients with CN AML, prognosis can be specified by mutational status of the genes *NPM1*, *FLT3*, and *CEBPA*. CN AML patients with *NPM1* mutation, but no *FLT3*-ITD, or with *CEBPA* mutation, have a favorable prognosis. In contrast, CN AML patients with *FLT3*-ITD mutation have a poor prognosis.

Recently a new class of mutations affecting genes for DNA methylation and post-translational histone modification was identified in AML. These mutations frequently occur in the DNA nucleotide methyltransferase 3A gene (*DNMT3A*) and isocitrate dehydrogenase 1/2 gene (*IDH1/2*). Different studies have shown a negative impact of *DNMT3A* mutations on outcomes in patients with AML. The prognostic effect is known to depend on certain biological factors as well as a combination of cytogenetics and other mutations such as those in *FLT3* and *NPM1.* In contrast, the impact of *IDH1/2* mutations on prognosis is not completely understood. It appears that prognosis may depend on specific patient populations and a combination with *NPM1* mutations.

Moreover, a growing number of recurrent mutations in additional genes have recently been identified. Increasing evidence suggests that AML develops throughout the process of branching evolution.

Keywords: AML, mutations, prognosis, *FLT3, NPM1, DNMT3A, IDH1/2*

1. Introduction

Acute myeloid leukemia (AML) is the most common type of leukemia among hematologic malignancies in adults. In the last years, progresses in molecular technologies have led to identify AML as a highly heterogeneous disorder. AML is a clonal hematopoietic disease that arises from multiple acquired genetic lesions accumulating in hematopoietic progenitors. The mutations give rise to a malignant clone [1]. In the initial development, Knudson's two-hit hypothesis has provided important insights into the pathogenesis of leukemia. Later studies using mouse models have confirmed that genetic abnormalities in leukemia could be divided into two classes. Class I mutations confer a proliferative or survival advantage to blast cells, while class II mutations block myeloid differentiation and give self-renewability [2-4]. Recently, next-generation sequencing methods provided more complete insight in oncogenic events. Early mutations may be present many years before disease develops [5]. Evidence from many murine models has confirmed that early mutations lead to clonal expansions by progenitor cells. Later, cooperating mutations would arise in cells that already contain initiating early mutations [6].

Karyotype analysis allows detecting genetic changes on a chromosomal level by visual assessment of chromosomal banding. Recurrent chromosomal abnormalities are found in about 55% of adults with AML. Some, not all, of the chromosomal aberrations are strong independent predictors of outcome and are the mainstay of the World Health Organization (WHO) classification of AML risk groups [7]. In AML patients with cytogenetically normal karyotype (CN AML) who have an intermediate-risk cytogenetics, clinical outcomes vary greatly. Identification of recurrent mutations in AML improved the understanding of the molecular pathogenesis. Later studies revealed recurrent genetic markers in more than 85% of CN AML patients [8]. Some of the mutations add important prognostic information and also indicate potential therapeutic targets. The more detailed insight into the genetic architecture of AML is challenging the established classification and prognostication systems [8]. Particular mutations have already been included in the latest WHO classification that was established in 2008 and in subsequent recommendations for diagnosis of AML by an international expert panel [9].

2. Nucleophosmin 1 (*NPM1*) mutations

The nucleophosmin/nucleoplasmin (NPM) family of chaperones has diverse functions in the cell. The *NPM1* gene maps to chromosome 5q35 and encodes a phosphoprotein that moves between the nucleus and the cytoplasm. The gene product involves a number of cellular processes such as chromatin remodeling, genome stability, ribosome biogenesis, DNA duplication, and transcriptional regulation. *NPM1* also interacts with a number of proteins at the mitotic spindle and in the nucleolus and includes in regulation of the ARF/ p53 pathway [10, 11]. *NPM1* is clearly having both growth promoting and tumor suppressive functions [11, 12].

In AML, there are some chromosomal translocations involving *NPM1* gene. These genetic alterations usually disturb the cellular transport of *NPM1* [13]. In AML carrying the t(3;5) (q25;q35) translocation, leukemic cells display fusion protein *NPM1–MLF1* (myelodysplasia/ myeloid leukemia factor 1) and show aberrant *NPM1* expression in cytoplasm [14]. In rare cases of acute promyelocytic leukemia carrying the translocation t(5;17), the *NPM1–RARα* fusion protein was detected [15]. The transforming role of partner genes in these cases is well established [13]. Nevertheless, *NPM1* moiety seems to be not only provides a dimerization substrate for the C-terminal onco-protein. *In vivo* studies using mouse model have shown that *NPM1* is a haploinsufficient tumor suppressor gene [16]. Therefore, loss of *NPM1* could also contribute to the pathogenesis of AML [17, 18].

Mutations in the *NPM1* gene represent one of the most common gene mutations in AML [19]. Approximately 25%–30% of AML patients and about 60%–85% of CN AML patients display *NPM1* mutation [13, 20]. *NPM1* mutations are heterogeneous; more than 50 different variants of mutations are identified. A more common variant of mutations is the insertion of four nucleotides at position 288-290 at exon 12. Mutations type A with insertion of "TCTG" at position 288 is the most frequent aberration (75%–80% of cases) [14, 19, 21]. In most cases (about 95%), three mutations types (A, B, and D) are found [13]. *NPM1* mutations result in common changes at the C-terminus end of the *NPM1* protein, that is, changes of tryptophans and insertion of a new nuclear export signal motif. These changes cause aberrant cytoplasmic accumulation of *NPM1* mutants, thus preventing or decreasing *NPM1* binding to the nucleolus. Aberrant *NPM1* expression in cytoplasm is easily detectable by immunohistochemistry [21, 22]. *NPM1* mutations often combined with other AML-associated mutations, especially with *FLT3* (fms-related tyrosine kinase 3), *DNMT3A* (DNA (cytosine-5-methyltransferase 3 alpha), *IDH1* and *IDH2* (isocitrate dehydrogenase 1 and 2 (NADP+)), *NRAS* (neuroblastoma RAS viral (v-ras) oncogene homolog), and others. Most likely, these mutations do not accumulate in a random order but instead could be allocated to early and late events in the transformation process [5, 23].

The prognostic status of *NPM1* depends on the presence of other concurrent genetic alterations. In the absence of *FLT3*-internal tandem duplication (ITD) mutations, *NPM1* mutations are associated with improved outcome for CN AML patients, even in those older than 60 years [9]. Current European Leukaemia Net (ELN) recommendations for diagnosis and treatment of AML determines CN AML with *NPM1* mutation without *FLT3* mutation as a favorable risk and does not recommend allogeneic stem cell transplantation (alloSCT) in first complete remission (CR) [9]. Recently, a beneficial prognostic effect of *NPM1* mutations was reported in AML patients with simultaneous mutations in *IDH1* or *IDH2* [8], whereas a worse prognosis of CN AML without *FLT3*-ITD but with mutations in *IDH1* or *IDH2* has also been described [24]. *NPM1* mutations inform treatment decisions also in elderly patients because it identifies those who might benefit from intensive chemotherapy.

NPM1 mutation provides a sensitive marker for minimal residual disease (MRD) detection by qPCR. Because of their stability in the course of disease and relative homogeneity of mutation pattern, *NPM1* represent a useful target for MRD monitoring, in particular in CN AML. The applicability of an RNA- or DNA-based q-PCR assay for *NPM1*mutation monitoring has been shown by several groups [25-28]. Many authors have shown that *NPM1* mutation as MRD marker is a relevant factor for the identification of patients at high and low risk of relapse [28].

3. *FLT3* mutations in AML

The *FLT3* gene in chromosome band 13q12 encodes a protein known as fms-like tyrosine kinase 3, which belongs to the family of receptor tyrosine kinases (RTK). RTKs transmit signals from the cell surface into the cell through a signal transduction. RTK3 family members are characterized by an extracellular domain comprised of 5 immunoglobulin-like domains and by a cytoplasmic domain with a split tyrosine kinase motif [29, 30]. The FLT3 protein is located in the membrane of certain cell types where FLT3 ligand binds it. *FLT3* is highly expressed in CD34+ hematopoietic progenitor cells and variable express in the more mature monocytic lineage. *FLT3* expression has been described in lymphohematopoietic organs such as the liver, spleen, thymus, and placenta [30, 31].

The binding with ligand activates the FLT3 protein, which subsequently activates a series of proteins inside the cell that are part of multiple signaling pathways and leads to receptor oligomerization and transphosphorylation of specific tyrosine residues, which activates the downstream signaling pathways including STAT5, RAS/mitogen-activated protein kinase, and phosphatidylinositol 3-kinase/AKT. The signaling pathways stimulated by the FLT3 protein control many important cellular processes such as the growth, proliferation, and survival of cells, particularly of hematopoietic progenitor cells [32, 33].

The *FLT3* receptor consists of an extracellular domain composed of a transmembrane region, a cytoplasmic juxtamembrane domain (JMD), and 2 cytoplasmic tyrosine kinase domains

(TKD; TKD1 and TKD2) interrupted by a short kinase insert. The JMD can be subdivided into 3 distinct parts: the binding motif, which is implicated in activation and in stabilizing the inactive kinase conformation; the switch motif, which consists of 2 phosphorylation sites and contains the STAT5-binding motif; and the linker/zipper peptide segment, which can undergo large amplitude rotations by pivoting about its attachment point [34].

Two predominant types of *FLT3*-activating mutations have been described in association with AML. The first involves ITD mutations that are found in about 25% of adults and 15% of pediatric AML cases [9, 35-37]. The *FLT3* mutations lead to constitutive activation by autophosphorylation of the *FLT3* RTK that could activate multiple signaling pathways and lead to cell proliferation [38, 39]. ITDs are located in exons 14 and 15 of the *FLT3* gene and show a broad variation in the position of insertion site, as well as in the number and sizes of the duplicated fragments. The length of the duplicated JMD region varies from 3 to 400 nucleotides but, despite this heterogeneity, the resultant transcripts are always in-frame [40]. These mutations are mostly located in the JMD. Localization outside the JMD is present in about 25% of the cases [41-43].

FLT3-ITD mutations have a significantly adverse impact on prognosis due to a high relapse rate, which translates into an inferior overall survival (OS) [23, 36, 44-46]. The effect on prognosis is modulated by the mutated to wild-type allele ratio, with inferior outcome in the presence of a higher load of ITDs in *FLT3*. The high *FLT3*-ITD/*FLT3*-WT ratio predict for low CR rate and OS [42-44]. Localization outside the JMD was associated with inferior outcome [42]. Many groups studied the role of alloSCT to overcome the negative impact of *FLT3*-ITD in AML patients. Some data suggest that *FLT3*-ITD positivity also outweighs other conventional prognostic markers in predicting relapse [47]. Recently published data from the German-Austrian AML Study Group showed that the high allelic ratio is a predictive factor for the beneficial effect of alloSCT [43].

The second type of *FLT3* mutation is point mutations, which most frequently occur in the activation loop of the TKD. *FLT3*-TKD mutations occur in 10% of both adult and pediatric AML patents [48]. These mutations also lead to constitutive tyrosine kinase activation. The most common TKD mutation occurs at codon 835, converting aspartic acid to tyrosine (D835Y). Also seen are mutations D835V, D835E, and D835H, converting aspartic acid to valine, glutamic acid, and histidine at residue 835, respectively. The rare mutations convert glycine to glutamic acid at residue 831 (G831E) and arginine to glutamine at residue 834 (R834Q), as well as the deletion of isoleucine at residue 836 [36, 45, 48]. TKD mutations differ from ITD in *FLT3* in their biologically transforming potency. Prognostic impact of FLT3-TKD mutations remains controversial [49, 50].

Specific gene expression signatures have been reported for CN AML with both *FLT3*-ITD and *FLT3*-TKD1 mutations. The *FLT3*-ITD signature predicts a less favorable outcome analogous to the *FLT3*-ITD mutation. High expression of wild-type *FLT3* also seems to adversely affect prognosis [51].

Sequencing studies show that *FLT3* mutations frequently occur together with mutations and alterations of other genes, especially *DNMT3A* (13.3%), *NPM1* (6.8%), Wilms tumor 1 (*WT1*,

5%), runt-related transcription factor 1 (*RUNX1*, 3.5%), mixed-lineage leukemia (*MLL*, 2.5%), CCAAT/enhancer binding protein alpha (*C/EBPα*, 1.5%), and core-binding factor (1.5%) [8, 52].

In addition, *FLT3*-ITD mutation status is different approximately in 30% of AML patients at the time of diagnosis and at relapse. *FLT3*-ITD mutations may be present in only a subset of leukemic blasts, consistent with a role in disease progression. This data suggest that *FLT3*-ITD may contribute as the initial transforming event in relapse of AML and it can reflect the selection and outgrowth of a mutant clone or evolution of a new clone harboring this mutation [53, 54].

Recent studies also show that both the *FLT3* mutations, as well as the collaborating mutations, can have prognostic significance. Recently published data submit that *FLT3*-ITD retains its negative prognostic impact in intermediate-risk AML, even in the context of other genetic abnormalities, such as *NPM1*, *DNMT3A*, and *TET2* [8, 55].

The prevalence and prognostic implications of *FLT3* mutations make them a promising therapeutic target in AML. A number of tyrosine kinase inhibitors (TKI) against *FLT3* are currently in clinical trials, with varying degrees of clinical responses, but even those patients who respond develop resistance to monotherapy [56]. One of the mechanisms of acquired resistance to several *FLT3* TKIs is the selection for *FLT3*-TKD mutations documented in relapsed patients [57]. Moreover, some data reported that *FLT3*-TKD AML blasts do not confer increased sensitivity to tyrosine kinase inhibition [58].

4. CCAAT/Enhancer-Binding Protein α (*C/EBPα*) mutations

The *C/EBPα* gene is localized on chromosome 19q13.1. This gene is intronless and it encodes a transcription factor that contains two transactivation domains: a dimerization leucine zipper region and a DNA-binding domain. It recognizes the CCAAT motif in the promoters of target genes [59]. Activity of this protein can modulate the expression of genes involved in cell cycle regulation. *C/EBPα* directly interacts with cyclin-dependent kinase 2 and 4 and arrests cell proliferation by blocking the association of these kinase with cyclins [60]. *C/EBPα* is involved in lineage specification as a transcription factor, it is crucial for the development of myeloid progenitors to the neutrophils. It is exclusively expressed in myelomonocytic cells. *C/EBPα* is specifically upregulated during granulocytic differentiation, and conditional expression of *C/EBPα* alone is sufficient to trigger neutrophil differentiation in bipotential precursors. In addition, C/EBPα is capable of arrest cell proliferation [61, 62]. C/EBPα regulates the expression of many myeloid genes, including genes encoding growth factor receptors (granulocyte-, macrophage-, and granulocyte-macrophage colony-stimulating factor) and the secondary granule proteins [59, 61]. Numerous studies suggest that *C/EBPα* is a general inhibitor of cell proliferation and a tumor suppressor [63, 64].

When *C/EBPα* gene is altered by mutations in AML, DNA-binding is altered or eliminated. *C/EBPα* mutation was first described by Pabst and colleagues in 2001 [65]. These mutations are detected in 10%–18% of CN AML patients and are predominantly found in M1 and M2 morphological subtypes of AML [65, 66]. Clinically, *C/EBPα* mutations are associated with lower leukocyte counts and lactate dehydrogenase levels and with aberrant expression of T-cell surface markers such as CD7 at presentation [67].

C/EBPα mutations can occur across the whole coding region with two main spots frequently involved, one of them affecting the N-terminus, another affecting the C-terminus. Mutations in the amino terminus truncate the full-length protein. N-terminal mutations are nonsense mutations leading to exert dominant-negative effects on the unmutated C/EBPα protein. As the mutant proteins block the binding of wild-type C/EBPα with DNA, occurs transactivation of granulocytes target genes and block of differentiation of myeloid progenitor cells. N-terminal C/EBPα mutations allow the development of committed myeloid progenitors, which represent templates for leukemia-initiating cells. C-terminal mutations are usually located between the basic region and the leucine zipper coding sequence resulting in disturbed DNA binding by the mutant protein as well as altered dimerization with its partner proteins [66]. C-terminus mutations increase the proliferation of premalignant stem cells and block myeloid lineage differentiation when homozygous. The majority of all mutations are homozygous mutations. Combination of both mutations is associated with accelerated disease development [59, 60, 66, 68]. The mechanism of C/EBPα-mutant leukemogenesis has been demonstrated in studies of C/EBPα knockout mice [69].

There is evidence that C/EBPα mutations are early events in the generation of leukemic clones. In contrast to *FLT3* mutation, in C/EBPα mutations, the majority of relapsed patients display the same mutations in both C/EBPα alleles [69]. Schin et al. demonstrated that 91% of *de novo* AML harboring *C/EBPα* mutations at diagnosis retained the identical mutant patterns but frequently changed in the allelic distribution at relapse [70].

Three different *C/EBPα* mutant patterns have been reported in AML patients. One half of patients carry single mutation on one allele (*C/EBPα*-sm), and these patients express wild type of C/EBPα. Second half of patients have double-mutated *C/EBPα* (*C/EBPα*-dm). In these cases, no wild-type *C/EBPα* protein is expressed. Some of *C/EBPα* mutated patients harbor bi-allelic mutations with an N-terminal frame-shift mutation on one allele and a C-terminal in-frame mutation on the other allele [71, 72]. Third variant of aberration is a homozygous *C/EBPα* mutation due to loss of heterozygosity, also no wild-type *C/EBPα* protein is expressed [73].

Expression profiling revealed that *C/EBPα* mutant cases cluster together, suggesting that they share similar gene expression signatures. Moreover, C-terminal *C/EBPα*-sm patients may be less distinct from *C/EBPα*-dm cases than N-terminal *C/EBPα*-sm patients [68, 71, 74]. Recent study suggest that homozygous *C/EBPα* mutations have a similar gene expression signature as *C/EBPα*-dm and thus may be considered as equivalent [75].

Most patients with *C/EBPα* mutations had a normal karyotype. Importantly, *C/EBPα* mutations have not been observed in patients with a favorable karyotype [76]. The association of deletion 9q and *C/EBPα* loss-of-function mutations could suggest that loss of a critical segment of 9q and disruption of *C/EBPα* function possibly cooperate in the pathogenesis of del(9q) AML [77]. Concurrent mutations are significantly less frequent in *C/EBPα*-dm compared with *C/EBPα*-sm AML. It is correct for *FLT3*-ITD and in particular for *NPM1*, which are essentially not present among C/EBPα-dm cases [68, 78, 79]. Recently, the mutation in transcription factor *GATA2* was found to have a strong association with *C/EBPα*-dm mutation [75].

The prognostic impact of *C/EBPα* mutations seems to be favorable. The most significant effect of mutation on clinical outcome is its association with better relapse-free survival or OS [80-84]. Recent data show that a favorable outcome is limited to double, not to single, *C/EBPα* mutations [71, 78]. These data suggest that only the *C/EBPα*-dm AML should be definitely designated as AML with the favorable risk of molecular abnormalities [84]. These results have important implications for the application of risk-stratified therapy and require confirmation. Given the evidence of the prognostic value of *C/EBPα* mutations, analysis of a possible interaction between *FLT3*-ITD and *C/EBPα* mutations is of particular interest. There are contradictory studies whether coexisting *FLT3*-ITD adversely affects the favorable prognosis of *C/EBPα* mutations. Some studies showed significantly worsened prognostic outcome in patients with *FLT3*-ITD and *C/EBPα* mutations [82, 85]. In contrast, in other study negative prognostic influence among patients with *C/EBPα* mutations were not found [81]. Obviously, further studies of numerous concurrent mutations analysis are necessary to determine the relationship between these molecular markers.

5. *RUNX1* mutations

The runt-related transcription factor 1 (*RUNX1*) gene is located on chromosome 21q22 and it consists of 10 exons. RUNX family proteins were found to have an essential role in the regulation of gene expression by temporal transcriptional repression and epigenetic silencing via chromatin alterations, especially in the context of chromosomal translocations. The protein encoded by *RUNX1* gene represents the alpha subunit of the core binding factor (CBF) and is found to be involved in the development of normal hematopoiesis. CBF is a heterodimeric transcription factor that binds to the core element of many enhancers and promoters [86]. RUNX1 protein consists of runt homology domain, transcription activation domain, and repression domain. The runt homology domain is a highly conserved protein motif, it is responsible for both DNA binding and heterodimerization with the beta-subunit of CBF. The transcription activation domain is responsible for the interaction with a transcription coactivator of RUNX1 [87]. The *RUNX1* gene is part of the t(8;21) fusion gene in CBF AML and is also affected by recurrent gene mutations in AML. The *RUNX1* gene is one of the most frequently deregulated genes in leukemia.

The reported incidence of *RUNX1* mutation in AML varied from 3% to 46% depending on the patient population selected, the regions of *RUNX1* screened, and the methods used [88-90]. The role of *RUNX1* mutation in the leukemogenesis of AML remains to be defined. *RUNX1* mutation, a class II mutation, has been implicated as the initiating event to block differentiation of hematopoietic cells, and the subsequent class I gene mutation would synergistically provide growth advantages of these cells and lead to the development of AML [88]. Most of *RUNX1*-mutated patients concurrently had other gene mutations and the majority simultaneously showed class I mutations, most commonly *FLT3/ITD*, *FLT3/TKD*, and *N-RAS*, which might result in hyperactivation of the receptor tyrosine kinase-RAS signaling pathways [88]. Interestingly, Tang et al. reported high coincidence of *RUNX1* mutations with *MLL/PTD*, and both *FLT3/ITD* and *FLT3/TKD* mutations [88].

RUNX1 mutations in AML are associated with poor outcomes, which contrast with the favorable prognostic effect of gene fusions involving *RUNX1* [88, 90]. Differential prognostic value of chromosomal damage and mutation in *RUNX1* consequences the importance of a complete assessment of genetic factors in the pathogenesis of AML.

RUNX1 mutations are less frequent in cytogenetic high-risk AML and rarely occur in CBF-AML and APL. Among intermediate-risk AML, *RUNX1* mutations are mostly associated with normal karyotype, with trisomy 8, and with trisomy 13 [90, 91]. With regard to the correlation with other molecular makers, in some studies, a higher frequency of coincidence of *FLT3* mutation and *RUNX1* mutations was reported [88, 92]. But data from Dicker et al. did not confirm that [89, 91]. Significant correlation of *RUNX1* mutations with *MLL*-PTD and *IDH* mutations and an inverse correlation with *NPM1* and *CEBPA* mutations was observed in a large cohort of AML patients [90]. Recently, rare coexistence of *RUNX1* and *NPM1* mutations in *de novo* intermediate risk karyotype AML was reported [93, 94]. In the first study, it was found that *RUNX1* mutations in these cases were structurally unusual when compared to *RUNX1* mutations observed in *NPM1* wild-type cases and located outside the *RUNX1* homology domain and were also present in the germline. However, later study did not confirm structurally unusual *RUNX1* mutations in *NPM1* mutated cases. These data could suggest that *FLT3*, *RUNX1*, *MLL*-PTD, and *IDH* mutations contribute to leukemogenesis by other mechanisms than do *NPM1* and *C/EBPα* mutations.

6. *RAS* mutations

The *RAS* oncogene family was the first human oncogene discovered in human cancer and has been extensively studied over the last 3 decades. RAS gene is named for "rat sarcoma." The *RAS* gene family is comprised of three homologues, *HRAS* (11p15.5), *KRAS* (12p12.1), and *NRAS* (1p13.2). The members of the RAS family are tyrosine kinase receptors that are important participants of many signaling pathways connected with functional control of a large variety of cellular effects including cell cycle progression, growth, migration, cytoskeletal changes, apoptosis, and senescence. The crosstalk between these multiple signaling pathways and others controlled by different sets of signaling molecules creates molecular networks whose balance is crucial to determine the final outcome of cellular responses in the cell [95, 96]. RAS proteins function as a conduit for signals received from RTK on the cell surface through downstream cell signaling partners to nuclear transcription factors regulating cell growth and cell-cycling proteins [97]. Under physiologic conditions, RAS activation is initiated by binding with ligand that induces RTK autophosphorylation, dimerization, and activation [98].

Mutations in *RAS* genes are frequent in AML and exemplify mutation Class I, initiating key downstream hyperproliferative signal transduction pathways. *NRAS* mutations are the most common. *NRAS* and *KRAS* mutations are present in about 25% and 15% of AML patients [52].

Constitutive activation of RAS originates from mutations in *RAS* itself or from mutation or overexpression of related RTK such as *FLT3* or *KIT*. Activated NRAS signals get through the several pathways to mediate oncogenic effects, especially the MAPK, PI3K–AKT, and Ral–GDS pathways [97, 98]. In contrast to other gene mutations frequently involved in AML, *NRAS* mutations are present much more often in patients with myelodysplastic syndromes (MDS) and secondary AML (sAML) arising from MDS. An analysis of samples from MDS patients and sAML identified only a modest increase in the frequency of *NRAS* mutations in the sAML cohort compared with the MDS group, suggesting that *NRAS* mutations may be an early event in MDS [89].

Despite being initially described almost 30 years ago, the prognostic implications of RAS mutations remain controversial. Several studies indicate that *RAS* mutation did not impact prognosis in CN AML patients [99, 100]. In contrast, *RAS* mutations have been linked to an inferior outcome in AML by some researchers [101]. In childhood AML, activating *NRAS* mutations commonly in cooperation with *NPM1* mutations occur frequently in the favorable risk population [102].

No association *NRAS* mutations with cytogenetic alterations have been identified. *NRAS* are similarly distributed among the major cytogenetic groups [102]. *NRAS* has been previously found to correlate with abnormalities of chromosomes 3 and 16 [100, 103]. However, this was not confirmed in the next study [102]. *RAS* mutations tend to occur together with *NPM1* mutations, while coexistence of *RAS* mutations with *FLT3-ITD*, *CEBPA*, or *WT1* appears to be less common [99, 102].

7. *KIT* (CD117) mutations

The *KIT* gene is located on chromosome 4q12 and encodes transmembrane glycoprotein that belongs to a family of the type III RTK. The structure of RTK consists of five immunoglobulin-like domains in the extracellular portion of the receptor, a transmembrane and juxtamembrane domain, and an intracellular kinase domain [104]. The KIT protein is found in the cell membrane and binds with ligand. This binding activates the KIT protein, which then activates other proteins inside the cell by adding a phosphate group at specific positions. This phosphorylation leads to the activation of a series of proteins in multiple signaling pathways. The signaling pathways stimulated by the KIT control cell growth, proliferation, survival, and migration of cells [104, 105]. The majority of stem cells in the bone marrow express CD117. KIT expression and intensity on normal blast cells in the bone marrow decrease during maturation as a strong negative regulation during hematopoiesis. *KIT* is expressed on the surface of leukemic blasts in 80% of AML patients.

Ligand-independent activation of *KIT* can be caused by gain-of-function mutations that have been reported in core binding factor (CBF) AML [106, 107]. In cytogenetically favorable CBF-AML, which is associated with t(8;21)(q22;q22) and inv(16)/t(16;16)(q13;q22), *KIT* mutation is found most frequently within exon 17, which encodes the *KIT* activation loop in the kinase domain, and in exon 8, which encodes a region in the extracellular portion of the *KIT* receptor

[104, 108, 109]. Mutations of *KIT* occur in 20%–25% of t(8;21) and in approximately 30% of inv(16) cases [106].

The clinical significance of *KIT* mutations in CBF-AML has been intensively studied. The clinical significance of c-*KIT* mutations in CBF-AML is potentially related to mutation type, patient age, and type of chromosomal translocation. Paschka et al. reported that *KIT* mutations confer higher relapse risk and adverse OS in AML with inv(16) and t(8;21) AML [106, 110]. Contrary to most published studies, in a single CBF AML group no association between c-KIT mutations and prognosis of AML was found [107]. Various further studies confirmed that *C-KIT* mutations linked to adverse outcome in patients with t(8;21) but not in inv(16)/t(16;16) AML [108, 111-113]. National Comprehensive Cancer Network (NCCN) guidelines have defined t(8;21) and inv(16) AML with *KIT* mutations as intermediate risk guidelines, whereas ELN has provided no further recommendation for those with a *KIT* mutation [9, 114].

8. *TET2* mutations

The TET (ten–eleven translocation) protein family includes three members (TET1, TET2, and TET3) and is involved in the epigenetic regulation, in particular, responsible for demethylation. *TET2* gene located on chromosome 4q24 and catalytic activity converts 5-methylcytosine to 5-hydroxymethylcytosine in an α-ketoglutarate-dependent reaction [115]. TET proteins further oxidize 5-hydroxymethylcytosine to formylcytosine and carboxylcytosine, which are replaced by unmodified cytosines through the DNA repair machinery [115]. The data published suggests a role for the TETs in the regulation of gene expression through modification of chromatin at promoter regions [116]. The *TET* family members have two highly conserved regions, an *N*-terminal cysteine-rich domain followed by a 2-oxoglutarate -Fe(II) oxygenase characteristic double-stranded b-helix [117]. Somatic loss-of-function mutations in *TET2* gene occur in a significant proportion of patients with myeloid malignancies. In AML, TET2 mutations affect 7%–10% of the adult and 1.5%–4% of pediatric patients [118-121].

TET2 mutations show loss-of-function phenotype [118, 122] and are anticipated to result in hypermethylation [123]. It was shown that *TET2* mutation samples display low levels of 5-hydroxymethylcytosine compared with normal controls, supporting a functional relevance of *TET2* mutation in leukemogenesis. *TET2* mutant AML displays increased promoter methylation [123]. In addition, it was shown that *TET2* mutants do not suppress the function of the wild-type protein and hence do not show dominant negative traits [118].

Several studies based on mouse model suggested that *TET2* mutation occurs in progenitor cells, which creates a predisposition to the development of myeloid malignancy. These studies confirm the role of *TET2* mutations in the pathogenesis of myeloid malignancies. Therefore, *TET2* mutation may exist as an early event, and in cooperation with secondary mutations, drives the phenotype of the disease [124, 125].

TET2 mutations were spread over all cytogenetic subgroups. It was reported that *TET2* alterations are associated with *NPM1* and *FLT3*-ITD mutations [119, 121, 126]. Recent data observed that *TET2* and *IDH1/2* mutations were mutually exclusive in a large, genetically annotated *de novo* AML cohort, suggesting that these lesions may be biologically redundant [123]. The high incidence of *DNMT3A* mutations in both of these groups was reported [118].

This could indicate of a cooperative mechanism through which mutations impairing DNA hydroxymethylation and DNA methylation contribute to leukemogenesis [118].

The prognostic relevance of *TET2* mutation is still not well established and remains controversial. In some studies no prognostic impact of *TET2* mutations on clinical outcome as well as in CN AML subtype was observed [121, 126]. A study of Cancer and Leukemia Group B Study with a large cohort of AML patients reported an adverse prognostic impact in the molecular favorable-risk cytogenetically CN AML group whereas there was no impact of mutation in the intermediate risk I group [120]. In a study by Chou et al., shorter OS was observed in patients with intermediate-risk cytogenetic [119]. An integrated genetic analysis revealed that mutations of *TET2* gene are associated with poor OS in intermediate risk patients, regardless of the presence of the *FLT3-ITD* mutation. Weissmann et al. also showed a negative impact of *TET2* mutations on survival in favorable risk AML patients with normal cytogenetics [127]. Most recently, the negative effect of *TET2* mutation on OS was confirmed in various risk groups in adult AML patients less than 60 years of age [118].

In addition, recently demonstrated low levels of *TET2* expression as a poor prognostic marker for patients without *TET2* or *IDH1* mutations can suggest that both loss of function mutations and low expression of *TET2* are markers of poor prognosis in AML [118]. The development of target therapies could be beneficial for these patients [118].

9. *IHD1* and *IDH2* mutations

Isocitrate dehydrogenases (IDH) 1 and 2 are NADP-dependent enzymes of the citrate cycle that convert isocitrate to α-ketoglutarate. *IDH1* and *IDH2* genes encode cytoplasmic/peroxisomal isocitrate dehydrogenase 1 and mitochondrial isocitrate dehydrogenase 2, respectively. These are homodimeric, NADP+-dependent enzymes that catalyze the oxidative decarboxylation of isocitrate to α-ketoglutarate (α-KG), generating NADPH from NADP+. NADPH is an important source of synthetic reducing power and has key functions in cellular detoxification processes. Both genes function in a crossroads of cellular metabolism, cellular defense against oxidative stress, oxidative respiration, and oxygen-sensing signal transduction [128].

Somatic mutations in *IDH1* and *IDH2* occur frequently (50%–80%) in adult glioma [129]. In *de novo* CN AML, *IDH1/2* mutations occur in 15% and in 20% in sAML [24, 123, 130]. The frequency is higher in CN AML and in elderly patients. In contrast with glioma, in AML, *IDH2* mutations occur more frequently than *IDH1* mutations, with *IDH2*-R140Q as the most common mutation [131, 132].

The typical *IDH1* mutation affects the evolutionary conserved arginine residue 132 (*IDH1* R132) and the analogous amino acids 172 (*IDH2* R172) and 140 (*IDH2* R140) of the *IDH2* gene [133]. A great variety of *IDH1/2* mutants were reported (*IDH1*-R132, *IDH2*-R140, *IDH2*-R172 and their variants). All of them possess varying enzymatic properties. The most common *IDH1/2* mutants in AML, *IDH2* R140Q, and another mutant *IDH1*-R132H are weak *D*-2HG producers, as compared with other variants. Different mutant, *IDH1* R132C, produces relatively high levels of *D*-2HG [129]. It has been hypothesized that in oncogenesis, the intracellular *D*-2HG concentration that gives the largest growth advantage varies depending on the tumor's cell type of origin. This could explain why each type of cancer has a specific *IDH1/2* mutation. In addition, an *IDH1/2* mutation and the subsequent high *D*-2HG levels may affect which specific type of cancer is being formed [129, 134]. Acquired somatic mutations of *IDH1* and *IDH2* genes contribute to abnormal metabolic processes. Despite these effects of 2-HG on DNA and histone methylation, there is a growing consensus that, while obviously important, IDH1/2 mutations are insufficient to drive neoplasia [134]. *IDH1* and *IDH2* missense mutations were infrequent in patients with preleukemic disorders, particularly in MDS, Paroxysmal nocturnal hemoglobinuria (PNH), and Aplastic anemia (AA) patients, suggesting that these genetic alterations may not be essential in the development and transformation of preleukemic disorders to AML [135].

In AML, *IDH1* mutations correlate with worse patient survival, whereas *IDH2*-R140Q mutations are associated with a moderately prolonged survival [136, 137]. Prognostic effect is known to depend on certain biological factors as well as a combination of cytogenetics and other mutations such as those in *FLT3* and *NPM1* [24, 130-132].

IDH mutations in AML are predominantly associated with CN AML and *NPM1* mutations.

IDH1 and *IDH2* mutations are mutually exclusive of each other, or with *TET2* mutations, which suggests functional redundancy [123].

10. *DNMT3A* mutations

Somatic mutations in the *DNMT3A* have been reported approximately in 22% of *de novo* AML and 36% of CN AML [138]. Mutations in *DNMT3A* were first described by Ley et al. using whole genome sequencing [139]. *DNMT3A* belongs to the mammalian methyltransferase gene family which is responsible for tissue-specific gene expression [140]. DNA methyltransferases are the key enzymes for genome methylation, which plays an important role in epigenetically regulated gene expression and repression. *DNMT3A* together with other methyltransferase conducts *de novo* methylation of cytosine residues in CpG islands by the enzymatic addition of methyl residues from S-adenosyl-L-methionine to the 5-carbon atom of the cytosine ring. CpG islands are often located proximate to gene promoters thereby regulating their activation. Actively transcribed genes display unmethylated CpG islands that supports the euchromatin structure whereas methylated CpG islands are associated with untranscribed genes stabilizing the heterochromatin structure [141, 142]. Cancer genomes are most commonly characterized by global DNA hypomethylation. However, cancer cells also typically exhibit distinct regions of DNA hypermethylation, which are particularly well characterized in the CpG islands of promoter regions of tumor-suppressor genes. *DNMT3A* mutations are typically heterogenous. More common, mutations affect residual R882 within the methyltransferase domain [139, 143].

The biology of *DNMT3A* is not fully understood. Holz-Schietinger et al. reported that mutations in *DNMT3A* could retard its function by multiple mechanisms as changes in the catalytic properties, its processivity, and the disruption of interaction with binding partners [144]. Furthermore, Russler-Germain et al. found that mutations in the position R882 inhibit the formation of active tetramers of *DNMT3A* [145]. The impaired function of mutated *DNMT3A* leads to a hypomethylated genome of myeloid cells possibly promoting leukemogenesis and influencing disease outcome [146]. *DNMT3A* mutations are typically heterozygous. Continued expression of both mutated and wild-type *DNMT3A* in heterozygous cells, observed *in vitro*, suggests a dominant negative or possibly a neomorphic gain of function role for *DNMT3A* mutations in AML [147].

Since the *DNMT3A* mutations are present in the early preleukemic cells, this alteration seems to be a "founder" mutation, which can be implicated as functional components of AML evolution [148, 149]. *DNMT3A* mutations are highly associated with *NPM1*, *FLT3*, *IDH1*, and *IDH2* [150, 151]. Patients with *DNMT3A* mutations are typically older than average, have a higher white cell count, and are more likely to have monocytic or myelomonocytic leukemia (FAB M4/M5) [8].

Several studies reported a negative prognostic impact of *DNMT3A* mutations [150-154]. Prognostic effect is known to depend on certain biological factors as well as a combination of cytogenetics and other mutations such as those in *FLT3* and *NPM1*.

Some authors have found stability of *DNMT3A* mutations during the course of disease; therefore those aberrations could be a potential marker for minimal residual disease (MRD). Furthermore, the presence of *DNMT3A* mutations seems to be associated with the incidence of *FLT3*-ITD-positive clones at relapse possibly influencing the responsiveness of *FLT3*-positive cases to chemotherapy [155, 156]. In contrast, Hou et al. reported persistence of *DNMT3A* mutations at CR in AML patients, which later achieved relapse and died of disease progression. These data could relate the persistence of *DNMT3A* mutations and high risk of relapse [156]. Recently, Pløen et al. have identified persistence of *DNMT3A* mutations in long-term remission of patients with AML that received cytoreduction or palliative therapy [157]. Using cell-sorting, the authors showed that *DNMT3A* mutations were present in T-cells and B-cells at diagnosis in some patients, and also in T-cells several years after diagnosis. The presence of *DNMT3A* in both B-cells and T-cells could lead to assumption that mutation had occurred in an early pre-leukemic stem cell prior to the acquisition of other genetic events, and could be resistant to chemotherapy [157]. Therefore, further exploration of the role of *DNMT3A* R882H mutations for the progression of AML disease is needed.

Recent discoveries utilizing whole-exome sequencing in a large cohort of persons unselected for cancer or hematologic phenotypes have demonstrated somatic mutations in significant proportion of persons particularly older than 65 years. Moreover, *DNMT3A* gene together with *TET2*, *ASXL1* (additional sex combs like transcriptional regulator 1), and *PPM1D* (Protein phosphatase 1D) had disproportionately high numbers of somatic mutations [5, 158]. The data suggest that mutations in pre-leukemic cells could precede leukemia. Furthermore, *DNMT3A* mutations could drive clonal expansions.

http://dx.doi.org/10.5772/60928

11. Conclusion

The whole gene analysis has revealed that leukemic cell carry hundreds of mutated genes. Most of them are "passenger" mutations, which do not provide a selective advantage, and a less number of mutations are "driver" mutations. The latter can cause the tumor. The simultaneous presence of genetic alterations with different functional effects on hematopoietic progenitors led to the concept of leukemogenesis as a multi-step process that ultimately gives rise to malignant transformation. Evidence from many murine models confirmed that a single genetic change is not sufficient for the occurrence of AML. Moreover, two modern studies have demonstrated that somatic mutations that drive clonal expansion of blood cells were a common finding in the elderly and most frequently involved *DNMT3A*, *TET2*, or *ASXL1*. The age-related clonal hematopoiesis is a common premalignant condition that is also associated with increased overall mortality [5, 158]. Overall this knowledge has provided useful elements to stratify AML patients into different subgroups, resulting in better prognosis and therapy.

Author details

Olga Blau*

Address all correspondence to: olga.blau@charite.de

Charité Universitätsmedizin Berlin, Department of Hematology, Oncology and Tumourimmunology, Berlin, Germany

References

[1] Renneville, A., et al., *Cooperating gene mutations in acute myeloid leukemia: a review of the literature*. Leukemia, 2008. 22(5): p. 915-931.

[2] Knudson, A.G., *Mutation and cancer: statistical study of retinoblastoma*. Proceedings of the National Academy of Sciences, 1971. 68(4): p. 820-823.

[3] Tucker, T. and J.M. Friedman, *Pathogenesis of hereditary tumors: beyond the "two-hit" hypothesis*. Clinical Genetics, 2002. 62(5): p. 345-357.

[4] Park, S., Y. Koh, and S.-S. Yoon, *Effects of somatic mutations are associated with SNP in the progression of individual acute myeloid leukemia patient: the two-hit theory explains inherited predisposition to pathogenesis*. Genomics Inform, 2013. 11(1): p. 34-37.

[5] Genovese, G., et al., *Clonal hematopoiesis and blood-cancer risk inferred from blood DNA sequence*. TheNew England Journal of Medicine, 2014. 371(26): p. 2477-2487.

[6] Reya, T., et al., *Stem cells, cancer, and cancer stem cells*. Nature, 2001. 414(6859): p. 105-111.

[7] Grimwade, D., *The changing paradigm of prognostic factors in acute myeloid leukaemia*. Best Practice & Research Clinical Haematology, 2012. 25(4): p. 419-25.

[8] Patel, J.P., et al., *Prognostic relevance of integrated genetic profiling in acute myeloid leukemia*. The New England Journal of Medicine, 2012. 366(12): p. 1079-1089.

[9] Döhner, H., et al., *Diagnosis and management of acute myeloid leukemia in adults: recommendations from an international expert panel, on behalf of the European LeukemiaNet*. Blood, 2010. 115(3): p. 453-474.

[10] Frehlick, L.J., J.M. Eirin-Lopez, and J. Ausio, *New insights into the nucleophosmin/nucleoplasmin family of nuclear chaperones*. Bioessays, 2007. 29: p. 49-59.

[11] Kurki, S., et al., *Nucleolar protein NPM interacts with HDM2 and protects tumor suppressor protein p53 from HDM2-mediated degradation*. Cell, 2004. 5: p. 465-475.

[12] Lindström, M.S., *NPM1/B23: a multifunctional chaperone in ribosome biogenesis and chromatin remodeling*. Biochemistry Research International, 2011. 2011: p. 16.

[13] Falini, B., et al., *Translocations and mutations involving the nucleophosmin (NPM1) gene in lymphomas and leukemias*. Haematologica, 2007. 92: p. 519-532.

[14] Falini, B., et al., *Aberrant subcellular expression of nucleophosmin and NPM-MLF1 fusion protein in acute myeloid leukaemia carrying t(3;5): a comparison with NPMc+ AML*. Leukemia, 2006. 20: p. 368-371.

[15] Redner, R., et al., *The t(5;17) variant of acute promyelocytic leukemia expresses a nucleophosmin-retinoic acid receptor fusion*. Blood, 1996. 87: p. 882-886.

[16] Sportoletti, P., et al., *Mouse models of NPM1-mutated acute myeloid leukemia: biological and clinical implications*. Leukemia, 2015. 29(2): p. 269-278.

[17] Grisendi, S., et al., *Nucleophosmin and cancer*. Nature Reviews Cancer, 2006. 6(7): p. 493-505.

[18] Sportoletti, P., et al., *Npm1 is a haploinsufficient suppressor of myeloid and lymphoid malignancies in the mouse*. Blood, 2008. 111: p. 3859-3862.

[19] Falini, B., et al., *Cytoplasmic nucleophosmin in acute myelogenous leukemia with a normal karyotype*. The New England Journal of Medicine, 2005. 352(3): p. 254-266.

[20] Ferrara, F. and C.A. Schiffer, *Acute myeloid leukaemia in adults*. The Lancet, 2013. 381(9865): p. 484-495.

[21] Falini, B., et al., *Molecular and alternative methods for diagnosis of acute myeloid leukemia with mutated NPM1: flexibility may help*. Haematologica, 2010. 95: p. 529-534.

[22] Falini, B., et al., *Aberrant cytoplasmic expression of C-terminal-truncated NPM leukaemic mutant is dictated by tryptophans loss and a new NES motif.* Leukemia, 2007. 21: p. 2052-2054.

[23] Schlenk, R.F., et al., *Mutations and treatment outcome in cytogenetically normal acute myeloid leukemia.* The New England Journal of Medicine, 2008. 358(18): p. 1909-1918.

[24] Paschka, P., et al., *IDH1 and IDH2 mutations are frequent genetic alterations in acute myeloid leukemia and confer adverse prognosis in cytogenetically normal acute myeloid leukemia with NPM1 mutation without FLT3 internal tandem duplication.* Journal of Clinical Oncology, 2010. 28(22): p. 3636-3643.

[25] Dvorakova, D., et al., *Monitoring of minimal residual disease in acute myeloid leukemia with frequent and rare patient-specific NPM1 mutations.* American Journal of Hematology, 2010. 85(12): p. 926-929.

[26] Schnittger, S., et al., *Minimal residual disease levels assessed by NPM1 mutation–specific RQ-PCR provide important prognostic information in AML.* Blood, 2009. 114: p. 2220-2231.

[27] Stahl, T., et al., *Minimal residual disease diagnostics in patients with acute myeloid leukemia in the post-transplant period: comparison of peripheral blood and bone marrow analysis.* Leukemia & Lymphoma, 2010. 51(10): p. 1837-43.

[28] Kronke, J., et al., *Monitoring of minimal residual disease in NPM1-mutated acute myeloid leukemia: a study from the German-Austrian acute myeloid leukemia study group.* Journal of Clinical Oncology, 2011. 29(19): p. 2709-2716.

[29] Rosnet, O., et al., *Human FLT3/FLK2 gene: cDNA cloning and expression in hematopoietic cells.* Blood, 1993. 82: p. 1110-1119.

[30] Meshinchi, S. and F.R. Appelbaum, *Structural and functional alterations of FLT3 in acute myeloid leukemia.* Clinical Cancer Research, 2009. 15(13): p. 4263-4269.

[31] Sitnicka, E., et al., *Human CD34+ hematopoietic stem cells capable of multilineage engrafting NOD/SCID mice express flt3: distinct flt3 and c-kit expression and response patterns on mouse and candidate human hematopoietic stem cells.* Blood, 2003. 102: p. 881-886.

[32] Gilliland, D.G. and J.D. Griffin, *The roles of FLT3 in hematopoiesis and leukemia.* Blood, 2002. 100, p. 1532-1542.

[33] Adolfsson, J., et al., *Upregulation of Flt3 expression within the bone marrow Lin−Sca1+c-kit+ stem cell compartment is accompanied by loss of self-renewal capacity.* Immunity, 2001. 15(4): p. 659-669.

[34] Griffith, J., et al., *The structural basis for autoinhibition of FLT3 by the juxtamembrane domain.* Molecular Cell, 2004. 13(2): p. 169-178.

[35] Gale, R.E., et al., *The impact of FLT3 internal tandem duplication mutant level, number, size and interaction with NPM1 mutations in a large cohort of young adult patients with acute myeloid leukemia.* Blood, 2008. 111: p. 2776-2784.

[36] Kottaridis, P.D., et al., *The presence of a FLT3 internal tandem duplication in patients with acute myeloid leukemia (AML) adds important prognostic information to cytogenetic risk group and response to the first cycle of chemotherapy: analysis of 854 patients from the United Kingdom Medical Research Council AML 10 and 12 trials.* Blood, 2001. 98: p. 1752-1759.

[37] Marcucci, G., T. Haferlach, and H. Dohner, *Molecular genetics of adult acute myeloid leukemia: prognostic and therapeutic implications.* Journal of Clinical Oncology, 2011. 29(5): p. 475-486.

[38] Rocnik, J.L., et al., *Roles of tyrosine 589 and 591 in STAT5 activation and transformation mediated by FLT3-ITD.* Blood, 2006. 108: p. 1339-1345.

[39] Gu, T.-l., et al., *Survey of activated FLT3 signaling in leukemia.* PLoS ONE, 2011. 6(4): p. e19169.

[40] Schnittger, S., et al., *Analysis of FLT3 length mutations in 1003 patients with acute myeloid leukemia: correlation to cytogenetics, FAB subtype, and prognosis in the AMLCG study and usefulness as a marker for the detection of minimal residual disease.* Presented in part at the 42nd annual meeting of the American Society of Hematology, December 1-5, 2000, San Francisco, CA (abstract 3569). Vol. 100. 2002. 59-66.

[41] Breitenbuecher, F., et al., *Identification of a novel type of ITD mutations located in nonjuxtamembrane domains of the FLT3 tyrosine kinase receptor.* Blood, 2009. 113: p. 4074-4077.

[42] Kayser, S., et al., *Insertion of FLT3 internal tandem duplication in the tyrosine kinase domain-1 is associated with resistance to chemotherapy and inferior outcome.* Blood, 2009. 114: p. 2386-2392.

[43] Schlenk, R.F., et al., *Differential impact of allelic ratio and insertion site in FLT3-ITD–positive AML with respect to allogeneic transplantation.* Blood, 2014. 124: p. 3441-3449.

[44] Blau, O., et al., *Molecular analysis of different FLT3-ITD mutations in acute myeloid leukemia.* Leukemia & Lymphoma, 2013. 54(1): p. 145-152.

[45] Fröhling, S., et al., *Prognostic significance of activating FLT3 mutations in younger adults (16 to 60 years) with acute myeloid leukemia and normal cytogenetics: a study of the AML Study Group Ulm.* Blood, 2002. 100: p. 4372-4380.

[46] Mrózek, K., et al., *Clinical relevance of mutations and gene-expression changes in adult acute myeloid leukemia with normal cytogenetics: are we ready for a prognostically prioritized molecular classification?* Blood, 2007. 109: p. 431-448.

[47] Sengsayadeth, S.M., et al., *Allo-SCT for high-risk AML-CR1 in the molecular era: impact of FLT3/ITD outweighs the conventional markers.* Bone Marrow Transplant, 2012. 47(12): p. 1535-1537.

[48] Yamamoto, Y., et al., *Activating mutation of D835 within the activation loop of FLT3 in human hematologic malignancies.* Blood, 2001. 97: p. 2434-2439.

[49] Mead, A.J., et al., *FLT3 tyrosine kinase domain mutations are biologically distinct from and have a significantly more favorable prognosis than FLT3 internal tandem duplications in patients with acute myeloid leukemia.* Blood, 2007. 110: 1262-1270.

[50] Whitman, S.P., et al., *FLT3 D835/I836 mutations are associated with poor disease-free survival and a distinct gene-expression signature among younger adults with de novo cytogenetically normal acute myeloid leukemia lacking FLT3 internal tandem duplications.* Blood, 2008. 111: p. 1552-1559.

[51] Ozeki, K., et al., *Biologic and clinical significance of the FLT3 transcript level in acute myeloid leukemia.* Blood, 2004. 103: p. 1901-1908.

[52] Cancer Genome Atlas Research Network. *Genomic and epigenomic landscapes of adult de novo acute myeloid leukemia.* The New England Journal of Medicine, 2013. 368(22): p. 2059-2074.

[53] Kottaridis, P.D., et al., *Studies of FLT3 mutations in paired presentation and relapse samples from patients with acute myeloid leukemia: implications for the role of FLT3 mutations in leukemogenesis, minimal residual disease detection, and possible therapy with FLT3 inhibitors.* Blood, 2002. 100: p. 2393-2398.

[54] Shih, L.-Y., et al., *Internal tandem duplication of FLT3 in relapsed acute myeloid leukemia: a comparative analysis of bone marrow samples from 108 adult patients at diagnosis and relapse.* Blood, 2002. 100: p. 2387-2392.

[55] Gaidzik, V.I., et al., *Clinical impact of DNMT3A mutations in younger adult patients with acute myeloid leukemia: results of the AML Study Group (AMLSG).* Blood, 2013. 121: p. 4769-4777.

[56] Chu, S.H. and D. Small, *Mechanisms of resistance to FLT3 inhibitors.* Drug Resistance Updates, 2009. 12(1–2): p. 8-16.

[57] Moore, A.S., et al., *Selective FLT3 inhibition of FLT3-ITD+ acute myeloid leukaemia resulting in secondary D835Y mutation: a model for emerging clinical resistance patterns.* Leukemia, 2012. 26(7): p. 1462-1470.

[58] Mead, A.J., et al., *Acute myeloid leukaemia blast cells with a tyrosine kinase domain mutation of FLT3 are less sensitive to lestaurtinib than those with a FLT3 internal tandem duplication.* British Journal of Haematology, 2008. 141(4): p. 454-460.

[59] Koschmieder, S., et al., *Dysregulation of the C/EBPα differentiation pathway in human cancer.* Journal of Clinical Oncology, 2009. 27(4): p. 619-628.

[60] Wang, H., et al., *C/EBPα arrests cell proliferation through direct inhibition of Cdk2 and Cdk4*. Molecular Cell, 2001. 8(4): p. 817-828.

[61] Radomska, H.S., et al., *CCAAT enhancer binding protein alpha is a regulatory switch sufficient for induction of granulocytic development from bipotential myeloid progenitors*. Molecular and Cellular Biology, 1998. 18(7): p. 4301-4314.

[62] Zhang, D.-E., et al., *Absence of granulocyte colony-stimulating factor signaling and neutrophil development in CCAAT enhancer binding protein α-deficient mice*. Proceedings of the National Academy of Sciences, 1997. 94(2): p. 569-574.

[63] Umek, R.M., A.D. Friedman, and S.L. McKnight, *CCAAT-enhancer binding-protein - a component of a differentiation switch*. Science, 1991. 251(4991): p. 288-292.

[64] Watkins, P.J., et al., *Proliferation and tumorigenicity induced by CCAAT/enhancer-binding protein*. Cancer Research, 1996. 56(5): p. 1063-1067.

[65] Pabst, T., et al., *Dominant-negative mutations of CEBPA, encoding CCAAT/enhancer binding protein-[alpha] (C/EBP[alpha]), in acute myeloid leukemia*. Nature Genetics, 2001. 27(3): p. 263-270.

[66] Nerlov, C., *C/EBP[alpha] mutations in acute myeloid leukaemias*. Nature Reviews Cancer, 2004. 4(5): p. 394-400.

[67] Wouters, B.J., et al., *Distinct gene expression profiles of acute myeloid/T-lymphoid leukemia with silenced CEBPA and mutations in NOTCH1*. Blood, 2007. 110: p. 3706-3714.

[68] Taskesen, E., et al., *Prognostic impact, concurrent genetic mutations, and gene expression features of AML with CEBPA mutations in a cohort of 1182 cytogenetically normal AML patients: further evidence for CEBPA double mutant AML as a distinctive disease entity*. Blood, 2011. 117: 2469-2475.

[69] Kirstetter, P., et al., *Modeling of C/EBPα mutant acute myeloid leukemia reveals a common expression signature of committed myeloid leukemia-initiating cells*. Cancer Cell, 2008. 13(4): p. 299-310.

[70] Shih, L.Y., et al., *AML patients with CEBP[alpha] mutations mostly retain identical mutant patterns but frequently change in allelic distribution at relapse: a comparative analysis on paired diagnosis and relapse samples*. Leukemia, 2006. 20(4): p. 604-609.

[71] Wouters, B.J., et al., *Double CEBPA mutations, but not single CEBPA mutations, define a subgroup of acute myeloid leukemia with a distinctive gene expression profile that is uniquely associated with a favorable outcome*. Blood, 2009. 113: p. 3088-3091.

[72] Cagnetta, A., et al., *Role of genotype-based approach in the clinical management of adult acute myeloid leukemia with normal cytogenetics*. Leukemia Research, 2014. 38(6): p. 649-659.

[73] Wouters, B.J., et al., *Segmental uniparental disomy as a recurrent mechanism for homozygous CEBPA mutations in acute myeloid leukemia*. Leukemia, 2007. 21(11): p. 2382-2384.

[74] Valk, P.J.M., et al., *Prognostically useful gene-expression profiles in acute myeloid leukemia.* The New England Journal of Medicine, 2004. 350(16): p. 1617-1628.

[75] Marceau-Renaut, A., et al., *Classification of CEBPA mutated acute myeloid leukemia by GATA2 mutations.* American Journal of Hematology, 2015. 90: p.E93-E94.

[76] Pabst, T. and B.U. Mueller, *Transcriptional dysregulation during myeloid transformation in AML.* Oncogene, 2007. 26(47): p. 6829-6837.

[77] Fröhling, S., et al., *Acute myeloid leukemia with deletion 9q within a noncomplex karyotype is associated with CEBPA loss-of-function mutations.* Genes, Chromosomes and Cancer, 2005. 42(4): p. 427-432.

[78] Green, C.L., et al., *Prognostic significance of CEBPA mutations in a large cohort of younger adult patients with acute myeloid leukemia: impact of double CEBPA mutations and the interaction with FLT3 and NPM1 mutations.* Journal of Clinical Oncology, 2010. 28(16): p. 2739-2747.

[79] Behdad, A., et al., *A clinical grade sequencing-based assay for CEBPA mutation testing: report of a large series of myeloid neoplasms.* The Journal of Molecular Diagnostics, 2015. 17(1): p. 76-84.

[80] Bienz, M., et al., *Risk assessment in patients with acute myeloid leukemia and a normal karyotype.* Clinical Cancer Research, 2005. 11(4): p. 1416-1424.

[81] Fröhling, S., et al., *CEBPA mutations in younger adults with acute myeloid leukemia and normal cytogenetics: prognostic relevance and analysis of cooperating mutations.* Journal of Clinical Oncology, 2004. 22(4): p. 624-633.

[82] Preudhomme, C., et al., *Favorable prognostic significance of CEBPA mutations in patients with de novo acute myeloid leukemia: a study from the Acute Leukemia French Association (ALFA).* Blood, 2002. 100: p. 2717-2723.

[83] Pastore, F., et al., *Long-term follow-up of cytogenetically normal CEBPA-mutated AML.* Journal of Hematology & Oncology, 2014. 7(1): p. 55.

[84] Wen, X.-M., et al., *Double CEBPA mutations are prognostically favorable in non-M3 acute myeloid leukemia patients with wild-type NPM1 and FLT3-ITD.* International Journal of Clinical and Experimental Pathology, 2014. 7(10): p. 6832-6840.

[85] Renneville, A., et al., *The favorable impact of CEBPA mutations in patients with acute myeloid leukemia is only observed in the absence of associated cytogenetic abnormalities and FLT3 internal duplication.* Blood, 2009. 113: p. 5090-5093.

[86] Taniuchi, I. and D.R. Littman, *Epigenetic gene silencing by Runx proteins.* Oncogene, 2004. 23(24): p. 4341-4345.

[87] Yoshida, H. and I. Kitabayashi, *Chromatin regulation by AML1 complex.* International Journal of Hematology, 2008. 87(1): p. 19-24.

[88] Tang, J.-L., et al., *AML1/RUNX1 mutations in 470 adult patients with de novo acute myeloid leukemia: prognostic implication and interaction with other gene alterations*. Blood, 2009. 114: p. 5352-5361.

[89] Dicker, F., et al., *Mutation analysis for RUNX1, MLL-PTD, FLT3-ITD, NPM1 and NRAS in 269 patients with MDS or secondary AML*. Leukemia, 2010. 24(8): p. 1528-1532.

[90] Gaidzik, V.I., et al., *RUNX1 mutations in acute myeloid leukemia: results from a comprehensive genetic and clinical analysis from the AML Study Group*. Journal of Clinical Oncology, 2011. 29(10): p. 1364-1372.

[91] Dicker, F., et al., *Trisomy 13 is strongly associated with AML1/RUNX1 mutations and increased FLT3 expression in acute myeloid leukemia*. Blood, 2007. 110: p. 1308-1316.

[92] Matsuno, N., et al., *Dual mutations in the AML1 and FLT3 genes are associated with leukemogenesis in acute myeloblastic leukemia of the M0 subtype*. Leukemia, 2003. 17(12): p. 2492-2499.

[93] Mendler, J.H., et al., *In rare acute myeloid leukemia patients harboring both RUNX1 and NPM1 mutations, RUNX1 mutations are unusual in structure and present in the germline*. Haenatologica, 2013. 98: p. e92-e94.

[94] Fasan, A., et al., *Rare coincident NPM1 and RUNX1 mutations in intermediate risk acute myeloid leukemia display similar patterns to single mutated cases*. Haematologica, 2014. 99: p. e20-e21.

[95] Fernández-Medarde, A., and E. Santos, *Ras in cancer and developmental diseases*. Genes & Cancer, 2011. 2(3): p. 344-358.

[96] Stites, E.C. and K.S. Ravichandran, *A systems perspective of Ras signaling in cancer*. Clinical Cancer Research, 2009. 15(5): p. 1510-1513.

[97] Johnson, D.B., K.S.M. Smalley, and J.A. Sosman, *Molecular pathways: targeting NRAS in melanoma and acute myelogenous leukemia*. Clinical Cancer Research, 2014. 20(16): p. 4186-4192.

[98] Fedorenko, I.V., G.T. Gibney, and K.S.M. Smalley, *NRAS mutant melanoma: biological behavior and future strategies for therapeutic management*. Oncogene, 2013. 32(25): p. 3009-3018.

[99] Reuter, C.M., et al., *Lack of noncanonical RAS mutations in cytogenetically normal acute myeloid leukemia*. Annals of Hematology, 2014. 93(6): p. 977-982.

[100] Bacher, U., et al., *Implications of NRAS mutations in AML: a study of 2502 patients*. Blood, 2006. 107: p. 3847-3853.

[101] Padua, R.A. and R.R. West, *Oncogene mutation and prognosis in the myelodysplastic syndromes*. British Journal of Haematology, 2000. 111(3): p. 873-874.

[102] Berman, J.N., et al., *Prevalence and clinical implications of NRAS mutations in childhood AML: a report from the Children's Oncology Group*. Leukemia, 2011. 25(6): p. 1039-1042.

[103] Bowen, D.T., et al., *RAS mutation in acute myeloid leukemia is associated with distinct cytogenetic subgroups but does not influence outcome in patients younger than 60 years*. Blood, 2005. 106: p. 2113-2119.

[104] Roskoski Jr, R., *Structure and regulation of Kit protein-tyrosine kinase—the stem cell factor receptor*. Biochemical and Biophysical Research Communications, 2005. 338(3): p. 1307-1315.

[105] Yarden, Y. and A. Ullrich, *Growth factor receptor tyrosine kinases*. Annual Review of Biochemistry, 1988. 57(1): p. 443-478.

[106] Paschka, P., et al., *Adverse prognostic significance of KIT mutations in adult acute myeloid leukemia with inv(16) and t(8;21): a Cancer and Leukemia Group B study*. Journal of Clinical Oncology, 2006. 24(24): p. 3904-3911.

[107] Riera, L., et al., *Core binding factor acute myeloid leukaemia and c-KIT mutations*. Oncology Reports, 2013. 29(5): p. 1867-1872.

[108] Cairoli, R., et al., *Prognostic impact of c-KIT mutations in core binding factor leukemias: an Italian retrospective study*. Blood, 2006. 107: p. 3463-3468.

[109] Park, S.H., et al., *Prognostic impact of c-KIT mutations in core binding factor acute myeloid leukemia*. Leukemia Research, 2011. 35(10): p. 1376-1383.

[110] Hoyos, M., et al., *Core binding factor acute myeloid leukemia: the impact of age, leukocyte count, molecular findings, and minimal residual disease*. European Journal of Haematology, 2013. 91(3): p. 209-218.

[111] Schnittger, S., et al., *KIT-D816 mutations in AML1-ETO-positive AML are associated with impaired event-free and overall survival*. Blood, 2006. 107: p. 1791-1799.

[112] Jiao, B., et al., *AML1-ETO9a is correlated with C-KIT overexpression/mutations and indicates poor disease outcome in t(8;21) acute myeloid leukemia-M2*. Leukemia, 2009. 23(9): p. 1598-1604.

[113] Qin, Y.-Z., et al., *Prevalence and prognostic significance of c-KIT mutations in core binding factor acute myeloid leukemia: a comprehensive large-scale study from a single Chinese center*. Leukemia Research, 2014. 38(12): p. 1435-1440.

[114] O'Donnell, M.R., et al., *Acute myeloid leukemia, version 2.2013*. Journal of the National Comprehensive Cancer Network, 2013. 11(9): p. 1047-1055.

[115] Ito, S., et al., *Role of Tet proteins in 5mC to 5hmC conversion, ES-cell self-renewal and inner cell mass specification*. Nature, 2010. 466(7310): p. 1129-1133.

[116] Chen, Q., et al., *TET2 promotes histone O-GlcNAcylation during gene transcription*. Nature, 2013. 493(7433): p. 561-564.

[117] Mohr, F., et al., *TET genes: new players in DNA demethylation and important determinants for stemness.* Experimental Hematology, 2011. 39(3): p. 272-281.

[118] Aslanyan, M., et al., *Clinical and biological impact of TET2 mutations and expression in younger adult AML patients treated within the EORTC/GIMEMA AML-12 clinical trial.* Annals of Hematology, 2014. 93(8): p. 1401-1412.

[119] Chou, W.-C., et al., *TET2 mutation is an unfavorable prognostic factor in acute myeloid leukemia patients with intermediate-risk cytogenetics.* Blood, 2011. 118: p. 3803-3810.

[120] Metzeler, K.H., et al., *TET2 mutations improve the new European LeukemiaNet risk classification of acute myeloid leukemia: a Cancer and Leukemia Group B study.* Journal of Clinical Oncology, 2011. 29(10): p. 1373-1381.

[121] Gaidzik, V.I., et al., *TET2 mutations in acute myeloid leukemia (AML): results from a comprehensive genetic and clinical analysis of the AML study group.* Journal of Clinical Oncology, 2012. 30(12): p. 1350-1357.

[122] Ko, M., et al., *Impaired hydroxylation of 5-methylcytosine in myeloid cancers with mutant TET2.* Nature, 2010. 468(7325): p. 839-843.

[123] Figueroa, M.E., et al., *Leukemic IDH1 and IDH2 mutations result in a hypermethylation phenotype, disrupt TET2 function, and impair hematopoietic differentiation.* Cancer Cell, 2010. 18(6): p. 553-567.

[124] Moran-Crusio, K., et al., *Tet2 loss leads to increased hematopoietic stem cell self-renewal and myeloid transformation.* Cancer Cell, 2011. 20(1): p. 11-24.

[125] Quivoron, C., et al., *TET2 inactivation results in pleiotropic hematopoietic abnormalities in mouse and is a recurrent event during human lymphomagenesis.* Cancer Cell, 2011. 20(1): p. 25-38.

[126] Nibourel, O., et al., *Incidence and prognostic value of TET2 alterations in de novo acute myeloid leukemia achieving complete remission.* Blood, 2010. 116: p. 1132-1135.

[127] Weissmann, S., et al., *Landscape of TET2 mutations in acute myeloid leukemia.* Leukemia, 2012. 26(5): p. 934-942.

[128] Reitman, Z.J. and H. Yan, *Isocitrate dehydrogenase 1 and 2 mutations in cancer: alterations at a crossroads of cellular metabolism.* Journal of the National Cancer Institute, 2010. 102(13): p. 932-941.

[129] Molenaar, R.J., et al., *The driver and passenger effects of isocitrate dehydrogenase 1 and 2 mutations in oncogenesis and survival prolongation.* Biochimica et Biophysica Acta (BBA) - Reviews on Cancer, 2014. 1846(2): p. 326-341.

[130] Emadi, A., et al., *Presence of isocitrate dehydrogenase (IDH) mutations may predict clinical response to hypomethylating agents in patients with acute myeloid leukemia (AML).* American Journal of Hematology, 2015. 90: p. E77-E79.

[131] Abbas, S., et al., *Acquired mutations in the genes encoding IDH1 and IDH2 both are recurrent aberrations in acute myeloid leukemia: prevalence and prognostic value*. Blood, 2010. 116: p. 2122-2126.

[132] Marcucci, G., et al., *IDH1 and IDH2 gene mutations identify novel molecular subsets within de novo cytogenetically normal acute myeloid leukemia: a Cancer and Leukemia Group B study*. Journal of Clinical Oncology, 2010. 28(14): p. 2348-2355.

[133] Dang, L., S. Jin, and S.M. Su, *IDH mutations in glioma and acute myeloid leukemia*. Trends in Molecular Medicine, 2010. 16(9): p. 387-397.

[134] Horbinski, C., *What do we know about IDH1/2 mutations so far, and how do we use it?* Acta Neuropathologica, 2013. 125(5): p. 621-636.

[135] Chotirat, S., et al., *Acquired somatic mutations of isocitrate dehydrogenases 1 and 2 (IDH1 and IDH2) in preleukemic disorders*. Blood Cells, Molecules, and Diseases, 2015. 54(3): p. 286-291.

[136] Green, C.L., et al., *The prognostic significance of IDH2 mutations in AML depends on the location of the mutation*. Blood, 2011. 118: p. 409-412.

[137] Zhou, K.-G., et al., *Potential application of IDH1 and IDH2 mutations as prognostic indicators in non-promyelocytic acute myeloid leukemia: a meta-analysis*. Leukemia & Lymphoma, 2012. 53(12): p. 2423-2429.

[138] Marcucci, G., et al., *Age-related prognostic impact of different types of DNMT3A mutations in adults with primary cytogenetically normal acute myeloid leukemia*. Journal of Clinical Oncology, 2012. 30(7): p. 742-750.

[139] Ley, T.J., et al., *DNMT3A mutations in acute myeloid leukemia*. The New England Journal of Medicine, 2010. 363(25): p. 2424-2433.

[140] Zhang, Y., et al., *Effects of DNMT1 silencing on malignant phenotype and methylated gene expression in cervical cancer cells*. Journal of Experimental & Clinical Cancer Research, 2011. 30: p. 98.

[141] Jasielec, J., V. Saloura, and L.A. Godley, *The mechanistic role of DNA methylation in myeloid leukemogenesis*. Leukemia, 2014. 28(9): p. 1765-1773.

[142] Li, K.K., et al., *DNA methyltransferases in hematologic malignancies*. Seminars in Hematology, 2013. 50(1): p. 48-60.

[143] O'Brien, E.C., J. Brewin, and T. Chevassut, *DNMT3A: the DioNysian MonsTer of acute myeloid leukaemia*. Therapeutic Advances in Hematology, 2014. 5(6): p. 187-196.

[144] Holz-Schietinger, C., D.M. Matje, and N.O. Reich, *Mutations in DNA methyltransferase (DNMT3A) observed in acute myeloid leukemia patients disrupt processive methylation*. The Journal of Biological Chemistry, 2012. 287(37): p. 30941-30951.

[145] Russler-Germain, D.A., et al., *The R882H DNMT3A mutation associated with AML dominantly inhibits wild-type DNMT3A by blocking its ability to form active tetramers.* Cancer Cell, 2014. 25(4): p. 442-454.

[146] McDevitt, M.A., *Clinical applications of epigenetic markers and epigenetic profiling in myeloid malignancies.* Seminars in Oncology, 2012. 39(1): p. 109-122.

[147] O'Brien, E.C., J. Brewin, and T. Chevassut, *DNMT3A: the DioNysian MonsTer of acute myeloid leukaemia.* Therapeutic Advances in Hematology, 2014. 5(6): p. 187-196.

[148] Shlush, L.I., et al., *Identification of pre-leukaemic haematopoietic stem cells in acute leukaemia.* Nature, 2014. 506(7488): p. 328-333.

[149] Corces-Zimmerman, M.R., et al., *Preleukemic mutations in human acute myeloid leukemia affect epigenetic regulators and persist in remission.* Proceedings of the National Academy of Sciences of the United States of America, 2014. 111(7): p. 2548-2553.

[150] Thol, F., et al., *Incidence and prognostic influence of DNMT3A mutations in acute myeloid leukemia.* Journal of Clinical Oncology, 2011. 29(21): p. 2889-96.

[151] Ribeiro, A.F., et al., *Mutant DNMT3A: a marker of poor prognosis in acute myeloid leukemia.* Blood, 2012. 119(24): p. 5824-5831.

[152] Ibrahem, L., et al., *Prognostic significance of DNMT3A mutations in patients with acute myeloid leukemia.* Blood Cells, Molecules & Diseases, 2014.

[153] Im, A.P., et al., *DNMT3A and IDH mutations in acute myeloid leukemia and other myeloid malignancies: associations with prognosis and potential treatment strategies.* Leukemia, 2014. 28(9): p. 1774-1783.

[154] Shivarov, V., et al., *DNMT3A mutation is a poor prognosis biomarker in AML: results of a meta-analysis of 4500 AML patients.* Leukemia Research, 2013. 37(11): p. 1445-1450.

[155] Wakita, S., et al., *Mutations of the epigenetics-modifying gene (DNMT3a, TET2, IDH1/2) at diagnosis may induce FLT3-ITD at relapse in de novo acute myeloid leukemia.* Leukemia, 2013. 27(5): p. 1044-1052.

[156] Hou, H.A., et al., *DNMT3A mutations in acute myeloid leukemia: stability during disease evolution and clinical implications.* Blood, 2012. 119(2): p. 559-568.

[157] Ploen, G.G., et al., *Persistence of DNMT3A mutations at long-term remission in adult patients with AML.* British Journal of Haematology, 2014. 167(4): p. 478-486.

[158] Jaiswal, S., et al., *Age-related clonal hematopoiesis associated with adverse outcomes.* The New England Journal of Medicine, 2014. 371(26): p. 2488-2498.

Chapter 5

Update on Non-M3 Acute Myeloid Leukemia — Etiology, Classification, Risk Stratification, Emergencies, Complications, Disease in Special Circumstances and Current and Future Therapeutics

Khalid Ahmed Al-Anazi

Additional information is available at the end of the chapter

http://dx.doi.org/10.5772/61827

Abstract

Acute myeloid leukemia (AML) is a heterogeneous condition characterized by clonal proliferation of myeloid precursors and accumulation of leukemic blasts in the bone marrow (BM), ultimately resulting in failure of the BM. It accounts for approximately 80% of cases of acute leukemia in adults. AML has several life-threatening complications.

After establishing the diagnosis of AML, classifying the disease into the appropriate subtype, stratifying the risk group and determining fitness of the patient for chemotherapy, induction treatment is usually commenced. For elderly individuals and those unfit for chemotherapy, several alternative therapeutic options are available. After achieving complete remission of the disease, the patient will either receive consolidation therapy or will be subjected to hematopoietic stem cell transplantation (HSCT). Autologous and allogeneic forms of HSCT have their own indications, inclusion as well as exclusion criteria. The recent advancements in the diagnostics and therapeutics have facilitated the introduction of personalized therapy in patients with AML. There are several targeted therapies for AML and their clinical use is increasing with time. Evaluation of minimal residual disease and determination of drug resistance are vital tools to improve the outcome of AML therapy.

Keywords: Acute myeloid leukemia, induction chemotherapy, hematopoietic stem cell transplantation, drug resistance and residual disease

1. Introduction

AML is a heterogeneous condition, or group of disorders, at both phenotypic and molecular levels with a variety of distinct genetic alterations that give rise to the disease [1]. It is characterized by clonal cells that exhibit maturation defect corresponding to the stages in hematopoietic differentiation [2]. Leukemic stem cells (LSCs) play a major role in the maintenance of AML, while the bone marrow (BM) microenvironment permits leukemogenesis as well as disease progression [2,3]. Various environmental exposures such as exposure to chemicals and radiation, and various infections in addition to hereditary factors can predispose vulnerable individuals to develop AML [2,4,5]. The two-hit hypothesis of leukemogenesis is characterized by two types of genetic mutations that evolve following certain environmental exposures [2].

AML accounts for approximately 80% of cases of acute leukemia in adults [6]. It is characterized by clonal proliferation of myeloid precursors and accumulation of leukemic blasts in the BM, ultimately resulting in various cytopenias due to BM failure [6-8]. After establishing the diagnosis of AML, the disease is classified into the appropriate type and cytotoxic chemotherapy is commenced in order to control the disease and restore BM function [6,8,9]. Currently, various induction regimens are available for AML patients belonging to various age groups [9-11]. Once the disease is controlled, patients usually receive post-remission therapy (PRT) and the choice of treatment depends on several factors including: age of the patient, performance status, comorbid medical conditions, availability of donors for HSCT and experience of the medical institution, particularly if stem cell therapy is considered [10-12].

This review on AML will cover the following aspects: insights into the pathogenesis of AML; complications of AML with particular attention to various infections; diagnosis, classification and risk stratification; AML in special situations such as: old age, pregnancy, Philadelphia chromosome positivity and therapy-related AML (t-AML). The available and future AML therapeutics will cover the following: induction, consolidation and maintenance therapies; drug resistance; treatment of relapsed and refractory disease; various forms of HSCTs; immunotherapies; and newly evolving targeted therapies in AML.

2. Etiology and pathogenesis of AML

The existence of cancer stem cells (CSCs) was established about two decades ago, following demonstration that only a small fraction of leukemic cells from AML patients were able to propagate the disease in xenografts [1]. AML appears to be maintained by LSCs or leukemia-initiating cells that are more immature than the majority of circulating leukemic cells and are capable of self-renewal [2]. Thus, the heterogeneity of AML extends to LSC compartment at both cellular and molecular levels [1]. Further identification of LSC-specific markers paves the way for novel therapeutic platforms, although no single marker has been found to be uniform for LSCs [1]. However, the following surface markers are expressed by LSCs: (1) strongly positive CD13, CD33, CD123, CD44, CD45, CD96 and TIM3, (2) positive CD25, CD32, CD45 RA and CLL-1, and (3) weakly positive CD34, CD38 and CD90 [reviewed in 1].

The two-hit hypothesis of leukemogenesis implies that AML is a consequence of at least 2 mutations: (1) class I mutations that confer a proliferative advantage, and (2) class II mutations that impair hematopoietic differentiation [2]. These leukemic mutations may occur following the exposure to: cytotoxic chemotherapy, ionizing radiation, chemical compounds and infection with retroviruses. Additionally, certain familial disorders are associated with increased incidence of AML [2].

The BM is a dynamic network of growth factors, cytokines and stromal cells that provide a permissive environment of leukemogenesis and tumor progression. The BM stroma and leukemic blasts promote angiogenesis which is enhanced in AML [3]. Vascular endothelial growth factor (VEGF), basic fibroblast growth factor and angioproteins are the main proangiogenic mediators in acute leukemia. Also, high expression of CXC chemokine ligand 4 (CXCR4) by leukemic blasts and activation of CXCR4-CXCR14 axis are involved in the disruption of normal hematopoiesis and progression of leukemia [3]. Tumor microenvironment has a major role in cancer progression and resistance to treatment and, recently, it has been receiving particular attention reflecting its vital importance in cancer progression. The interaction between leukemic cells, BM microenvironment stromal cells and soluble mediators plays a critical role in blast survival, disease progression and resistance to chemotherapy [3].

Hematopoietic stem cells (HSCs) are a unique population of somatic stem cells that are capable of self-renewal and differentiating into myeloid and lymphoid lineages [4]. The accumulation of genetic mutations and cytogenetic abnormalities, within partially differentiated cells belonging to the myeloid lineage, following the exposure to benzene and cytotoxic anticancer agents can give rise to malignancies such as AML [4]. However, the etiology of AML is multifactorial and the following can predispose to the development of AML: (1) exposure to ionizing radiation and chemicals, (2) long-term exposure to benzene, (3) exposure to cytotoxic chemotherapy in t-AML, (4) infection with retroviruses, (5) familial forms of AML, (6) secondary to myelodysplastic syndrome (MDS), (7) secondary to congenital disorders of DNA repair such as Fanconi anemia, and (8) secondary to chronic myeloproliferative neoplasms (MPNs) such as: polycythemia rubra vera, chronic myeloid leukemia (CML), essential thrombocythemia and primary myelofibrosis [2,4,5]. Thus, AML is a heterogeneous disease in terms of the underlying chromosomal or molecular aberrations [13]. However, despite genetic heterogeneity, there is increasing evidence for common molecular and biological mechanisms in AML [13].

3. Diagnosis and classification of AML

AML refers to a group of hematopoietic neoplasms involving cells committed to the myeloid line of cellular development [7]. It is characterized by a clonal proliferation of myeloid precursors and reduced capacity to differentiate into more mature cellular elements [7]. AML should be suspected in any patient presenting with varying combinations of the following: (1) manifestations of anemia such as fatigue, dyspnea, dizziness and pallor; thrombocytopenia such as bruising and excessive bleeding; and neutropenia or neutrophils dysfunction such as various infectious complications, (2) marked reduction in red blood cells, platelets and mature neutrophils on complete blood count, and (3) the presence of leukemic blasts on peripheral blood, BM and other tissues [6]. AML is diagnosed by BM biopsy using morphologic, cytochemical, immunophenotypic and cytogenetic analyses and molecular assays. Blasts should account for at least 20% of the total cellularity of the BM biopsy sample, except in leukemia with certain cytogenetic abnormalities and myeloid sarcoma which are diagnostic of AML regardless of the proportion of blast cells [6]. The blast forms must be identified as cells belonging to the myeloid, not the lymphoid, lineage. AML blasts express the following surface markers: CD13, CD32, CD33, CD34, CD38, CD64, CD11b, CD4 dim and HLA-DR [6]. After establishing the diagnosis of AML, the disease should be classified into the appropriate subtype according to the World Health Organization (WHO) classification scheme and/or the French-American-British (FAB) classification as shown in Tables 1 and 2 [6,14,15]. The subtype of AML is essential for prognostic scoring and therapeutic interventions [6]. The WHO classification system of AML is based on: morphology, immunophenotyping, genetics and clinical grounds and thus the 4 main subgroups of AML include: (1) AML with recurrent genetic mutations that accounts for 11% of all cases of AML, (2) AML with MDS-related features (6%), (3) t-AML and therapy-related MDS (t-MDS) (2%), and (4) AML, not otherwise specified, accounting for 81% of all cases as shown in Table 1 [6,8,14].

(1) AML with recurrent genetic abnormalities:
(a) AML with t(8,21) (q22, q22) RUNX1-RUNX1T1 (CBFA-ETO)
(b) AML with inv 16 (p3q22) or t(16,16) (p3q22) CBFB-MYH11
(c) APL with t(15,17) (q22,q12) PML-RARA
(d) AML with t(9,11) (q22,q23) MLLT3-MLL and other balanced translocations of 11q23 (MLL)
(e) AML with t (6,9) (p23,q34) DEK-NUP214
(f) AML with inv(3) (q21q26.2) or t(3,3)(q21,q26.2) RPNI-EV11
(g) AML (megakaryoblastic) with t(1,22)(p13,q13) RBM15-MKL1
(h) AML with mutated NPM (provisional entity)
(i) AML with mutated CEBPA (provisional entity)
(2) AML with myelodysplasia-related changes
(3) Therapy-related myeloid neoplasms; t-MDS and t-AML
(4) AML; NOS; not otherwise specified:
(a) AML with minimal differentiation
(b) AML without maturation
(c) AML with maturation
(d) Acute myelomonocytic leukemia
(e) Acute monoblastic/monocytic leukemia

http://dx.doi.org/10.5772/61827

(f) Acute erythroid leukemia (erythroid/myeloid and pure erythroleukemia)
(g) Acute megakaryoblastic leukemia
(h) Acute basophilic leukemia
(i) Acute panmyelosis with myelofibrosis
(5) Myeloid Sarcoma
(6) Myeloid proliferation related to Down syndrome (+21);
- Transient abnormal myelopoiesis
- Myeloid leukemia associated with Down syndrome
(7) Blastic plasmacytoid dendritic cell neoplasms
WHO: World Health Organization

Table 1. WHO classification of AML related tumors

FAB subtype	Morphological classification	Percentage of all AML cases
AML - M_0	Undifferentiated acute myeloid leukemia	5%
AML - M_1	Acute myeloid leukemia with minimal maturation	15%
AML - M_2	Acute myeloid leukemia with maturation	25%
AML - M_3	Acute promyelocytic leukemia	10%
AML - M_4	Acute myelomonocytic leukemia	20%
AML - $M_{4\ e05}$	Acute myelomonocytic leukemia with eosinophilia	5%
AML - M_5	Acute monocytic leukemia	10%
AML - M_6	Acute erythroid leukemia	5%
AML - M_7	Acute megakaryocytic leukemia	5%

FAB: French – American - British

AML: acute myeloid leukemia

Table 2. FAB classification of acute myeloid leukemia

Several cytogenetic abnormalities and genetic mutations have been reported in patients with AML as shown in Tables 3 and 4 [12,15]. In AML patients with normal cytogenetics, certain mutational abnormalities are present and these molecular mutations have their impact not only on the response to chemotherapeutic regimens, but also on the overall prognosis of patients as shown in Tables 5 and 6 [12,16-22]. According to their cytogenetic abnormalities and their molecular profiles, patients with AML are stratified into 4 risk groups, namely favorable, intermediate I, intermediate II or unfavorable as shown in Table 6 [12,21,22].

Translocation or chromosomal Abnormality	Oncofusion protein involved	Frequency of occurrence in AML
t (8,21)	AML1 - ETO	10%
t (15,17)	PML - RARA	10%
inv (16)	CBF - MYH11	5%
der (11q 23)	MLL - fusions	4%
t (9,22)	BCR - ABL	2%
t (6,9)	DEK - CAN	<1%
t (1,22)	OTT - MAL	<1%
t (8,16)	MOZ - CBP	<1%
t (7,11)	NUP 98 - HOX A9	<1%
t (12,22)	MN1 - TEL	<1%
inv (3)	RPN - EV11	<1%
t (16,21)	FUS - ERG	<1%

Table 3. Chromosomal abnormalities and their frequencies in AML

Category	Frequency	Examples	
Transcription factor fusions	18%	- PML / RARA - CBFB / MYH11 - RUNX1 / RUNX1T1 - PICALM – MLLT10	
NPM1 mutations	27%	-	
Tumor suppresser genes	16%	- TP 53 - WT1 - PHF 6	
DNA methylation	44%	- DNMT3A - DNMT3B - DNMT1	- TET1 - TET2 - IDH1 - IDH2
Activated signals	59%	- FLT3 - KIT - Other tyrosine kinases - Serin-theonine kinases - PTP: protein tyrosine phosphatases	- KRAS - NRAS
Myeloid transcription factors	22%	- RUNX1 - CEBPA - Other myeloid transcription factors	
Chromatin modifiers	30%	- MLL fusions - MLL - PTD - NUP 98 – NSD1	- ASXL1 - EZH2 - KDM6A
Cohesion complex	13%	-	
Spliceosome complex	14%	-	

Table 4. Gene mutations in acute myeloid leukemia

Genetic mutation	Chromosome involved	Frequency in CN - AML	Prognostic impact	
NPM1	5q35	45-60%	Favorable	* Higher CR rates * Better OS, EFS and DFS
CEBPA	19q13.1	10-15%	Favorable	* Better OS, EFS and DFS
IDH1	2q33	7.6-13.6%	Unfavorable	* Worse DFS * High risk of relapse
IDH2	15p26	8.7-19%	Unfavorable	* Shorter OS and lower remission rates * High frequency of induction failure
WT-1	11q13	10-13%	Unfavorable	* Shorter OS and DFS * Lower CR rates and higher relapse rates
FLT-ITD	13q12	25-35%	Unfavorable	* Worse OS and DFS
MLL-PTD	11q23	11%	Unfavorable	* Worse median survival and RFS * Shorter duration of remission
DNMT3A	2p23.3	15-36.1%	Unfavorable in young and older patients	* Worse OS, EFS and risk free survival * Lower CR rates
TET2	4 q 24	7 - 34%	Unfavorable in young and older patients	* Worse OS and EFS * Lower CR rates * Poorer prognosis in favorable risk CN-AML
ASX1 -1	20 q11	5.3 - 17.2%	Unfavorable	* Worse OS and EFS * Poorer prognosis in favorable risk CN-AML
RUNX 1	8 q 22	6.3 - 13.2%	Unfavorable	
EZH 2	-	Occasional in AML	Unfavorable	* Carries poor prognosis in AML secondary to: MDS, CMML and primary myelofibrosis.
BAALC	8 q 22.3	19 - 50%	Unfavorable	* Worse OS and DFS * Greater disease resistance to treatment
MN1	22 q 12.1	50%	Unfavorable	* Worse OS and risk free survival * High relapse rates and poor response to therapy
ERG-1	21 q22.3	25 - 37%	Unfavorable	* Worse OS and higher relapse rates

Genetic mutation	Chromosome involved	Frequency in CN - AML	Prognostic impact	
NRAS	1 p13	9.1 - 13%	Neutral	*May be favorable when other genetic aberrations are considered * May sensitize to cytarabine
CKIT	4 q12	17%	Unfavorable	* Poor prognosis
MIR - 181q	9q33.3	-		** Favorable outcome
MIR - 191	3p 21.31	-		** Poor prognosis
MIR-199a	19p13.2	-		** Poor prognosis

OS: overall survival

MDS: myelodysplastic syndrome

EFS: event free survival

CMML: chronic myelomonocytic leukemia

DFS: disease free survival

CR: complete remission

RFS: relapse free survival

Table 5. Genetic mutations in AML with normal cytogenetics and their impact on prognosis

Risk category	percentage	Subsets and examples	
Favorable	27%	- t(8,21) (q22,q22) - inv 16 (p13.1,q22) or t(16,16) (p13.1,q22) - Mutated NPM_1 without FLT_3 - ITD (CN - AML) - Mutated CEBPA (CN-AML)	RUNX1 - RUNX 1T1 (AML-ETO) CBFB - MYH 11
Intermediate I	31%	- Mutated NPM_1 and FLT_3 - ITD - Wild-type NPM1 and FLT3 - ITD - Wild-type NPM_1 without FLT_3 - ITD	(CN - AML) (CN - AML) (CN-AML)
Intermediate II	19%	- t (9,11) (p22, q23) - Cytogenetic abnormality not classified as favorable or adverse	MLL T3 - MLL
Unfavorable	23%	- inv 3 (q21, q 26.2) or t (3,3) (q21, q 26.2) - t (6,9) (p23, q34) - t (v,11) (v1q233) - -5 or del (5q) ; -7, abnormal ((17p) ; complex karyotype	RPN_1 - EV11 DEK - NUP 214 (CAN) MLL - rearranged

Table 6. Risk stratification of AML according to cytogenetics and molecular genetics

After establishing the diagnosis of AML and classifying the disease into the appropriate subtype, all patients should undergo a thorough evaluation in order to determine their fitness for the treatment [23,24]. Particular attention should be given to older patients who are likely to have comorbid medical conditions and decreased performance status which may limit their chances to have the standard therapies [23,24]. When compared to younger individuals, older adults with AML are likely to develop more complications related to chemotherapy and thus have diminished survival rates [23]. The pre-treatment assessment of older patients with AML includes specific investigations to evaluate their physical function and their comorbid conditions [23]. Patients with age-related chronic cardiac, pulmonary, renal, and hepatic disorders in addition to diabetes mellitus suffer greater toxicity of chemotherapy and radiotherapy. However, therapeutic decisions should be individualized and tailored according to the conditions of each patient taking into consideration: the age, performance status, comorbidity index and cytogenetic as well as molecular profiles [23].

4. Complications of AML

AML has numerous complications and these include: (1) anemia [25], (2) infectious complications including neutropenic colitis [25-27], (3) bleeding diathesis due to thrombocytopenia and disseminated intravascular coagulation [25], (4) leukostasis and hyperleukocytosis [25,26,28], (5) metabolic and electrolytic disturbances that include: lactic acidosis, hyperphosphatemia, hypokalemia, hyperuricemia, hypercalcemia, hypocalcemia, hyperkalemia, and tumor lysis syndrome following the administration of chemotherapy [25,26,29,30], (6) venous thromboembolism [25,26], (7) extramedullary involvement including: myeloid sarcomas, central nervous system (CNS), ocular involvement as well as skin and joint involvement [25,26], (8) acute pulmonary failure and pericardial effusions [25], and (9) oral complications including mucositis, mouth ulcerations and gingival hypertrophy [25].

4.1. Infectious complications in patients with AML

Despite the significant advances in supportive care, infectious complications remain a significant cause of morbidity and mortality in patients with leukemia [31]. The risk factors for infectious complications in patients with acute leukemia include: (1) impaired cellular and humoral immunity caused by the underlying disease, (2) the utilization of more intensive chemotherapeutic regimens in induction and salvage therapies, (3) the incorporation of monoclonal antibodies, (4) the use of consolidation and maintenance strategies, (5) profound neutropenia, (6) severe mucositis, (7) the increased use of indwelling vascular catheters, and (8) the degree of hemorrhagic diathesis of skin and mucosal tissues [31,32]. However, studies have shown that: (1) the addition of cladrabine to standard induction chemotherapy in patients with newly diagnosed AML, aimed at increasing the response rate to chemotherapy, has no impact on the incidence and spectrum of infectious complications, and (2) in AML patients younger than 65 years, fludarabine-based induction chemotherapy is not associated with an increase in the incidence of infections, particularly invasive fungal infections (IFIs), compared to conventional regimens that are commonly used in AML induction treatment [32,33]. The early utilization of empirical antimicrobial therapy and the maintenance of proper hygiene are the most effective strategies to combat infectious complications and to reduce mortality in hospitalized AML patients, while delayed recognition of infections and late administration of antimicrobial therapy not only increase morbidity and mortality but also potentially increase the economic burden associated with infections in patient with leukemia [31,34].

Neutropenic fever is an important cause of mortality and morbidity in patients with AML receiving intensive chemotherapy [35]. The implementation of empirical antibacterial therapy in patients with febrile neutropenia has led to a dramatic reduction in infection-associated mortality in patients with hematological malignancies [31]. Careful selection of antibiotics and early institution of antifungal treatment in addition to consideration of endemic infections such as tuberculosis may help in reducing morbidity and mortality during AML treatment [35]. However, the emergence of multidrug-resistant microorganisms is a real concern [31]. Therefore, medical institutions should evaluate antibacterial resistance routinely and regularly in order to select appropriate empirical antibiotic therapy [35]. Additionally, timely diagnosis and early initiation of appropriate antimicrobial therapy are crucial in combating infections in these immunocompromised hosts [31].

Gram-negative bacterial infections are still among the most important causes of mortality during neutropenia in patients with hematological malignancies, especially when related to *Pseudomonas aeruginosa* [36]. Due to its potent anti-pseudomonas activity, ceftazidime represents one of the antibiotics of choice for the empirical therapy of bacterial infections in high-risk febrile neutropenic patients. In these immunocompromised patients, blood concentrations of the drug 4 - 5 times the minimum inhibitory concentration may be required for maximal bacterial efficacy with ceftazidime [36].

Fluoroquinolone prophylaxis is frequently used in high-risk neutropenic patients world-wide. In particular, levofloxacin prophylaxis during neutropenia in high-risk patients was shown to be effective in preventing infectious complications in a study published in 2005 by GIMEMA group and was confirmed by a Cochrane systemic review in 2012 [37]. In a retrospective study performed in Italy that included 81 patients with AML diagnosed and treated between 2001 and 2007, the following results were obtained: Gram-positive bacterial infections predominated during the induction phase of chemotherapy, while Gram-negative bacterial infections predominated during the consolidation phase of chemotherapy, and a high rate of bacterial resistance to levofloxacin was encountered during the consolidation therapy [37]. Therefore, constant monitoring for fluoroquinolone resistance among Gram-negative bacterial isolates is recommended to preserve the efficacy of levofloxacin prophylaxis [37]. In a randomized prospective study, which included 95 patients with AML, conducted in South Korea between March and July 1999, it was found that antibiotic prophylaxis did not reduce the incidence of infections or infection-associated deaths in patients with AML on intensive chemotherapy. The authors recommended that routine use of antibiotic prophylaxis should be reconsidered taking into consideration the increased incidence of Gram-positive bacterial infections, and the high level of resistance to fluoroquinolones and macrolides [38].

In patients with AML receiving cytotoxic chemotherapy, sepsis remains a serious complication of neutropenia as it is associated with significant morbidity and mortality [34,39]. Risk factors for bloodstream infections (BSIs) in patients with AML include: (1) intensive chemotherapeutic regimens, (2) prolonged neutropenia, (3) neutropenic enterocolitis, (4) lower respiratory tract infections, (5) uncontrolled hematological malignancy, (6) cellulitis, (7) mucositis, (8) central venous catheter (CVC) infections, and (9) IFIs [40,41]. The expression of Toll-like receptors has been found to be an independent risk factor for the development of sepsis in patients with AML following the administration of intensive induction chemotherapy. Toll-like receptors play an important role in host defense against microorganisms [39].

In a French multicenter study that included 459 younger patients with AML: 1369 febrile neutropenic episodes were encountered, no identifiable cause for fever was found in 23% of patients, and clinically and microbiologically documented infections were identified in 77% of patients [42]. BSIs were reported in 314 episodes (29% of patients), Gram-positive organisms were cultured in 129 episodes (12%) and Gram-negative organisms were cultured in 144 episodes (14%). Pulmonary infections were documented in 14% of episodes while IFIs were documented in 11% of episodes of febrile neutropenia [42]. In another study that included 129 febrile episodes experienced by 42 patients with AML receiving chemotherapy and antibiotic prophylaxis; non-infectious sources of fever accounted for 17.8% of febrile episodes, Gram-positive microorganisms accounted for 75.8% of BSIs, while Gram-negative bacteria accounted for 12.1% of BSIs [41].

Despite the broad use of primary antifungal prophylaxis (PAP), IFIs particularly mold infections remain an important cause of treatment failure in patients with acute leukemia and a leading cause of morbidity and mortality in patients with AML, predominantly during the remission-induction phase of chemotherapy [43-45]. The incidence of IFIs has increased dramatically over the past few decades [43]. In the USA, the incidence of fungal sepsis has doubled between 1979 and 2000 due to the following reasons: (1) the extended survival of patients with acute leukemia, (2) the recent advances in supportive care, (3) the improvement in controlling bacterial infections, (4) the use of more intensive chemotherapy, (5) the utilization of potent immunosuppressive agents, and (6) the increase in the performance of HSCT [43]. The risk factors for IFIs in patients with acute leukemia include: (1) the primary disease such as AML, (2) cytotoxic chemotherapy including high-dose cytarabine and fludarabine, (3) indwelling devices including CVCs, (4) colonization with *Candida* species, (5) neutropenia, (6) old age, (7) use of total body irradiation (TBI) in pre-transplant conditioning therapy, (8) HSCT, particularly allogeneic grafts and mismatched donors, (9) graft versus host disease (GVHD) and (10) corticosteroid therapy [43]. Patients with acute leukemia can be stratified into 3 risk categories for IFIs: low risk, intermediate risk and high risk depending on a variety of factors that include: (1) host factors: age, fitness and comorbid conditions, (2) factors related to the primary disease: responsive or refractory to chemotherapy, and (3) other factors including the use of aggressive cytotoxic chemotherapy and immunosuppressive treatment, organ function and prior fungal infection or exposure to antifungal therapy [45].

In patients with AML, treatment of IFIs faces the following challenges: (1) the changing epidemiology of fungal infections, (2) early and correct diagnosis of fungal infections is usually difficult, and (3) monotherapy with antifungal agents is often unsuccessful [46]. The management of IFIs in patients with acute leukemia is further complicated by the recent increase in the frequency of infections by non-*Aspergillus* molds such as zygomycosis and the emergence of drug-resistant fungal pathogens [43]. Therefore, despite the recent and rapid expansion in antifungal armamentarium over the past few decades, the mortality associated with IFIs in patients with acute leukemia is still high [43]. Early diagnosis of IFIs in neutropenic patients has the potential to increase antifungal therapeutic response [47]. In patients with AML, the following chemotherapy-independent factors influence the onset of invasive mold infections: (1) hospital-independent exposure to infectious agents, (2) comorbidities, and (3) personal habits [48]. The recognition of these risk factors at the time of hospital admission helps to define the risk category of the patient and improve targeted prophylactic strategies [48]. The gold standard diagnostic tests are histopathological demonstration of organisms in tissue specimens and growth of fungal agents in culture media [47]. Blood cultures are positive in 50% of patients with invasive *Candida* or *Fusarium* infections, but are rarely positive in patients having invasive aspergillosis. Unfortunately, obtaining specimens for histopathology or culture may be difficult [47]. The glutacell serum β-glucan detection assay is highly sensitive and specific as a diagnostic test for IFIs in patients with AML [47]. Advancements in the diagnostic techniques are the following: (1) non-culture-based serum biomarkers such as β-glucan and *Aspergillus* galactomannan, (2) molecular tests such as polymerase chain reaction (PCR) for fungal DNA, and (3) high resolution radiological imaging such as computed axial tomography (CAT) scans that have improved the early detection of fungal infections and facilitated prompt pre-emptive antifungal therapy [43].

In patients with acute leukemia, the following factors influence decisions regarding the initiation of antifungal therapy and the choice of antifungal treatment: (1) the net state of immunosuppression, (2) the risk stratification of the primary disease such as AML, (3) the disease status such as high risk, relapsed or refractory AML, (4) the concomitant comorbidities, (5) the presence or absence of organ dysfunction, (6) the local fungal epidemiological patterns, (7) the pharmacological profile of antifungal agents, (8) exposure to pathogenic fungi, (9) drug-drug interaction, (10) the overall cost, (11) the presence of CVCs, (12) old age, and (13) neutropenia [43-45]. The following immunocompromised patients are at risk of invasive aspergillosis: (1) patients with AML during remission induction, (2) recipients of HSCT, and (3) patients having severe and prolonged immunosuppression [43-45,49]. The risk factors for invasive candidiasis include: (1) hematological malignancy such as AML, (2) extremes of age: < 1 month and > 65 years, (3) neutropenia, and (4) recent abdominal surgery [43-45,50]. In patients with leukemia having documented or presumed IFIs, the following factors influence the decision making of antifungal therapy: (1) the presence of active leukemia and plans for HSCT, (2) the type of chemotherapy: induction, consolidation or palliative, (3) certainty of diagnosis of fungal infection, (4) the type of fungus, (5) the site of infection, (6) prior antifungal exposure, (7) refractory IFI or previous lines of antifungal therapies, (8) concomitant infection such as cytomegalovirus or bacteria and their treatments, (9) risk of nephrotoxicity, (10) liver dysfunction, (11) infected CVCs, (12) ability to take oral medications, (13) interactions between antifungal agents and other medications, (14) compliance of the patients, (15) outpatient versus inpatient treatment, and (16) preference of the patient and the ability to cover medication costs [31,43-46,50].

http://dx.doi.org/10.5772/61827

The recent advances in the diagnostic modalities such as *Aspergillus* galactomannan test, 1,3-β-D-glucan test and PCR for fungal DNA, and antifungal therapeutics have facilitated an early diagnosis of IFIs and improved the response to treatment, ultimately resulting in improved outcome [50,51]. Strategies that improve survival of patients with AML having mold infections include: the preemptive initiation of antifungal therapy at the first sign of invasive aspergillosis on CAT scans, and antifungal prophylaxis with posaconazole and other drugs [49,51].

In patients with AML, management of fungal infections, particularly IFIs, requires an individualized treatment plan and a multimodal approach that includes: the use of more effective antifungal agents such as combination therapies or high-dose treatments, and the use of agents to enhance the immune response of the host [46]. Strategies that are utilized to enhance the immunity of cancer patients having opportunistic infections include: donor granulocyte transfusions, growth factors such as granulocyte-colony stimulating factor (G-CSF), and interferon-δ [46].

In patients with IFIs, early initiation of antifungal therapy has a profound impact on mortality rates, but reliable diagnostic tests are lacking [49]. In patients with febrile neutropenia suspected to have fungal infection, empirical therapy includes caspofungin as the first choice and liposomal amphotericin-B (ambisome) as the second choice [49]. In AML patients undergoing induction chemotherapy, 200 mg of prophylactic oral fluconazole twice daily is safe and well tolerated and results in trends towards reduced incidences of lung infiltrates and hepatosplenic candidiasis [51]. In the setting of consolidation therapy for AML, fluconazole is the most cost-effective approach to antifungal prophylaxis compared to posaconazole or voriconazole [52]. During the induction phase of AML, posaconazole was found to reduce the incidence of proven or probable breakthrough IFI, particularly aspergillosis, in a real life setting [53]. Hence, in patients at risk of invasive aspergillosis, posaconazole prophylaxis is recommended [49]. In patients with AML subjected to remission-induction chemotherapy, echinocandin-based primary antifungal prophylaxis has been associated with a higher risk of breakthrough IFIs than patients receiving azoles [44,54]. Isavuconazole is a novel, broad-spectrum, triazole antifungal agent which has recently been proven to be safe and tolerable at doses of 200-400 mg daily when used as prophylaxis in immunocompromised patients at high-risk of fungal infections [55]. In patients with AML receiving induction chemotherapy, a single high dose of ambisome [15 mg/kg] is safe and feasible when used as antifungal prophylaxis [56]. The mortality rate of IFIs in neutropenic individuals having *Candida* infection may reach 50% and those having aspergillosis, fusariosis and trichosporonosis may reach 100% [47].

4.2. Emergencies in AML

The following emergencies can be encountered in patients with AML: (1) tumor-lysis syndrome that occurs mainly in patients presenting with high white blood cell (WBC) count and high tumor load. It manifests with hyperkalemia, hyperuricemia, hypocalcemia, and hyperphosphatemia. It requires urgent treatment with aggressive hydration, correction of electrolytic abnormalities and reduction of elevated uric acid levels [26,29,30]. (2) Hyperleukocytosis and leukostasis which can predispose to thromboembolic manifestations, paradoxical bleeding as well as respiratory distress. Management can be in the form of leukapheresis if the WBC is more than 50,000 in symptomatic patients or more than 100,000 in asymptomatic patients as well as early initiation of chemotherapy [26,28]. (3) Neutropenic complications that include: febrile neutropenia; bacteremia, fungemia and septic shock; IFIs; and enterocolitis which manifests as fever, abdominal pain and thick bowel wall. Neutropenic colitis can be treated by: bowel rest, intravenous fluids, total parenteral nutrition in addition to intravenous antimicrobials with appropriate anaerobic cover [26,28]. (4) Transfusion-related acute GVHD which is a rare complication, but mortality rate may exceed 95%. It occurs 1-4 weeks after blood transfusion and manifests with fever, skin rash, diarrhea and hepatitis or elevated bilirubin and liver enzymes. This rare complication can be managed with corticosteroids and other immunosuppressive therapies but can be prevented by irradiation, leukodepletion and leukofiltration of blood products [26]. (5) Leukemic meningitis, which requires specific interventions including intrathecal chemotherapy [26]. (6) Cytarabine-induced cerebellar toxicity that requires replacement of cytarabine by another cytotoxic agent. (7) Finally, life-threatening hemorrhagic tendency [26].

4.3. AML in old age

The management of older patients with AML is a real therapeutic challenge because of the following reasons: (1) these patients are more likely to have comorbid medical conditions that limit their treatment options, (2) their clinical condition and their performance status may not allow the application of intensive chemotherapeutic regimens, (3) their disease is more likely to be resistant to chemotherapy, and (4) they have more frequent unfavorable AML subtypes [10]. Once AML is diagnosed in older subjects, physicians should make a therapeutic plan and try to adhere to it as much as possible, although therapeutic modifications may become justified under certain circumstances [11]. The same therapeutic principles that apply in younger adults can be followed provided the clinical circumstances of the patients allow the delivery of intensive induction chemotherapy [11]. The molecular features that characterize the risk of AML in middle-aged adults also apply to older patients with AML although the incidence of unfavorable genotype is significantly higher in older patients [11]. Numerous new drugs including targeted therapies and monoclonal antibodies are emerging from the development pipeline. Some of these drugs may be more tolerable and more efficacious in elderly patients than the standard induction regimens [11]. Otherwise healthy older patients with AML having good performance status can be subjected to standard induction chemotherapeutic regimens that include anthracyclines and cytarabine [10]. For older patients with: indolent AML, high comorbidity index, poor performance state and unfavorable risk disease, it is justifiable to offer them supportive care alone and/or less intensive chemotherapy rather than the standard induction chemotherapy which is associated with high treatment-related mortality (TRM) [10]. These patients can be offered: (1) transfusion of blood components, (2) various antimicrobials to treat their infectious complications, and (3) less intensive therapies such as: hydroxyurea, decitabine and low-dose cytarabine [10]. Although growth factors, such as G-CSF, may be beneficial in patients having neutropenia and sepsis, randomized trials have found no benefit to the routine use of G-CSF during remission induction in older patients with AML [10]. Older patients with AML should be encouraged to participate in well-designed clinical trials in order to draw conclusions on the safety and efficacy of the agents used in this

http://dx.doi.org/10.5772/61827

age group [10,11]. Also, older patients with AML achieving complete remission (CR) of their disease, but are not eligible for standard myeloablative HSCT, should be offered either a reduced intensity conditioning (RIC)-allogeneic HSCT or a clinical trial for post-induction or maintenance therapy [10,11].

The available therapeutic options for older patients with AML include: (1) standard induction therapy with 7+3 regimen, (2) hypomethylating agents such as azacitidine and decitabine, (3) nucleoside analogs such as clofarabine and sapacitabine, (4) immunomodulatory agents such as lenalidomide, (5) farnesyl transferase inhibitors such as tipifarnib, (6) monoclonal antibodies such as gemtuzumab ozogamicin (GO, myelotarg), (7) low-dose cytarabine, and (8) the best supportive care with blood product transfusions, antimicrobials as needed and oral cytotoxic drugs such as hydroxyurea [10,11,57,58].

In general, the median age for AML is in the 6th decade of life, but in certain countries like Sweden, most patients with AML are on the old side and the median age for AML is 71 years [59]. However, survival in patients with AML decreases with age, most patients with AML who are younger than 75 - 80 years, in certain geographic locations, tolerate and benefit from induction chemotherapy [59]. As AML induction chemotherapy is cost-effective in elderly individuals, all AML patients younger than 80 years without specific contraindications should be considered candidates for remission induction [60].

In AML patients older than 60 years of age, doubling the dose of daunorubicin in the induction phase of chemotherapy has been associated with a more rapid response and a higher response rate than the conventional dose without having significant adverse toxic effects [61]. Additionally, decitabine is well tolerated in older patients with AML who are medically unfit to have intensive chemotherapy, but myelosuppression related to the use of decitabine is the major toxicity encountered [62]. Interestingly, the response rate to decitabine and the overall survival (OS) are not adversely influenced by poor risk cytogenetics and preceding MDS [62].

In a study in patients with AML older than 60 years of age, the addition of bortezomib at doses of 1.3 mg/m^2 to the standard induction therapy, 7+3 regimen, and consolidation therapy with intermediate dose cytarabine has been shown to be associated with encouraging remission rates. Additionally, that study showed effectiveness and tolerability of bortezomib [63]. Also, in older AML patients, who are medically fit, the farnesyl transferase inhibitor tipifarnib, can be safely administered at a dose of 600 mg twice daily for 10 days in combination with the standard 7+3 induction regimen with severe gastrointestinal toxicity as the chief limiting factor [64].

Clofarabine, a nucleoside analog, may be an appropriate alternative to intensive induction regimens in certain subsets of older patients with newly diagnosed AML, particularly those with decreased performance status and history of cardiovascular disease [65]. Clofarabine has been shown to be an active drug in the treatment of older patients with AML as a single agent or in combination with other drugs [66]. It produces similar responses and potentially decreased mortality when compared to the traditional 7+3 induction chemotherapy [66]. Clofarabine use in combination with DNA methyltransferase inhibitors such as decitabine is a promising approach in older patients with AML who are not eligible for intensive chemotherapy [66]. The use of clofarabine therapy in the induction treatment of older AML patients, who are not suitable for intensive chemotherapy, has produced superior CR rates compared to low-dose cytarabine, but survival may be either similar to or even superior to low-dose cytarabine [67,68]. Sapacitabine, a novel oral nucleoside analog, has shown promising clinical efficacy and favorable toxicity once used in treating AML in older subjects [69].

GO is an anti-CD33 monoclonal antibody which has been shown to be effective in the treatment of older patients with CD33 positive AML in first relapse and it has acceptable toxicity. Unfortunately, the duration of remission is relatively short [57]. Also, in patients with CD33 positive in relapsed or refractory setting, the combination of: GO, intermediate-dose cytarabine and mitoxantrone has been shown to be an effective salvage regimen with 2-year rates of overall survival, event-free survival (EFS) and disease-free survival (DFS) of 41%, 33% and 53% respectively [70]. Once GO is used in combination with induction therapies in older AML patients, it reduces the risk of relapse and improves survival with slight increase in toxicity as revealed by a meta-analysis that included 2228 patients in the United Kingdom [71]. A randomized phase II study has shown that the addition of GO to the 7+3 induction regimen did not show significant superiority over the standard 7+3 regimen. In fact, death during the induction phase of chemotherapy was higher in the GO group due to venoocclusive disease (VOD) [72]. However, the addition of GO to: fludarabine, cytarabine and idarubicin induction therapy in CD33-positive AML in patients younger than 65 years has shown higher CR rates and lower mortality rates during the induction phase of chemotherapy [73].

5. Philadelphia chromosome positive AML

Studies have shown that the incidence of Philadelphia chromosome positivity in de novo AML is extremely rare and that Philadelphia chromosome positive AML accounts for only 0.3-3.0% of all newly diagnosed cases of de novo AML [74-77]. However, Philadelphia chromosome positive AML has to be distinguished from: CML in blast cell crisis, mixed phenotype leukemia and secondary AML with positive Philadelphia chromosome [75,76,78].

The following features have been reported in Philadelphia chromosome positive de novo AML: (1) lack of splenomegaly, (2) lack of history of abnormal hemogram, (3) lack of history of chronic phase CML, (4) lack of significant peripheral blood basophilia, (5) frequent expression of lymphoid markers, (6) lower cellularity and lower myeloid/erythroid ratio on BM examination, (7) presence of monosomy 7, inversion 16 and chromosome 10 deletion, (8) predominance of p210 rather than p190 fusion protein, and (9) return to normal karyotype after induction chemotherapy [75-78]. On the contrary, CML in myeloid blast cell crisis presents in patients with history of an abnormal hemogram and chronic phase CML in addition to splenomegaly on physical examination. Also, trisomy 8, trisomy 19 and iso-chromosome 17q as well as return to chronic phase CML after induction therapy are in favor of CML in myeloid blast cell crisis [75-79].

The available therapeutic interventions in patients with Philadelphia chromosome positive AML include: induction chemotherapy using various chemotherapeutic regimens, tyrosine kinase inhibitors (TKIs) such as imatinib and dasatinib as well as allogeneic HSCT with its graft versus leukemia (GVL) effect which constitute the only potentially curative therapeutic modality [74,75,80]. Prognosis of Philadelphia chromosome-positive AML is usually poor as the disease is aggressive, relapse rates are high and durations of responses are rather short. Additionally, responses to anthracyclines and cytarabine are poor and the median survival is limited to 6-9 months [74,75,77,80]. However, complete molecular responses have been reported after conventional chemotherapy and imatinib and tetraploidy have been reported in a patient with Philadelphia chromosome-positive AML [74,81]. As the disease is insufficiently studied, further epidemiological studies and large-scale registries may contribute not only to a better understanding of the disease but also to more efficacious therapeutic interventions [75,76,80].

5.1. Therapy-related AML

Therapy-related myeloid neoplasms (t-MNs) account for approximately 10-20% of all cases of: AML, MDS, MSD/MPNs [82]. The incidence of t-MNs among patients treated with cytotoxic chemotherapy varies according to the underlying disease, specific agents used, timing of exposure and doses of chemotherapeutic agents used [82,83]. The median age for t-MNs is 61 years, although they can develop at any age [82]. The risk of t-MNs associated with the use of alkylating agents and radiation appears to increase with age, while the risk of t-MNs associated with the use of topoisomerase II inhibitors appears to be constant across all ages [82]. The latency period between the first exposure to cytotoxic therapy and the development of t-MNS ranges from 1 to 10 years [82,83]. Patients usually present with complications of pancytopenia and they should have thorough clinical and laboratory evaluation [82,83]. However, therapeutic recommendations depend on: (1) age of the patient, (2) comorbidities, (3) performance status, (4) status of the primary disease, (5) presence of complications from the primary disease, and (6) clonal abnormalities present in t-AML cells [83].

t-AML is an important disease entity to be studied for several reasons: (1) it represents the most serious complication of current cancer treatment, (2) it is directly induced by chemotherapeutic agents and irradiation, (3) t-AMLs presenting with the same chromosomal abnormalities and genetic mutations that are present in de novo AML are particularly suited for studies on leukemogenesis and leukemia biology, (4) t-AML may be preceded by a transient phase of t-MDS and cytopenias and this stage is suited for further studies and comparison with de novo MDS transforming into AML, (5) there is still no consensus on the therapeutic management of t-AML, and (6) t-AML stimulates scientists to study the safety of various therapeutic modalities that are used in the treatment of various cancers in order to replace these treatments by safer ones in the future [83].

t-AML can occur at any age and it represents 5-14% of all newly diagnosed cases of AML [83]. The primary disease in t-AML can be: (1) a hematological malignancy such as acute lymphoblastic leukemia (ALL), chronic lymphocytic leukemia, Hodgkin's disease, non-Hodgkin lymphoma, multiple myeloma or acute promyelocytic leukemia, (2) a solid tumor such as small cell lung cancer, germ cell tumor and cancers of ovaries, breast, testis or prostate, and (3) an autoimmune disease such as rheumatoid arthritis, systemic lupus erythromatosis, multiple sclerosis, ulcerative colitis and Wegener's granulomatosis [83,84]. The use of the following drugs and chemotherapeutic agents is associated with the development of t-AML: (1) alkylating agents such as: busulfan, melphalan, chlorambucil, cyclophosphamide, procarbazine as well as mitomycin-C, (2) topoisomerase II inhibitors such as: etoposide, mitoxantrone, doxorubicin and dactinomycin, (3) antimetabolites such as methotrexate, 6-mercaptopurine in addition to fludarabine, (4) antimicrotubules such as vincristine and paclitaxel, (5) growth factors such as G-CSF, and (6) immunomodulators such as azathioprine [82-92].

Studies have shown that the use of alkylating agents is associated with the development of t-MDS and unbalanced chromosomal aberrations such as: 5q-, -5, 7q-, -7, 17p13 (TP53) and unarranged mixed lineage leukemia (MLL) gene mutation, while the use of topoisomerase II inhibitors is associated with the evolution of balanced chromosomal aberrations such as: 11q23, 21q22, 16q22, rearranged MLL, AML_1, CBFB and retinoic acid receptor-alpha (RARA) [89]. A study that included 761 patients analyzed between 1976 and 1993 and 5098 patients reported in literature between 1974 and 2001 revealed that: exposure to radiation was associated with the development of t-MDS and 5q- chromosomal abnormality, exposure to alkylating agents was associated with the evolution of t-MDS and t-AML with monosomy 7, while exposure to topoisomerase II inhibitors was associated with the development of t-AML and t11q23 [86]. The cytogenetic abnormalities and the genetic mutations that have been reported in patients with t-AML are included in Table 7 [83,86,88,89]. The genetic mutations that are involved in t-AML can be classified into: (1) class I mutations that can be sub-classified into: (a) tyrosine kinases such as FMS-like tyrosine kinase 3-internal tandem duplication (FLT3-ITD) point mutations, c-Kit point mutations and cFMS and Janus Kinase 2 (JAK-2) point mutations, and (b) genes in the RAS/BRAF pathway such as: KRAS or NRAS point mutations and BRAF and PTPN11 point mutations, and (2) class II mutations that can be divided further into: (a) transcription factors that include: AML1/CBFB chimerically rearranged, AML1 point mutations, MLL chimerically rearranged, MLL-ITD, chimerically rearranged RARA and EV11 in addition to CEBPA and nucleophosmin-1 (NPM1) point mutations, and (b) tumor suppressor genes such as P53 point mutations [87].

Clinical data obtained from 4 major cohorts on t-AML that included a total of 395 patient revealed the following: the mean age for the development of t-AML was 53.5 - 58 years, the median latency period to develop t-AML was 48 - 55 months, the mean WBC count at presentation was 6.7 - 27.4 $x10^9/L$, CR rates ranged between 23.8 and 63.0% and the median OS was 7 - 12 months [83].

The diagnosis of t-AML identifies a group of high-risk patients with multiple and varied poor prognostic features [84,90]. The spectrum of cytogenetic abnormalities in t-AML is similar to de novo AML, but the frequency of unfavorable cytogenetics such as complex karyotype or deletion or loss of chromosomes 5 and 7 is higher in t-AML. In t-AML survival varies according to cytogenetic risk group with better outcomes observed in patients with favorable-risk karyotype [84,90].

Abnormal response to DNA damage is a common finding in t-AML. TP53 aberrations are one of the most common mutations in t-AML and are usually associated with complex karyotypes. AML having complex karyotype accounts for 70% of cases of AML and has a high degree of

Cytogenetic abnormalities	(%)	Mutational abnormalities			(%)
t (8,21)	6.4%	TP53	18-25%	TET 2	9%
t (15,17)	5.4%	WT1	17%	IDH1/IDH2	3-12%
inv (16) , t (16,16)	14%	NPM1	12-16%	EV 11	0.2-1.0%
11 q 23	12.9%	KRAS	-	RUN X-1	2.9%
t (9,11)	-	NRAS	11-12%	AML 1	
inv(3), t (3,3)	-	BRAF	6%		
17 p deletion	-				
t (11,19)	-	FLT3-ITD	7-12%	PML-RARA	2.3%
- 7, 7q-	-				
- 5, 5q-	-	FLT3-TKD	2-2.5%	C-KIT	1-4%
- 17	-	CEBPA	0-6%	C-FMS	-
- 21	-	DNMT3A	16%	JAK 2	Rare
- 18	-	MLLT3-MLL	4-12%	CBF β- NYH 11	1.8%
t (1,3)	-				
Normal cytogenetics	14%	MLL-PTD	2-4%	PTPN 11	4%
Complex cytogenetics	26.39%				

Table 7. Cytogenetic and mutational abnormalities encountered in therapy-related AML

genomic complexity and is associated with interior OS [93]. The most common chromosomal translocation associated with topoisomerase-II inhibitor-induced t-AML is t(9,11) (p22, q23). MLL gene located on chromosome 11 at band q23 is the gene most commonly involved in secondary acute leukemias (ALL and AML) related to the use of topoisomerase II inhibitors [92]. t-AML having t(8,21) shares many features, including morphologic and immunophenotypic features as well as the characteristic AML-ETO (RUNX1-RUNX1T1) fusion, with de novo AML having t(8,21) (q22,q22), but affected individuals have a relatively worse outcome [94]. The poor prognosis and the rather aggressive behavior of t(8,21) t-AML may be explained by: (1) the older age of patients, and (2) the presence of active primary cancer at the time of diagnosis of t-AML with t(8,21) [94]. In t-AML, cytogenetic profile is an important prognostic parameter, while the age of patient and the WBC count at presentation have no impact on OS [89]. In general, survival and prognosis of t-AML is often poor despite prompt diagnosis and early institution of therapy [83]. CR rates of t-AML range between 24 and 63% and are interior to those of de novo AML (65-80%) [83]. However, within certain cytogenetically defined subgroups, the prognosis of t-AML does not differ significantly from their de novo AML counterparts [83,84,90]. Standard chemotherapy and allogeneic HSCT as well as experimental therapies are used in the treatment of t-AML [83,84,90]. Several studies have shown that therapeutic outcomes of t-AML patients after induction phase of treatment are not different from those of de novo AML [83]. In patients older than 60 years of age having t-AML, significantly greater relapse rates, mainly due to lower doses of chemotherapeutic agents used compared to those given to younger patients, have been encountered [83]. However, intensive induction chemotherapy should not be withheld in patients with t-AML provided they are fit to receive it [83,84,90]. Novel HSCT strategies using RIC regimens as well as targeted therapies await clinical evaluation in patients with t-AML and these may prove to have a positive impact on the prognosis of affected individuals [83]. Studies have shown that allogeneic HSCT can cure some patients with t-AML. Finally, patients with t-AML should be enrolled in front-line chemotherapeutic trials that are appropriate for patients with de novo AML with similar disease characteristics [84,90].

6. Prognosis in AML

The response to treatment and the OS of AML patients are very variable [7,8,83]. A number of prognostic factors related to the patient and the tumor characteristics have been described and they include age, performance status, comorbid medical conditions, cytogenetic profile, molecular or genetic profile, history of MDS or chronic MPNs, and history of receiving cytotoxic chemotherapy or ionizing radiation. Amongst these prognostic factors, the following have a direct effect on treatment outcome: age at diagnosis, performance status and karyotype [7,8,83,84].

The clinical role of gene mutational analysis, gene expression profiling, and micro-RNA profiling remains uncertain at this time, although a number of mutations and changes in the levels of certain proteins have been shown to have prognostic impact and will likely become part of the routine characterization of AML in the near future [7,8,83,84].

6.1. Induction therapy for AML

Once the diagnosis of AML is established, induction chemotherapy will be commenced in order to rapidly restore normal BM function [9]. The goal of the initial intensive course of combination chemotherapy is to obtain a CR [9,95]. Induction chemotherapy aims to reduce the total body leukemia cell population from 10^{12} to below the cytologically detectable level of approximately 10^9 cells [9,95]. A series of pre-1985 studies performed by the Cancer and Leukemia Group-B [CALG-B] established 7+3 regimen, which is composed of cytarabine and daunorubicin, as the standard of care in induction therapy of AML [96]. However, various induction regimens of chemotherapy are available for younger and older AML patients [9,96-100]. In younger patients with AML, the following induction chemotherapeutic regimens are used: (1) the classical or standard 7+3 regimen, which produces remission rate of 60-80%, comprises continuous intravenous (IV) infusion of 100-200 mg/m^2 of cytarabine for 7 days and 60-90 mg/m^2 IV push of daunorubicin daily for 3 days, (2) high-dose cytarabine (HiDAC) + daunorubicin regimen, which produces remission rate of 90%, comprises 1-3 g/m^2 of cytarabine IV infusion over 3 hours twice daily for 6 days, and (3) cytarabine + idarubicin regimen, which produces remission rate of 88%, is composed of 100-200 mg/m^2 of cytarabine daily by continuous IV infusion for 7 days and 12-13 mg/m^2 IV push of idarubicin daily for 3 days [9,96,97].

Throughout the years, many studies have been performed with the intent to improve on the outcome of 7+3 induction regimen for AML and the following are examples of these attempts: (1) replacement of daunorubicin by idarubicin, (2) replacement of daunorubicin by mitoxantrone, (3) escalation of daunorubicin dose, (4) addition of etoposide to the 7+3 regimen, (5) addition of thioguanine to the 7+3 regimen, (6) replacement of daunorubicin by amsacrine and gemtuzumab ozogamicin, (7) the use of HiDAC alone or in combination with fludarabine and/or G-CSF as induction therapy, and (8) incorporation of new agents such as cladarabine, clofarabine, lomustine, AC-220 and sorafenib [96,97,100].

Age is an important factor for the treatment outcomes demonstrated in numerous studies [7,9-11,23,24,58-69,71,73]. In patients with AML, younger than 46 years of age, HiDAC (3 g/m^2 IV twice daily for 4 days) in addition to daunorubicin and etoposide produces higher remission and survival rates compared to a standard dose cytarabine [100]. In AML patients who are ≥ 50 years of age, idarubicin has produced superior long-term outcome compared to high-dose daunorubicin in a French study that included 727 patients with AML [98]. In older patients with AML, the following factors can predict a better long-term outcome: favorable-risk AML, idarubicin treatment rather than daunorubicin, and belonging to a younger age as studies have shown that the younger the age of the patient the better the response to chemotherapy [98]. In patients with AML who are ineligible for intensive chemotherapy, volasertib (adenosine triphosphate competitive kinase inhibitor) and low-dose cytarabine produce responses across all AML genetic subgroups, improve survival and have clinically manageable safety profile [101]. In AML patients who are ≥ 60 years of age, the following induction therapies have been used: (1) single dose daunorubicin; 45 or 90 mg / m^2 IV or liposomal daunorubicin, (2) hypomethylating agents such as azacytidine or decitabine, (3) immunomodulatory agents such as lenalidomide, (4) clofarabine, and (5) other agents such as: plerixafor, flavoperidol, *Diphtheria* toxin linked to interleukin-3 (IL-3) and all trans-retinoic acid (ATRA) [99]. Recent studies have shown that doubling the dose of daunorubicin (90 mg/m^2 instead of 45mg/m^2) produces significantly higher CR rates in selected groups of AML patients, regardless of the age. Patients with favorable- or intermediate-risk cytogenetics have achieved better responses than patients with unfavorable karyotype or high-risk disease [96]. The following circumstances require unique therapeutic implications: Philadelphia chromosome positive AML, mixed-phenotype leukemia, AML with extramedullary involvement, t-AML, and AML in pregnancy [9].

Seven to ten days after completion of induction chemotherapy, response to chemotherapy is usually evaluated by a BM aspiration and trephine biopsy [9]. After achieving CR_1 of AML, PRT starts with either consolidation chemotherapy or HSCT in transplant-eligible patients [9]. Based on a landmark CALG-B study, the standard consolidation therapy for AML in CR_1 is 4 cycles of HiDAC (3 g/m^2 IV Q 12 hourly on days 1,3 and 5) [97]. Improving the quality of remission may reduce the risk of relapse in patients with AML [97]. Several emerging prognostic factors may enable a more personalized approach to post-induction therapy that takes into consideration the category of patients who should be offered allogeneic HSCT in CR1 [97].

6.2. Response to treatment in AML

Definition of CR in AML according to the criteria developed by the International Working Group includes: (1) Normal values for absolute neutrophil count >1000 × 10^9/L and platelet count >100 × 10^9/L in addition to independence from red blood cell transfusions. (2) BM biopsy that reveals no clusters or collections of blasts. Also, extramedullary leukemia such as CNS and soft tissue involvement must be absent. (3) BM aspiration reveals normal maturation of all cellular components; namely erythrocytic, granulocytic and megakaryotic series. However, there is no requirement for BM cellularity. (4) Less than 5% blasts in the BM and none can have a leukemia phenotype such as Auer rods. (5) The absence of a previously detected clonal cytogenetic abnormality, that is, complete cytogenetic remission (CRc) which confirms the morphologic diagnosis of CR but is not a criterion for CR in AML. The conversion from an abnormal karyotype at the time of first CR is an important prognostic indicator, supporting the use of CRc as a criterion for CR in AML [95,102].

A substantial burden of leukemia cells persist undetected referred to as minimal residual disease (MRD) leading to relapse within weeks to months if no further PRT is administered [95]. Response criteria in AML patients can be categorized as follows: (1) CR, (2) CR with incomplete recovery, (3) morphologic leukemia-free status, (4) partial remission, (5) cytogenetic remission, and (6) molecular remission. Treatment failure in AML can be classified as follows: (1) resistant or refractory disease, (2) disease relapse, (3) death in aplasia, and (4) death from an indeterminate cause [8]. The following methods are used in detecting MRD: (1) multiparameter flow cytometry (MFC), (2) quantitative, real time, polymerase chain reaction (Q-RT-PCR), and (3) gene expression analysis [95,102-104]. The evaluation of MRD in AML has the following advantages: (1) high-resolution determination of response to treatment, (2) allowing target-driven titration of dose as well as duration of therapy, (3) stratification of the risk of relapse after induction to allow triage of the optimal consolidation therapy, (4) determination of prognosis after completion of standard treatment, (5) sparing toxicity and cost of HSCT in patients with low risk of relapse, and (6) assignment to maintenance treatment after completion of standard therapy [102]. In patients with AML, assessment of MRD by flow cytometry after induction and consolidation chemotherapy has been shown to provide independent prognostic information. Early flow cytometry MRD assessment can improve the current risk stratification approaches by the prediction of relapse-free survival (RFS) in AML and may facilitate the adaptation of PRT for patients at high-risk of relapse [103]. MRD by flow cytometry offers high sensitivity [up to 10^{-4}] and is applicable in more than 90% of all AML cases. The individual choice of PRT requires a comprehensive knowledge of the risk profiles of patients in order to avoid overtreatment or undertreatment. MRD levels constitute a prognostic factor that combines disease-specific as well as patient-specific characteristics thus reflecting sensitivity to chemotherapy [103]. Also, MRD before myeloablative HSCT is associated with an adverse outcome in AML in CR1. The negative impact of pre-transplant MRD is similar for AML in CR1 and CR2 as even minute levels ($\leq 0.1\%$) are associated with adverse outcome [105].

http://dx.doi.org/10.5772/61827

Early blast clearance in AML is an essential indicator of response to chemotherapy [106]. Day 16 blasts represent a highly independent and sensitive prognostic factor and may be used for stratification of therapy early enough before the second course of chemotherapy, that is, salvage chemotherapy, re-induction or double induction. Day 16 blasts allow refinement but not replacement of the most important system for a prognostically based classification of patients with AML which is grouping according to karyotypic abnormalities [106]. Monitoring of early reduction of the leukemia cell burden may be further improved by techniques that are more sensitive and more reproducible than cytomorphology such as immunophenotyping using MFC. The prognostic significance of day 16 blasts is independent of pre-therapeutic parameters and predicts outcome even in patients achieving a CR [106]. Response rates and subsequent therapeutic recommendations for AML patients classified according to their prognostic groups are shown in Table 8 [22].

Prognostic Group	CR rate	Relapse rate	Response and non-relapse mortality	Induction	Post-remission	HSCT comorbidity index
Favorable	> 80-90%	35-40%	* Rapid CR * No MRD < 10-15%	- 3+7 regimen - Consider: FLAG + Idarubicin if age < 60-65 years	- Ara -C at 1.0-1.5g/m^2 daily for 6 doses, total of 2 cycles - Possibly preceded by 1 course of: FLAG + idarubicin	< 1%
Intermediate I	50-80%	50-60%	- Rapid CR - No MRD < 20-25%	- 3+7 regimen - Consider: FLAG + Idarubicin if age < 60-60 years or clinical trial	- HSCT from MSD if risk of NRM < 20-25% - If not candidate for HSCT: FLAG + Ida then Ara-C (as above) or clinical trial	≥ 2%
Intermediate II	40-80%	70-80%	- slow CR - CRp-CRi - MRD < 40%	- 3+7 regimen - Consider: FLAG + Idarubicin if age < 60-65 years - Clinical trial combining chemotherapy and FLT3 inhibitors	- HSCT from MSD or MUD if risk of NRM < 30%, otherwise as intermediate I. - If FLT3 positive, consider FLT3 inhibitors post HSCT.	≥ 3-4%
Unfavorable	< 50%	> 90%	- Slow CR - CRp-CRi - MRD < 40%	Clinical trial	- HSCT from MSD or MUD if risk of NRM < 40%	≥ 5%

Prognostic Group	CR rate	Relapse rate	Response and non-relapse mortality	Induction	Post-remission	HSCT comorbidity index
					- Consider post-HSCT trial - If not candidate for HSCT, consider clinical trial	

Ara-C: cytarabine

MSD: matched sibling donors

HSCT: hematopoietic stem cell transplantation

CR: complete remission

MUD: matched unrelated donor

FLAG: fludarabine, cytarabine, growth factors

MRD: minimal residual disease

NRM: non-relapse mortality

AML: acute myeloid leukemia

Table 8. Response rates and therapy recommendations for AML classified according to prognostic group

6.3. Drug resistance in AML

For the management of AML, the following general options are available: (1) standard chemotherapy, (2) investigational therapy, and (3) best supportive care without intensive chemotherapy [107]. Initial treatment for remission induction is still based on cytarabine and anthracyclines (7+3 regimen) which were introduced into the treatment of AML more than 40 years ago [108]. Given the natural history of AML and the uncertainty about the outcome of investigational therapy, 7+3 regimen is still the preferable standard treatment for most of the patients. The principal predictor of response to standard therapy is the duration of first CR [107].

Therapeutic resistance, defined as either failure to achieve initial CR or relapse after achievement of CR, remains the main problem in adult AML. It is widely appreciated that the likelihood of resistance to chemotherapy differs significantly from one individual to another [109]. Resistance to chemotherapy, not TRM, is the chief cause of treatment failure in AML. Drug resistance occurs in 71% of AML patients younger than 56 years, 61% of patients between 66 and 75 years of age and 54% of AML patients older than 75 years [107]. In an analysis that included 4601 AML patients, the following factors were independently associated with failure to achieve remission: (1) age of the patient, (2) performance status, (3) the WBC count at presentation, (4) secondary disease, (5) cytogenetic risk, and (6) presence of certain genetic mutations such as FLT3-ITD. Another study revealed that the presence of multidrug-resistant (MDR) phenotype such as MDR-gene-1 (mdr-1) is associated with drug resistance in AML [109,110].

The ability to accurately forecast drug resistance could have a tremendous impact on the management of AML and evaluation of new drugs [109]. Unfortunately, our ability to predict chemotherapeutic resistance on the basis of the routinely available clinical covariates, even with the inclusion of commonly used molecular data such as FLT3 and NPM1 is relatively limited [109]. In case of failure to respond to 7+3 regimen, alternative salvage therapies include: (1) fludarabine, cytarabine and G-CSF (FLAG) regimen, (2) mitoxantrone and etoposide, or (3) investigational agents [107]. In general, management of drug resistance in AML can be summarized as follows: (1) in case of lower drug resistance and lower TRM, current therapy should be intensified, (2) in case of higher drug resistance and lower TRM, new high-intensity therapy needs to be added, (3) in case of lower drug resistance and higher TRM, new low-intensity therapy, such as ATRA or azacytidine needs to be added, and (4) in case of higher drug resistance and higher TRM, new low intensity therapy should be used [107]. Chemomodulation of sequential HiDAC and idarubicin by fludarabine improves the anti-leukemic efficacy but only at a modest rate [108]. Given the efficacy of chemomodulation of cytarabine, even in a relapsed setting, incorporation of fludarabine into first-line therapy of AML seems warranted and may help to improve the outcome of AML patients [108]. The addition of cladrabine to daunorubicin and cytarabine induction regimen increases the anti-leukemic effect or potency of 7+3 regimen resulting in higher CR rates without causing additional toxicity [111]. The combination of azacytidine and lenalidomide improves the outcome of patients with high-risk MDS or AML. This regimen is well tolerated and is not associated with major toxicities apart from neutropenia and thrombocytopenia [112].

Valspodar (PSC833) can not only reverse MDR in patients with hematologic malignancies but alters the pharmacokinetics of concomitant anticancer agents [110]. A phase I study has shown that valspodar and MEC (mitoxantrone, etoposide and cytarabine) combination is safe and effective when administered early in relapsed or refractory AML [110].

A previous phase II study from the Borden laboratory had shown that ribavirin produced initial responses, including remissions in patients who had relapsed after cytarabine treatment, but all patients eventually developed drug resistance and relapsed [113]. A new study from the same group has shown that resistance to cytarabine and ribavirin is due to the sonic hedgehog pathway transcription factor glioma-associated oncogene [113]. However, the best modality to overcome drug resistance in AML patients is allogeneic HSCT, but unfortunately this therapy of choice can only be performed in a minority of patients [108].

7. PRT in AML

The preferred type of PRT in patients with AML in CR_1 is a subject of continued debate, especially in patients at high risk of non-relapse mortality (NRM) including patients above 40 years of age [114]. PRT is applied for the prevention of relapse and may include the following therapeutic options: (1) consolidation chemotherapy with HiDAC, (2) autologous HSCT, and

(3) allogeneic HSCT [12,114,115]. HiDAC at 2-3 g/m^2 IV-twice daily on days 1, 3 and 5 remains the standard of care for intensive PRT in AML [12,96,97,115]. Identification of the best therapeutic option for each patient regarding the best PRT, allogeneic HSCT versus intensive chemotherapy, should weigh the risk of relapse against the risk of NRM [12]. MRD assessment should be performed at regular intervals or once needed in patients receiving PRT in order to adjust therapeutic options before overt relapse [12,102,115,116].

In individuals at high risk of relapse and after completion of consolidation chemotherapy, maintenance therapy that includes the following agents can be administered: (1) azacytidine and decitabine, (2) lenalidomide, (3) dasatinib and imatinib, (4) bortezomib, (5) panobinostat, (6) midostaurin, (7) sorafenib, (8) AC-220, and (9) IL-2 [116-119]. In recent years, maintenance therapy with demethylating agents and TKIs is under evaluation in clinical trials. The combination of intensive chemotherapy and targeted therapies including TKIs or demethylating agents is currently under clinical evaluation as PRT in AML patients [12,119].

Allogeneic HSCT is preferred over chemotherapy as PRT in patients with intermediate- and poor- risk AML aged 40-60 years, whereas autologous HSCT remains a treatment option to be considered in patients with intermediate-risk disease [114]. Although allogeneic HSCT offers the most effective anti-leukemic therapy, increased NRM may compromise its favorable effects. RIC-allogeneic HSCT in patients above 40 years of age reduces NRM while maintaining the GVL effect. Given the potent GVL effect and the limited toxicity profile associated with the use of RIC-allogeneic HSCT, further evaluation of this form of HSCT in AML patients younger than 40 years is warranted [114]. In AML patients at high-risk of relapse, allogeneic HSCT with grafts obtained from matched-related donor (MRD) or matched-unrelated donor (MUD) is still the gold standard of care, while in patients at low-risk of relapse, autologous HSCT has shown promising results [12].

7.1. PRT for AML in younger adults

Young adult and adolescent patients (15 - 35 years) deserve special attention due to the specific medical and social needs. Approximately 60 - 80% of patients newly diagnosed with AML achieve CR with intensive chemotherapy. Without additional cytotoxic chemotherapy, virtually all of these patients will eventually relapse within 4 - 8 months [115,119]. However, the choice of PRT in these patients depends on a number of factors that include: (1) the expected rate of relapse with consolidation chemotherapy alone, influenced by karyotype, (2) the expected mortality and morbidity associated with each option as determined by age and comorbidities of patients, and (3) the available salvage therapy in case of disease relapse [115]. Although it is essential to maintain CR in AML patients responding to chemotherapy, maintenance therapy is not yet a standard AML treatment as it is still under evaluation [119]. According to risk stratification, the recommended PRT is as follows: (1) favorable cytogenetics such as t(8,21), inv(16) and t(16,16): 3 or more cycles of consolidation chemotherapy with HiDAC rather than standard dose cytarabine, alternative chemotherapeutic agents or early HSCT, (2) intermediate risk cytogenetics including normal karyotype: decision on option either HSCT or chemotherapy should be based on individual patient features such as age, comorbidities, initial WBC count and MRD, patient preference, HSCT donor availability and access to specific clinical trials, and (3) unfavorable cytogenetics: allogeneic HSCT is preferred over conventional chemotherapy and autologous HSCT [115].

8. Treatment of relapsed / refractory AML

Relapse after achieving CR is one of the most important obstacles in improving the outcome of patients with AML [120]. Approximately 70-75% of AML patients younger than 65 years will achieve CR if treated with standard induction chemotherapy [121]. TRM associated with induction chemotherapy has dropped to less than 5% with modern supportive care [121]. The prognostic scores and the risk factors for relapse in AML include: (1) adverse cytogenetics, (2) age at relapse, worst in patients more than 45 years old, (3) FLT3 mutation status, and (4) duration of first CR, worst if ≤ 6 months [122]. Also, adenine-adenine polymorphism in the cytotoxic T-lymphocyte antigen 4 (CTLA4) gene polymorphisms have higher relapse rates than adenine-guanine polymorphisms [122].

Therapeutic options that are available for patients having relapsed or refractory AML include: (1) salvage therapies that include various combinations of chemotherapeutic agents as shown in Table 9 [119,123], (2) chemotherapy and donor lymphocyte infusion (DLI) [123,124], (3) myeloablative allogeneic HSCT, RIC-allogeneic HSCT and second allogeneic HSCT [119,122,123], (4) novel and targeted therapies including: (a) immunomodulatory agents such as lenalidomide, (b) aminopeptidase inhibitors such as tosedostat, (c) purine analogs such as clofarabine, (d) mTOR inhibitors such as sirolimus and everolimus, (e) hypomethylating agents such as azacytidine and decitabine, (f) histone deacetylase (HDAC) inhibitors such as vorinostat, (g) farnesyl transferase inhibitors such as tipifarnib, (h) FLT3 inhibitors such as quizartinib, sorafenib and lestaurtinib, (i) CXCR4 antagonists such as plerixafor, (j) combination of azacytidine and sorafenib, and (k) monoclonal antibodies such as GO, lintuzumab, avastin and bevacizumab [122,123,125,126], (5) appropriate clinical trials, and (6) palliative care and supportive measures [122].

The following will improve the outcome of relapse: (1) improved understanding of the biology of AML, (2) molecular characterization of the subtype of AML, and (3) the development of new targeted and novel therapies [34]. Improvements in the outcome of patients with relapsed AML can be attributed to the following: (1) improvement in supportive care such as blood products and antimicrobials, (2) availability of better salvage therapies, (3) improvement in HSCT techniques, and (4) the introduction of new targeted therapies [120].

Despite the availability of multiple novel agents, prognosis of patients with relapsed AML remains poor [119,125]. The personalized approach is promising but will bring about new challenges for treating physicians [125]. Molecular tests may contribute to future personalized therapy, ultimately resulting in improved outcome [125]. In patients with relapsed/refractory AML, the dose of lenalidomide escalated to 50 mg/day for 21 days, every 4 weeks is safe, active and has low toxicity [126]. The immunomodulatory effect of lenalidomide can bring AML relapsing after HSCT into CR2 [126]. More than 20% of patients with newly diagnosed AML who fail induction therapy can still be cured, particularly if they are fit to have allogeneic HSCT

Regimen	Main adverse effects	Response rates
Reinduction with cytarabine and daunorubicin	Fever, gastrointestinal (GIT) upset, arrhythmias and daunorubicin-induced reactions	Complete remission (CR): 50%
HiDAC High dose cytarabine	Fever, GIT upset, cerebellar toxicity, chemical keratitis and conjunctivitis	CR: 35-40%
HAM High dose cytarabine and mitoxantrone	Fever, infections, stomatitis, arrhythmias and heart failure	Higher response rates than HiDAC alone
High dose cytarabine and etoposide	Fever, anaphylaxis and peripheral neuropathy	Similar responses to HiDAC alone
Mitoxantrone and etoposide	Fever, infections, heart failure, arrhythmias and Stomatitis	CR: 40%
MEC Mitoxantrone, etoposide and cytarabine	Fever, infections, hepatic dysfunction, arrhythmias and heart failure	Higher CR rates in patients < 60 years and those with unfavorable risk
FLAG; fludarabine, cytarabine and G-CSF (granulocyte monocyte colony stimulating factor)	Mucositis and infections	CR: 45-55%
CLAG Cladrabine, cytarabine and G-CSF	Fever, infections, mucositis and GIT upset	CR: 50%
Cyclophosphamide and high dose etoposide	Fever, infection, hemorrhagic cystitis, mucositis and liver dysfunction.	CR: 42%

Table 9. Chemotherapeutic regimens that are used in the treatment of relapsed / refractory AML

[121]. Thus, early human leukocyte antigen (HLA)-typing and donor identification are important components of the initial therapy of AML [121].

In patients with AML receiving allogeneic HSCT, relapse remains the main cause of treatment failure and is associated with poor prognosis [124]. Most treatments are of limited utility in AML patients relapsing after HSCT [124]. Re-induction chemotherapy can induce CR2 in 30 - 40% of AML patients relapsing following allogeneic HSCT, but remissions are usually of short duration and most of these patients ultimately relapse and die [124]. DLI alone may induce remission in 15-20% of patients, but long-term remissions are rare, while chemotherapy and DLI could induce durable remissions in a considerable proportion of patients with relapsed AML following HSCT [124]. Isolated extra-medullary relapse (EMR) is common after DLI and chemotherapy and it requires particular attention in future studies. Second allogeneic HSCT is associated with long-term overall survival of 10-35% and TRM of 40-50% [124].

8.1. Allogeneic HSCT for AML

Allogeneic HSCT is a potentially curative therapeutic option for many patients with AML [127-130]. Currently, AML is the most common indication for allogeneic HSCT [128,131,132]. Over the last decade, safety, effectiveness and the number of allogeneic HSCT procedures performed for patients with AML have increased substantially [128]. The ability to select candidates who benefit from allogeneic HSCT has improved due to an increased understanding of the biology of AML and implementation of risk stratification of AML based on cytogenetic and molecular markers [128,133].

In adult patients with AML, allogeneic HSCT is indicated in the following situations: (1) AML refractory to induction chemotherapy; all patients with AML who failed initial induction treatment and are: younger than 65 years, having available donor and an acceptable comorbidity index should be subjected to allogeneic HSCT, (2) AML in CR2; all patients who are younger than 75 years of age, having appropriate donor and a comorbidity index of ≤ 5 should be offered HSCT, (3) AML patients relapsing after induction or consolidation chemotherapy, (4) all AML patients with intermediate- or high-risk disease such as complex cytogenetics, monosomal karyotype or Philadelphia chromosome, (5) AML secondary to MDS or chronic MPNs, (6) t-AML not having favorable cytogenetics, and (7) AML with extramedullary disease such as CNS involvement [127,128,134-137]. The curative effect of HSCT results from both: (1) the radiation and/or chemotherapy used in the conditioning regimen administered prior to HSCT, and (2) the GVL effect obtained from the donor immune system [128]. The conditioning therapies administered before stem cell infusions can be divided into the following types: (1) conventional intensity conditioning (CIC) or standard myeloablative preparatory regimens which cause prolonged and irreversible pancytopenia and require stem cell rescue, otherwise leading to death, (2) minimally intensive conditioning (MIC) that cause cytopenias, but do not require stem cell rescue, and (3) RIC regimens which include all other conditioning therapies that do not qualify for either CIC or MIC [138]. In the latter form of conditioning therapies, peripheral blood counts may recover only after many weeks and these regimens require stem cell support to be clinically useful [138]. In patients with AML, the following conditioning therapies have commonly been used: (1) cyclophosphamide and total body irradiation, (2) busulfan and cyclophosphamide, (3) total lymphoid irradiation and anti-thymocyte globulin (ATG), (4) fludarabine, busulfan or treosulfan, and (5) clofarabine and busulfan [131,136]. However, myeloablative conditioning therapies, such as TBI and cyclophosphamide or busulfan and cyclophosphamide, cannot be administered to patients who are more than 50 years of age or have comorbidities because of high rate of TRM and toxicity [136].

Allogeneic HSCT has been established as an effective consolidation treatment in AML patients in first or subsequent remissions [134]. Allogeneic HSCT may be restricted to AML patients at a relatively high-risk of relapse such as intermediate and poor risk cytogenetics [134]. One of the main reasons for adopting allogeneic HSCT in the treatment of AML is the proven curative potential of GVL effect associated with allografting [131]. Unfortunately, GVL effect and GVHD are intimately linked [131]. Although allogeneic HSCT can effectively prevent relapse of AML, TRM associated with allogeneic HSCT may compromise that beneficial effect [130,134]. A significant reduction in TRM has been achieved during the last 3 decades and the ongoing developments may add to that improvement [134].

Achieving a cure for AML even in younger adult patients with de novo AML remains a challenge [139]. Despite being a curative therapeutic option for younger patients with AML in CR1, allogeneic HSCT with myeloablative conditioning therapy carries significant toxicity that limits its utilization. Alternative therapeutic options include intensive consolidation chemotherapy and autologous HSCT [139]. The potentially fatal complications of allogeneic HSCT include: (1) GVHD, (2) opportunistic infections, (3) VOD of the liver, (4) interstitial pneumonitis, and (5) organ failure [134]. Compared with non-allogeneic HSCT therapies, allografting has significant RFS and overall survival benefit for intermediate- and poor-risk AML, but not for good risk AML in CR1 according to a meta-analysis that was based on 24 prospective clinical trials which included 6007 AML patients [139]. Studies have shown that the factors determining the outcome of allogeneic HSCT in AML patients include: (1) age of the patient, (2) comorbidity index (3) number of induction cycles of chemotherapy administered to achieve morphological remission, (4) the type of consolidation chemotherapy given, (5) the cytogenetic risk group: favorable, intermediate or unfavorable, (6) pre-transplant karyotype, (7) pre-HSCT peripheral blood count recovery, (8) status of MRD prior to HSCT, and (9) the preparative conditioning therapy; myeloablative versus non-myeloablative [134,135,140]. The following developments or changes in the clinical management of patients with AML subjected to allogeneic HSCT have contributed to the improved survival: (1) improved prevention and treatment of GVHD by methotrexate, cyclosporine-A, mycophenolate mofetil as well as other immunosuppressive therapies, (2) transplantation or infusion of higher doses of hematopoietic progenitor cells, (3) molecular monitoring of viruses such as cytomegalovirus as well as Epstein-Barr virus and subsequent pre-emptive therapy in patients with viral infections, (4) improved detection and treatment of fungal infections, (5) introduction of high-resolution HLA-typing and the increased number of pre-transplant and procedure-related factors, which allow risk assessment and thereby may guide transplant policies that affect transplantation outcome, (6) the application of new techniques that assess the risk of relapse after HSCT such as MRD and chimerism, (7) the recent progress in transplant procedures such as: the use of alternative donors, RIC-allogeneic HSCT with its new conditioning therapies, and novel therapies in maintenance therapy after HSCT to prevent relapse of AML, and (8) improvement in supportive care, treatment of bacterial infections, provision of safer blood products and appropriate utilization of intensive care facilities [128,129,133,134].

In patients with AML, CNS involvement is rare and is associated with poor prognosis, hence allogeneic HSCT is indicated in AML patients with CNS disease [137]. In adults with AML having CNS involvement and subjected to allogeneic HSCT, the independent risk factors for survival include chronic GVHD, disease status and cytogenetic risk category [137].

Allogeneic HSCT in AML patients with monosomal karyotype particularly (-5/5q-) in CR_1 is associated with a significant reduction in relapse rate and an improvement in survival [141,142]. The role of allogeneic HSCT in AML patients with abnormal 17p is questionable as it is associated with poor outcome and a 2 year EFS of only 12% [142]. Hierarchical classification of adverse-risk karyotypes, according to distinct genetic lesions, is effective prognostically in detecting the outcome of allogeneic HSCT in AML patients [142]. Patients with AML who harbor FLT3-ITD genetic mutations carry a poor prognosis. Although allogeneic HSCT may improve the outcomes of these patients, relapses occur frequently [143]. Two management interventions may improve the outcome of allogeneic HSCT in patients with AML having FLT3-ITDs: (1) early detection of MRD following HSCT may allow early intervention, and (2) maintenance therapy with sorafenib and other agents may prevent or delay relapse [143,144].

In older patients with AML, allogeneic HSCT is a feasible therapeutic option and can provide approximately 40% survival at 2 years in appropriately selected patients [145]. Although increasing age is associated with poorer survival, higher comorbidities and poor performance status have more negative impact than age per se [145]. The increasing number and experience with alternative donors will facilitate allogeneic HSCT and make it a more achievable therapeutic option for elderly AML patients [119,145]. Also, the advent of RIC regimens made allogeneic HSCT an available treatment option with curative intent for older AML patients [114,146]. Recent studies on the role of allogeneic HSCT in AML patients have revealed: (1) little impact of age on the outcome of HSCT, and (2) greater impact of the following on HSCT outcome: (a) the recipient health status; comorbidity index and performance status, (b) the AML disease status; CR1 or CR2 at the time of transplantation, and (c) the associated chromosomal aberrations; favorable versus intermediate or unfavorable cytogenetics [146]. RIC-allogeneic HSCT has resulted in better survival among older patients with AML than autologous HSCT or conventional chemotherapy [146]. Despite the acceptable outcomes of alternative donors and the reports of equivalent outcomes of MRD and MUD allografts, grafts obtained from HLA-identical siblings continue to be associated with the most favorable outcomes after allogeneic HSCT [119,146].

Strategies that can speed up immune reconstitution following allogeneic HSCT for AML include: (1) infusion of genetically modified lymphocytes, (2) in vivo T-cell depletion, (3) rapamycin to promote T-regulatory cell expansion in vivo, and (4) cyclophosphamide, on day 3 after stem cell infusion, to reduce alloreactive lymphocytes [136]. There are new strategies to enhance and maintain the GVL effect of DLIs while minimizing GVHD and these strategies include: (1) pre-emptive DLI before overt relapse, (2) co-stimulation with cytokines or dendritic cells (DCs), and (3) the use of leukemia-specific antibodies and other immunotherapies including: (a) monoclonal antibodies such as GO, (b) hypomethylating agents such as azacytidine and decitabine, (c) proteasome inhibitors such as bortezomib, (d) immunomodulatory agents such as lenalidomide, and (e) HDAC inhibitors [130,147].

The main causes of treatment failure in allogeneic HSCT for AML are disease relapse and treatment toxicity [130,140,147,148]. Relapse after allogeneic HSCT in AML patients remains a major obstacle to survival as it accounts for 20-50% of the primary causes of death [147]. Factors that predict an increased risk of relapse in AML patients subjected to allogeneic HSCT include: (1) disease status at transplant, (2) adverse cytogenetics at diagnosis, and (3) increased intensity of post-transplant immunosuppression [136]. In AML patients relapsing following allogeneic HSCT, the following treatment options are available: (1) intensive chemotherapy and/or DLI, (2) second allogeneic HSCT after withdrawal of immunosuppression or (3) the best supportive care [147,148]. When relapse is the most common concern for treatment failure associated with allogeneic HSCT, a female donor for a male recipient may be beneficial in decreasing the incidence of relapse rate following HSCT [149]. However, AML relapse following allogeneic HSCT predicts a poor survival [148]. Patients who relapse ≥ 6 months after initial allogeneic HSCT have better survival and may benefit from intensive chemotherapy or a second allograft with or without DLI [148]. The use of alternative donor HSCT is increasing as the transplantation-eligible population ages and as sibling donors become less available [150]. A recently published study that included 414 patients with AML, treated at 2 institutions in the USA and France, evaluated the donor source of stem cells on the outcome of allogeneic HSCT [MRD: 187 patients; MUD: 76 patients; and umbilical cord blood (UCB): 151 patients] revealed that: (1) the 6-year overall survival was similar across all donor types, and (2) the TRM was also similar across all donor types. The data obtained from this study support the use of alternative donors as a graft source with myeloablative or RIC allogeneic HSCT for patients with AML when a sibling donor is not available [150].

In younger patients with high-risk AML, allogeneic HSCT has a significant positive impact on the outcome. In this group of patients, allografts from MRD or MUD yield similar results [151]. In AML patients relapsing after autologous HSCT, allogeneic HSCT using MUD is a feasible option that results in 20% long-term leukemia-free survival [152]. In patients with AML in CR1, without available identical donor, the possible transplantation options are: (1) haploidentical HSCT using T-cell depleted grafts, and (2) autologous HSCT but the choice depends on the experience of the transplant center [153]. Survival of older patients with AML undergoing allogeneic HSCT with grafts obtained from younger unrelated donors has improved compared to allografts obtained from older related donors [132]. UCB-HSCT has provided an alternative transplantation option for patients with high-risk AML lacking MRD and MUD, but it is associated with high risk of relapse which limits its use in this category of patients [154]. Risk factors for extramedullary relapse in patients with AML receiving haploidentical allogeneic HSCT include failure to achieve CR prior to HSCT and absence of chronic GVHD after allografts [155]. The GVL effect may help to prevent and eradicate EMR following allogeneic HSCT [155]. Haploidentical donors can safely extend transplantation options for AML patients without HLA matched siblings or unrelated donors [156,157]. HLA-haploidentical HSCT is an effective and immediate therapeutic modality for high-risk AML patients who lack matched donors [158]. The use of fractionated 800 cGy-TBI-based conditioning therapy and unmanipulated peripheral blood stem cell grafts seems feasible and can result in favorable outcomes for adult patients with AML in CR undergoing haploidentical HSCT [159]. However, relapse remains a leading cause of death in high-risk AML patients subjected to haploidentical HSCT [158]. Achievement of CR before transplantation and recombinant human G-CSF priming of conditioning therapy can improve the outcome of patients with high-risk AML receiving haploidentical allografts [158,160].

8.2. RIC-allogeneic HSCT for AML

The frequency of fatal toxicities in the course of myeloablative allogeneic HSCT for AML patients increases with age [138]. Unfortunately, the vast majority of patients with AML, who would benefit from an allograft, are older and therefore usually ineligible for such therapy [138]. RIC-allogeneic HSCT was introduced more than a decade ago for patients who were older, had significant comorbid conditions as well as poorer performance status [161]. This form of HSCT has improved the accessibility to transplant patients with AML or other hematological malignancies who are not eligible for standard conditioning therapy for allogeneic HSCT [162]. However, RIC-allogeneic HSCT appears to be safe and permits durable donor engraftment [162]. The antineoplastic potency of RIC-allogeneic HSCT relies primarily on the GVL effect of the allograft rather than ablating all residual leukemia disease [161]. The anti-leukemic GVL effect is derived from the donor cells infused [138]. TRM appears to be less with RIC-allogeneic HSCT than that observed with conventional myeloablative allogeneic HSCT [138]. RIC-allogeneic HSCT for AML has the following limitations: (1) insufficient anti-leukemic effect in the preparative conditioning therapy, (2) high relapse rates, (3) possible higher incidence of engraftment failure, (4) unclear benefit of using conventional pre-transplant cytoreductive treatment, (5) incidence and severity rates of chronic GVHD similar to myeloablative transplants, and (6) most of the available data have been obtained from small single-center reports or larger but retrospective multicenter studies rather than prospective trials [138].

In patients with high-risk AML ineligible for conventional allogeneic HSCT, RIC regimen can result in long-term remissions and chronic GVHD that reduces relapse rate and improves OS as well as DFS [163]. In these patients, novel approaches are also required to reduce post-HSCT relapses [163]. Allogeneic HSCT from related or unrelated donors after conditioning therapy with low-dose TBI and fludarabine relies almost exclusively on GVL effects and can result in long-term remissions in older patients and in patients who are medically unfit for the standard-myeloablative conditioning therapy [164]. Compared to fludarabine, cytarabine and idarubicin nonablative conditioning regimen, the more myelosuppressive conditioning therapy with fludarabine and melphalan provided better disease control, but higher TRM and morbidity in patients with high-risk MDS and AML subjected to allogeneic HSCT [165]. RIC-allogeneic HSCT using fludarabine, busulfan and alemtuzumab conditioning treatment is safe and has minimal toxicity even in high risk patients with advanced disease in whom conventional myeloablative conditioning therapy is contraindicated [162].

In a four arm clinical study that included 51 patients who were followed up for at least 100 days, RIC-allogeneic HSCT in these patients with AML using clofarabine and/or fludarabine in addition to IV busulfan daily conditioning therapy, the following results were obtained: (1) clofarabine had sufficient immunosuppressive capacity to consistently support the engraftment of allogeneic progenitor cells, (2) clofarabine and IV busulfan ± ATG appeared to be a highly active conditioning regimen in patients with advanced largely chemotherapy-refractory myeloid leukemia, (3) the use of fludarabine and clofarabine in addition to busulfan was safe, and (4) in pre-transplant conditioning therapy, a combination of 2 nucleoside analogs (fludarabine and clofarabine) may synergistically increase anti-leukemic efficacy without a concomitant increase in clinical toxicity [166].

Treosulfan in combination with fludarabine as RIC therapy for allogeneic HSCT in patients with secondary AML or MDS is a feasible and an effective regimen that enables engraftment in almost all patients subjected to transplantation [167]. Achieving a stringent CR in AML patients is critical for the success of RIC-allogeneic HSCT [161]. However, the definition of CR was updated in 2003 and the new definition requires no evidence of leukemia by flow cytometry in addition to having morphological remission [161]. Despite being associated with GVHD, TRM and relapse, RIC-allogeneic HSCT produces outcomes similar to allogeneic HSCT using myeloablative regimens [138].

8.3. Autologous HSCT

Autologous HSCT is an effective therapeutic modality in AML with the possibility of long-term survival, particularly in patients with standard-risk AML [168,169]. Several historical randomized trials have reported significantly lower relapse rates after autologous HSCT than after conventional chemotherapy [170,171]. Autologous HSCT has the following advantages: (1) faster hematological engraftment reflected by the recovery of blood indices, (2) the possibility of applying this form of transplant in older patients, (3) lower incidences of transplant-related complications, (4) faster immune reconstitution, and (5) absence of GVHD [169]. However, autologous HSCT has few disadvantages including: lack of GVL effect, insufficient number of peripheral stem cells at mobilization, and higher incidence of relapse [169]. Faster recovery of blood counts following autologous HSCT has the following advantages: shorter duration of hospitalization, decreased need for blood product transfusion, and reduction in the days of IV antimicrobials [172].

Oral busulfan is the historical backbone of the busulfan-cyclophosphamide conditioning regimen for autologous HSCT [170]. The use of IV busulfan, instead of the oral form, simplifies the autograft procedure and confirms the usefulness of autologous HSCT in AML. As in allogeneic HSCT, IV busulfan is associated with the uncommon complication of VOD in the autologous transplant setting [170].

BM is the traditional source of stem cells for HSCT [172]. Since 1994, the use of peripheral blood stem cells has resulted in more rapid engraftment kinetics and lower rates of NRM [170]. The use of G-CSF-mobilized peripheral blood stem cells use has been associated with more rapid engraftment presumably due to the higher number of infused CD34+ cells and with reduced morbidity and TRM compared to autologous BM transplantation [172,173]. Therefore, autologous peripheral blood HSCT has recently replaced autologous BM transplantation based on reduction in morbidity, resource utilization and duration of hospitalization [174]. Nevertheless, the outcomes of peripherally collected autologous stem cells and autologous stem cells collected by BM harvesting are similar [172].

Phase I and II studies have shown that patients with favorable- risk cytogenetics benefit from autologous HSCT with a reduction in relapse rate and improvement in leukemia-free survival [174]. However, in patients with high-risk AML, autologous HSCT is not a valuable option, while allogeneic HSCT is a valid therapeutic potential provided CR or control of the disease is achieved [175]. In elderly individuals with AML, there are limitations to the utilization of autologous HSCT [176]. Fortunately several new agents that can be used alone or in combinations may become more useful that autologous HSCT in this age group [176].

In elderly patients with AML, autologous HSCT has been performed, but the published studies lack randomization and have included highly selected patients [177]. However acceptable toxicity and relatively low TRM have been reported [177]. Relapses following autologous

HSCT were also the main cause of treatment failure [177]. In patients with de novo AML belonging to the age group of 60 - 70 years: more than 25% of patients benefit from standard intensive chemotherapy and autologous HSCT has a tolerable toxicity and may have a positive impact on leukemia-free survival [178].

The outcome of autologous HSCT widely varies among patients with AML [179]. Delayed hematological recovery in patients with AML in CR1, subjected to autologous HSCT, is associated with favorable outcome, that is, longer OS and longer time to progression [179]. A two-step approach to autologous HSCT is as follows: (1) HiDAC consolidation, and (2) conditioning therapy with busulfan and etoposide followed by infusion of peripherally collected autologous stem cells has produced excellent stem cell yields and has allowed a high proportion of patients to receive this intended therapy [180].

9. Maintenance therapy following HSCT

Disease recurrence is a major cause of treatment failure after HSCT for AML [117]. Disease relapse post-HSCT is a devastating event for patients with hematologic malignancies [116]. Maintenance therapy following HSCT offers the possibility of avoiding or delaying relapse, but its role remains unclear in most diseases treated by HSCT [116]. GVHD is a major cause for NRM and morbidity after HSCT. Decitabine maintenance after HSCT may eradicate MRD and facilitate a GVL effect. Lower doses of decitabine (15 mg/m^2 for 5 days every 6 weeks) are well tolerated after HSCT [117]. Decitabine maintenance may have a favorable effect on the incidence of GVHD by enhancing the effect of T-regulatory lymphocytes [117]. One study has shown that approximately 43% of patients are able to tolerate 8 cycles of low dose decitabine maintenance following HSCT. The lower incidence of GVHD and the lack of decitabine toxicity indicate that a longer period of administration may be required [117]. Methods that are used to monitor MRD following HSCT include: (1) MFC, (2) PCR for gene overexpression (PCR-GE) in disease compared to healthy tissue, (3) PCR for sequence, somatic mutation or splice variant specific to tumor (PCR-NUT), and (4) next-generation sequencing (NGS) [95,102-104,116].

9.1. Immunotherapy in AML

Myeloid forms of leukemia are particularly suited for immunotherapeutic interventions because of the following reasons: (1) myeloid leukemias express both HLA class I and class II molecules and their down-regulation is infrequently observed in leukemic blasts, (2) leukemic blasts typically exist in physical niches within the BM microenvironment and/or peripheral blood components that are relatively accessible to antigen-specific T-cells and other non-antigen-specific immunocytes, (3) myeloid disorders are often characterized by chromosomal translocations that result in chimeric proteins which are unique leukemia antigens that may offer target specificity, and (4) the window of immune recovery or reconstitution following cytotoxic-based induction therapy or HSCT offers a unique opportunity to prime an immune response or circumvent potential leukemia-induced peripheral tolerance [181]. The following are the types of immunotherapies that are available for AML patients: (1) allogeneic HSCT including RIC-allogeneic HSCT, (2) DLIs as well as GVL effects of HSCT and DLI, (3) autologous anti-leukemic T-cell infusions, (4) adoptive transfer of allogeneic or autologous T-cells and natural killer (NK) cells, (5) vaccination with leukemic cells, (6) use of peptides and DNA vaccines such as: peptide vaccines, granulocyte monocyte-colony stimulating factor (GM-CSF) secreting tumor vaccines and whole tumor cell vaccines, (7) use of immunomodulatory drugs, (8) DC immunotherapy including: monocyte or BM-derived-DCs and leukemia-derived-DCs, (9) treatment with cytokines such as IL-2, (10) administration of monoclonal antibodies such as GO, and (11) WT_1 antigen targeting [182-187].

Cytotoxic chemotherapy can successfully induce remissions in adult patients with AML, but such remissions are not usually sustained as the disease has high probability of relapse [182]. In AML patients durable remissions can be achieved in less than 30% of patients as most of these patients respond initially to combination chemotherapy, but relapse later on [182,183]. At relapse, blast cells are usually resistant to the drugs to which the patient has been exposed and also frequently to other cytotoxic agents. In such cases, immunological mechanisms for blast killing appear crucial [183]. There is evidence; obtained from tissue culture, animal and clinical studies, that stimulated donor T-cells can recognize and kill leukemic blasts through the recognition of alloantigens, differentiation antigens or leukemia-specific antigens as targets [183].

Strategies to prevent relapse of AML include: consolidation chemotherapy, HSCT and immunotherapy [182]. The principle of anti-leukemic adoptive immunotherapy, as coined by Georges Mathe in 1965, is an activity of allogeneic immunologically competent cells against the host leukemic cells [188]. The best known model and the most commonly used method of anti-leukemic adoptive immunotherapy is allogeneic HSCT [188]. The following provide evidence supporting the GVL effects of allogeneic HSCT: (1) lower relapse rate amongst recipients of HLA-identical sibling transplants than recipients of syngeneic transplants, (2) lower relapse rate among patients who develop GVHD following allogeneic HSCT, (3) decreased GVHD but increased relapse rate after T-cell depleted allografts, (4) anti-leukemic effect and curative potential of DLI in patients with leukemia who relapse after HSCT, and (5) the effectiveness of non-myeloablative allogeneic HSCT [188]. Wider application of immunotherapies such as allogeneic HSCT and RIC therapy has altered the landscape and could offer a potential for cure to an increasing number of older patients with AML [186]. RIC-allogeneic HSCT in older AML patients, after achievement of CR, is feasible and has improved DFS over conventional chemotherapy [186].

Immunotherapeutic approaches such as improvement in pre-HSCT conditioning regimens and the use of DLI to induce GVL effect will ultimately improve the outcome of HSCT and decrease the burden of AML [182]. The GVL effect of HSCT has shown that the immune system is capable of eradicating AML [189]. Allogeneic HSCT and DLI have the potential to eradicate leukemic cells by means of allogeneic T-cells [185]. Adoptive immunotherapy has the potential to provide long-term survival and even cure in patients with leukemia [188]. Novel approaches using NK cells and T-cells have been developed to provide more direct anti-leukemic therapy while sparing the risk of toxicity to normal tissues [188].

Emerging clinical data indicate that GO is efficacious not only in acute promyelocytic leukemia but also, once combined with conventional chemotherapy, in favorable and intermediate risk AMLs [190]. Data from several cooperative groups indicate that older patients with AML benefit from the incorporation of GO into the induction therapy [186]. Also, the clinical results of GO strongly support the utility of CD33 targeted therapeutics [190]. The early recognition that some AMLs may predominantly or entirely involve committed myeloid progenitor cells led to efforts underlying LSCs with antibodies recognizing the CD33 differentiation antigen [190]. Targeted therapy with GO has produced remissions in relapsed AML and the drug appears promising when used in combination with the standard chemotherapy for the treatment of newly diagnosed AML [191].

Targeted alpha-particle immunotherapy offers the potential of more efficient tumor cell killing, while sparing the surrounding normal cells, than beta-particles [192]. Clinical studies on alpha particle immunotherapy for AML have focused on the myeloid cell surface antigen CD33 as a target using the humanized monoclonal antibody lintuzumab. Studies have demonstrated the safety and efficacy of bismuth-213 labeled lintuzumab in the treatment of AML as it has produced remissions in some patients with AML after partial cytoreduction with cytarabine [192]. The second generation construct that contains actinium-225 (225 Ac-lintuzumab) has also been shown to have significant anti-leukemic activity even in elder patients with low-dose cytarabine [192]. Preclinical studies have shown that anti-CD45 monoclonal antibodies, as part of conditioning therapy prior to HSCT, are useful [192]. MRD reflected by the persistence of LSCs below the detection limit by conventional methods, causes a high rate of disease relapses [187]. Assessment of MRD is critical in monitoring the effectiveness of immunotherapy in AML patients as the ultimate goal of AML treatment is the eradication of MRD [182,187].

Four decades after the initial attempts at vaccination for AML, using bacilli Calmette-Guerin and irradiated autologous leukemic cells, interest in immunotherapy in AML has been revived [182,193,194]. Phase I and II studies using different DC vaccination protocols have been designed [187]. DC-based vaccination has resulted in the induction of potent anti-leukemic cytotoxic T cells, but with limited clinical efficacy [187]. To improve the effectiveness of DC-based vaccination, the optimal timing of vaccination during the course of AML has to be determined, although current literature and cumulative experience indicate that immunotherapy may be most effective in the state of MRD following induction and post-remission chemotherapy [187].

The development of antigen-targeted immunotherapy of AML has been accelerated by: (1) the GVL effect of HSCT on residual leukemic cells, and (2) the identification of leukemia associated antigens (LAAs) that can serve as potential targets for immunotherapy [189]. There are several LAAs and these together with other molecules that may serve as potential targets in AML immunotherapy are included in Table 10 [185,187,195,196]. Criteria that should be met for selection of ideal LAAs which can be used in AML targeted therapy include that they should: (1) be leukemia specific as they are expressed in leukemia cells with minimal or no expression in normal tissues, (2) display high and homogeneous expression in most leukemic blasts including LSCs, (3) play a defined oncogenic role and are important for the leukemia phenotype, (4) be immunogenic as they possess strong immunogenic properties, (5) demonstrate clinical utility and effectiveness, (6) show expression in hematopoietic stem cells and (7) display expression in T-cells particularly activated T cells [189,195].

Antigen or molecules	(percentage)	Antigen or molecule	(percentage)
AURKA (Aurora kinase A)	(37%)	CD 25 ; IL-2 receptor α	-
PRAME (preferentially exposed antigen in melanoma)	(32%)	CD 33 ; siglec - 3	> 80%
PHAMM (CD 168, receptor of hyaluronic mediated motility)	(60-70%)	CD 44 ; H-CAM	100%
WT_1 (Wilms tumor 1)	(73-100%)	CD 45	-
CLL-1 (c-type lectin-like molecule)	(92%)	CD 47 (integrin-associated protein immunoglobulin superfamily)	100%
MUC (mucin-1)	(67-70%)	CD 96 (tactile Ig superfamily)	30%
mHAgs (minor histocompatibility antigens)	-	CD 123 (IL-3 receptor α)	100%
HBG-2	(42%)	h Tert	
CCNA-1	(82%)	HSJ 2	
BAALC	(30%)	MPP 11	
PRTN-3	(48%)	NE (neutrophil elastase)	
RBPJk	-	PR_1	
Proteinase 3	-	DRAP and cyclin A_1	

Table 10. Leukemia-associated antigens and other molecules that the potential targets in AML immunotherapy

Improved understanding of NK cell biology has provided insights on selection of donors for HSCT and on the immunotherapeutic options in non-HSCT settings [186]. Novel immunotherapeutic approaches and identification of novel target antigens and improved donor selection for allogeneic HSCT hold promise for a variety of treatment options for older patients having AML in the near future [186]. The identification of LAAs and the observation that administration of allogeneic T- cells can mediate a GVL effect paved the way to develop active and passive immunotherapeutic strategies respectively [185]. Promising targeted passive immunotherapy approaches include: the administration of anti-CD33 antibodies and the adoptive transfer of LAA-specific T cell or KIR ligand-mismatched NK cells [185]. Whole tumor cell vaccines or DC-based vaccines also hold promise in boosting the immune system for the induction of anti-leukemia immune responses. The aim of these immunotherapeutic strategies is the eradication of AML blasts by the immune system [185]. Treatment of older patients with AML is slowly but steadily changing with emphasis on supportive care and potentially curative therapeutic approaches such as certain forms of allogeneic HSCT [186].

Recent advances in immunology and identification of promising LAAs open the possibilities of eradicating MRD by antigen-specific immunotherapy following the administration of cytotoxic chemotherapy [184]. Progress in inducing antitumor immune responses together with strategies to attenuate immunosuppressive factors will establish immunotherapy as an important armament to combat AML [184]. Although immunotherapeutic trials have shown improvement in immunogenicity and clinical outcomes, severe adverse events have been encountered in highly avid engineered T-cell therapies indicating the importance of having a balance between effectiveness and adverse effects related to the use of advanced immunotherapy. Such a balance between clinical efficacy and safety will become a main issue in the era of advanced future immunotherapy [184].

9.2. Novel and targeted therapies in AML

Development of effective targeted cancer therapeutic depends upon distinguishing disease-associated or driver mutations, which have causative roles in the pathogenesis of malignancy, from passenger mutations that are dispensable for cancer initiation maintenance [197]. Therapeutic strategies in AML are shown in Table 11 [15]. Molecular targeted therapies and novel agents that are being evaluated in clinical trials are included in Table 12 [17,58,198-213].

Number	Therapeutic approach	Examples
(1)	Epigenetic regulation	(a) histone deacetylase inhibitors: vorinostat, panobinostat and belinostat (b) DNA methyltransferase inhibitors: azacytidine and decitabine
(2)	Induction of differentiation	(a) Arsenic trioxide (b) Retinoid X receptor agonists: ATRA
(3)	Inhibition of angiogenesis	a- Thalidomide b- Lenalidomide c- Bortezomab
(4)	Modulation of drug resistance	(a) Valspodar (b) Zosuquidar
(5)	Modification of traditional chemotherapeutics	(a) Nucleoside analogs: clofarabine, sapacitabine and elacytarabine (b) Alkylating agents: irofulven, temodar and onrigin (c) Topoisomerase II inhibitor: hycamtin
(6)	Immunotherapy	a- Monoclonal antibodies: myelotarg, lintuzumab and avastin b- T-cell targeted therapies
(7)	Inhibition of signaling pathways	(a) Tyrosine kinase inhibitors: sorafinib, modostaurin and lestaurtinib. (b) Cell cycle inhibitors: ONO 1910. Na (c) Farnesyl transferase inhibitors: sarasar and zarnestra (d) mTOR inhibitors: afinitor, temsirolimus, PI-103 and GSK 21110183 (e) PARP inhibitors: ABT-888 (f) MEK 1/2 inhibitors: AZD 6244, GSK1120212, AS703026 and PD98059 (g) Bcl2 inhibitors: Obatoclax, Oblimersen and ABT-263 (h) XIAP inhibitors: AEG -35156 (i) Aminopeptidase inhibitors: tosedostat

Table 11. Therapeutic strategies in patients with acute myeloid leukemia

10. Small molecule inhibitors in AML

Many patients with AML who initially respond to induction chemotherapy will eventually relapse or develop refractory disease [115,213]. Targeted therapy with small molecule inhibitors (SMIs) represents a new therapeutic intervention that has been successful in treating several cancers [213]. Examples of SMIs that include inhibitors of the targets: FLT3, HDAC, heat shock protein, CXCR4, proteasomes and Aurora kinases are shown in Table 12 [213-233]. There has been great interest in generating selective SMIs that target critical pathways of proliferation and survival of blasts in AML. SMIs have been developed to modulate the activity of proteins encoded by mutated or over-expressed genes in patients with AML [213]. Clonal evolution and pharmacodynamics are potential obstacles to the clinical development of SMIs for the treatment of AML. Multi-targeted agents and the combination of SMIs with cytotoxic chemotherapy may improve the efficacy of treatment [213]. The analysis of patient samples is an important tool to investigate resistance mechanisms, and discover and validate biological markers that could be used for the prediction and assessment of treatment response [213].

Molecular target	Phase of study	Small molecule inhibitors or new drugs in clinical trials	
Aurora kinase	I	* Alisertib * AMG 900	
Farnesyl transferase	1/2	- Tipifarnib - Lestaurtinib	
Histone deacetylase	1/2/3	- Valproic acid - Panobinostat - Vorinostat - Entinostat	
Proteasome inhibitor	2	- Bortezomib - Ixazomib	
$CXCR_4$	1/2	* Plerixafor * BL- 8040 * BMS - 936564	
HSP 90	1/2	- Ganetespid	
FLT 3	1/2/3	- Crenolanib - Sorafenib - Midostaurin	- Quizartinib - Sunitinib - Listaurtinib
C-Kit	1/2	- Nilotinib - Dasatinib	
Hedgehog pathway	1/2	PF - 04449913	
WTN pathway	1	* PRI-728	

Molecular target	Phase of study	Small molecule inhibitors or new drugs in clinical trials	
		* CWP - 232291	
IDH 1/2	1	* AG - 120 * AG - 221	
Molecular target		**Small molecule inhibitors or new drugs in clinical trials**	
mTOR pathway		- Rapamycin - Everolimus - Temsirolimus	
Nucleoside analogs		- Clofarabine - Sapacitabine	
DNA hypomethylating agents		- Azacytidine - Decitabine	
Immunomodulatory agents		- Lenalidomide	
Monoclonal antibodies		- Gemtuzumab	
Bcl-2		* ABT - 199 * ABT - 737	
Retinoids		- ATRA	
MEK1		- E 6201	
Alkylating agents		- Bendamustine	
Statins		- Pravastatin	
Mitochondrial translation inhibitor		- Tigecycline	
EGFR inhibitor		- Erlotinib	
Oncogene elF4 E inhibitor		- Ribavirin	
VEGFR inhibitor		- Pazopanib	
CDK inhibitor		- Flavoperidol	
RAS mutation		- GSK1120212	- MSC 19363698
JAK 2 mutations		INCB 018424	

Table 12. Molecular targeted therapies and new drugs in AML clinical trials

10.1. FLT3 inhibitors

FLT3-ITD activating mutations are present in one fifth to one third of adult patients with AML and they are associated with poor prognosis [197,203,204]. FLT3-ITD mutations represent a driver lesion and can be a valid therapeutic target in AML [197]. Agents that target FLT3 mutations are under development for the treatment of patients with AML and they may offer a potential paradigm change in the current standard treatment of AML [17]. The introduction of FLT3 inhibitors for the treatment of AML may be the start of a new era in the treatment of AML after many years of exclusive dependency on cytotoxic chemotherapy [17]. Examples of FLT3 inhibitors include: sorafenib, midostaurin, sunitinib and lestaurtinib [17]. Early FLT3 inhibitors including midostaurin, sunitinib and lestaurtinib have demonstrated significant promise in preclinical models of FLT3 mutant AML. Unfortunately, in early clinical trials, many of these agents had failed to achieve robust and sustained FLT3 inhibition as they caused only transient decreases in peripheral blast counts [204]. The second-generation FLT3 inhibitors, such as quizartinib, have demonstrated enhanced FLT3 specificity and have been well tolerated in early clinical trials. Several FLT3 inhibitors have reached phase III clinical trials and a variety of phase I and II trials in order to explore the role of these novel agents in conjunction with conventional chemotherapy and HSCT [204]. Molecular insights provided by FLT3 inhibitors have shed light on the various mechanisms of drug resistance and have provided a rationale supporting the use of combinations of conventional chemotherapeutic regimens and novel targeted treatments [204].

Most patients with FLT3-ITD-positive AML show initial favorable response to FLT3 inhibitors followed by the development of drug resistance [203]. After the use of FLT3 inhibitors in patients with single FLT3-ITD-mutated AML, a new tyrosine kinase mutation may arise, a phenomenon that is associated with the evolution of drug resistance [205]. Acquired resistance to selective FLT3-ITD-positive AML is an emerging clinical problem in the treatment of FLT3-ITD and this resistance is associated with poor prognosis [203,205,206]. There are several mechanisms of resistance to FLT3 inhibitors and they include: (1) FLT3 receptor and ligand expression, (2) up-regulation of the compensatory signaling pathways, (3) acquired mutations in the tyrosine kinase domain (TKD) of FLT3, (4) mutations in other kinase genes, and (5) up-regulation of anti-apoptotic proteins [203]. One of the most common mechanisms of resistance to inhibitors is the acquisition of secondary FLT3-TKD mutations which primarily consist of point mutations in the activation loop TKD_2 and in the ATP-binding pocket of TKD [203].

Midostaurin and lestaurtinib are multi-targeted kinase inhibitors that include FLT3 as one of their targets [207]. They are more appropriate for the treatment of newly diagnosed AML as they are broad-spectrum agents [207]. Quizartinib is a highly selective FLT3 inhibitor and is less toxic to FLT3-ITD AML primary samples in vitro. It may be useful in relapsed patients in whom high FLT3 ligand levels may necessitate a highly potent agent that is able to prevent ligand binding to FLT3 [207]. In patients with relapsed/refractory AML, particularly those harboring FLT3-ITD mutations, quizartinib has shown clinical activity with acceptable toxicity profile [208]. Quizartinib is a potent and selective FLT3-TKI with activity against both FLT3-mutant and wild-type AML [209]. However, the quality and duration of responses achieved are suboptimal [209]. The combination of quizartinib and chemotherapy may improve the outcome, while the combination of quizartinib and agents that tackle BM microenvironment may enhance response rates [209]. Sunitinib has anti-leukemic activity in patients who become resistant to sorafenib indicating that sequential therapy with different FLT3 inhibitors may provide clinical benefit [203]. Clinical activity of sorafenib monotherapy in FLT3-ITD- positive adult AML patients including induction of CRs has been described [203]. However, clinical responses have not been durable in most patients [203].

Ponatinib is a multikinase inhibitor that has demonstrated clinical efficacy in patients with chemotherapy resistant AML having with FLT3-ITD mutations [210]. It exhibits activity against AC-220-resistant FLT3-ITD/F691 gatekeeper mutation, but it is highly ineffective against FLT3-ITD activation loop mutations, particularly at the D835 residue [210]. Crenolanib is a novel TKI that has demonstrated an inhibitory activity against drug-resistant AML primary blasts with FLT3-ITD and D835H/Y mutations [211]. It is effective against FLT3-ITD containing secondary kinase domain mutations, suggesting that crenolanib may be a useful therapeutic agent against TKI-naive and drug-resistant FLT3-ITD-positive AML [211].

The dual Aurora-B/FLT3 inhibitors represent a significant development in the treatment of AML [212]. These dual inhibitors may overcome FLT3 inhibitor resistance, partly due to inhibition of Aurora kinase, and thus may benefit patients with FLT3-mutated AML [206]. Orally bioavailable dual FLT3-Aurora kinase inhibitors with improved properties are currently under development [206]. More potent novel therapies that are useful in the management of relapsed or heavily pretreated AML having high circulating levels of FLT3 ligand include: FLT3-ITD-specific small molecules and monoclonal antibodies that target FLT3. Also, the use of sensitive methods to monitor FLT3 mutations during treatment may allow individualized treatment with the currently available kinase inhibitors [207].

10.2. HDAC inhibitors

In t(8,21) AML, the AML_1/ETO fusion protein promotes leukemogenesis by recruiting class I HDAC-containing repressor complex to the promoter AML1 target genes [214]. Recruitment of HDACs is an important epigenetic mechanism of transcriptional dysregulation and gene silencing in AML [215]. Modulation of protein lysine acetylation through the inhibition of HDACs is one of the therapeutic strategies to treat AML patients who are unfit for intensive chemotherapy [216]. HDAC-inhibitor-mediated differentiation therapy is a potent and molecularly rational therapeutic strategy in t(8,21) AML. Epigenetic modifying enzymes such as: HDACs, P300 and PRMT1 are recruited by AML-1/ETO thus providing a molecular rationale for targeting these enzymes to treat AML with t(8,21) [217]. Although early phase clinical assessment indicated that treatment with HDAC inhibitors may be effective in t (8,21) AML, rigorous preclinical studies to identify the molecular and biological events which may determine therapeutic responses have not been established [217]. The only HDAC inhibitors that have been investigated in clinical trials of AML are butyrate derivatives, valproic acid (VPA) and desipeptide [218]. HDAC inhibitors can mediate anti-leukemic effects in AML, but their clinical benefits are limited, thus further studies including combination therapies are warranted [218]. VPA is a HDAC inhibitor that is being utilized as a disease-stabilizing therapy as it improves normal blood values and has a minimal risk of clinically relevant toxicity [216]. However, VPA has not been investigated in randomized clinical trials [216]. VPA has been shown to cause growth arrest and induce differentiation of malignant cells via HDAC inhibition [214]. VPA may effectively target AML1/ETO-driven leukemogenesis through disruption of aberrant HDAC inhibitor function. Therefore, VPA should be integrated in the novel therapeutic approaches for AML_1/ETO-positive AML [214].

Autophagy is a catabolic pathway that is upregulated during times of nutrition limitations or stress to maintain cellular metabolism and organelle integrity [219]. In AML1/ETO- positive AML cells, HDAC inhibitors induce autophagy which acts as a pro-survival signal to limit HDAC-induced cell death. In contrast to the fusion oncoproteins, promyelocytic leukemia-RARA (PML-RARA) and breakpoint cluster region-abelson, AML1/ETO is not degraded by either basal or drug-induced autophagy [219]. Combined treatment with HDAC inhibitors and autophagy inhibitors such as chloroquine has resulted in a massive accumulation of ubiquitinated proteins that correlated with increased cell death [219]. The combination of VPA induced autophagy in the cells of patients with t (8,21) AML and chloroquine therapy has enhanced cell death. Because VPA and chloroquine are well-tolerated drugs, their combination could represent an attractive treatment option for AML1-ETO- positive leukemia [219].

10.3. Heat shock proteins

Heat shock proteins (HSPs) such as HSP-90 are often over expressed in AML and are involved in the regulation of apoptosis, proliferation, autophagy and cell cycle progression. Hence, they are considered as possible therapeutic targets in the management of AML [220]. Phase I and II clinical trials have revealed that HSP-90 inhibition can mediate anti-leukemic effects in vivo. Further studies including their combination with conventional chemotherapy are needed to clarify their efficacy and toxicity in the future treatment of AML [220].

11. Targeted therapies for CBF-AML

Core binding factor (CBF)-AML is a favorable AML subset defined cytogenetically by t (8,21) or inv (16) / t (16,16) rearrangement disrupting RUNX1 or CBFB transcription factor functions [221]. The receptor tyrosine kinase (KIT) is expressed in the vast majority of AML subsets and frequent activations of KIT gene mutations have been associated with a higher risk of relapse [221]. Romidepsin has differential anti-leukemic and molecular activity in CBF-AML [215]. The development of romidepsin in the treatment of CBF-AML should focus on drug combinations that target related mechanisms of gene silencing such as DNA methylation [215].

A phase II study evaluated dasatinib as maintenance therapy in 26 patients with high-risk CBF-AML with KIT mutations in first CR showing that dasatinib can be safely administered as single-agent maintenance in AML patients in CR, but does not seem to prevent relapse, because the activity of dasatinib may be impaired by spontaneous and/or dasatinib-driven clonal devolution [221].

11.1. Clofarabine

Clofarabine is a second generation purine nucleoside analog that incorporates the characteristics of 2 other purine analogs: fludarabine and cladrabine [222,223]. It inhibits DNA polymerases and ribonucleotide reductase, thus inducing apoptosis in cycling and non-cycling cells [222]. Clinical trials have shown the activity of clofarabine in adult AML both as a single agent and in combination with other cytotoxic drugs [223]. Clofarabine has also been used as front-line therapy combined with standard induction treatment, idarubicin and cytarabine, in newly diagnosed AML and its use has been shown to be effective (longer OS and EFS compared to chemotherapy alone) and relatively safe [224,225]. Clofarabine is cytotoxic to leukemic cells that are resistant to cytarabine [226].

11.2. Lenalidomide

The highly encouraging results of lenalidomide in the treatment of del (5q) in low-risk MDS have not been reproduced in del (5q) AML. However, in a study that included 33 patients, ≥ 60 years without del (5q) and having low circulating blasts at diagnosis, lenalidomide had produced CR rates of 50% [227]. The clear activity of lenalidomide in a subset of AML patients should promote efforts to identify patients who are likely to respond to the drug, thus allowing the rational use of this agent either alone or in combination with other drugs [227].

11.3. Obatoclax

Over-expression of Bcl-1, Bcl-xL and/or Mcl-1 has been associated with resistance to chemotherapy in AML cell lines and ultimately poor clinical outcome [228]. Obatoclax (a novel inhibitor of anti-apoptotic Bcl-2 family proteins and a pan-Bcl-2 inhibitor) enhances cytarabine-induced apoptosis by enhancing DNA damage or double strand breaks and improves outcome in AML patients harboring Bcl-2 proteins [228]. In a small cohort of elderly AML patients with primary chemorefractory disease, a combination of low-dose azacytidine, ATRA and pioglitazone (peroxisome proliferator-activated receptor γ ligand) has induced CRs, thus bimodulatory therapy may bypass genetically based chemotherapy resistance in AML [229].

11.4. CXCR4 antagonists

The chemokine receptor (CXCR4) and its ligand stromal derived factor-1 (SDF-1) are important key players in the cross-talk between leukemia cells and BM microenvironment or stroma niche [230-232]. SDF-1 regulates the process of homing and engraftment of LSCs into the BM and inhibition of its receptor CXRC4 induces mobilization of leukemic cells into the circulation [232]. CXRC4 expression is associated with poor prognosis in AML patients with or without FLT3 genetic mutations [231]. SDF-1α / - CXCR4 interactions contribute to the resistance of leukemic cells to signal transduction inhibitor-and chemotherapy-induced apoptosis in systems that mimic the physiologic microenvironment [233]. Disruption of these interactions with CXRC4 inhibitors represents a novel strategy of sensitizing leukemia cells by targeting their protective BM microenvironment [233]. Preclinical and clinical studies using CXCR4 antagonists in combination with chemotherapy have demonstrated that blocking CXCR4 is a novel promising approach in the treatment of AML [230-232].

11.5. Monoclonal antibodies

Approximately 87.8% of AML cells express CD33 and 9.7% of AML cells express CD123, without concomitant CD33 expression. Therefore, nearly all AMLs can be treated with monoclonal antibodies directed against CD33 and CD123 [234]. Identification of targets or antigens on the cell surface of leukemic cells, particularly LSCs, has recently attracted particular attention and new targeted therapies are under development. Tailored immunotherapy targeting CD33 and CD123 is likely to enhance treatment efficacy in the majority of AML patients [234].

CD33 is present on the leukemic blasts from the majority of patients with AML and MDS [235]. GO is a humanized anti-CD33 monoclonal antibody that was approved by the food and drug authority (FDA) in the USA in 2000 for the treatment of AML in first relapse in patients older than 60 years who are unfit for more intensive chemotherapy [235,236]. In recipients of HSCT, the main adverse effects of GO treatment are anaphylactic reactions, adult respiratory distress syndrome, hepatotoxicity and VOD [235-238]. GO has been shown to be effective in CD33 positive de novo AML even in younger adults and children either a single agent or in combination with conventional induction chemotherapy. However, its use has not improved OS and some studies have shown significant early TRM [237,239-241].

The IL-3 receptor α chain (CD123) has been identified as a potential immunotherapeutic target because it is overexpressed in AML compared to normal HSCs [242]. CD123 chimeric antigen receptor (CAR) T-cells specifically target CD123 positive AML cells [242]. AML patient-driven T cells can be genetically modified to lyse autologous tumor cells. CD123-CAR-T cells are a promising immunotherapy for treating high-risk AML [242]. CD123-specific CARs strongly enhance anti-AML-CIK (cytokine-induced killer) functions, while sparing normal HSCs/ progenitor cells thus paving the way to develop novel immunotherapeutic approaches for the treatment of AML [243]. The strategy of redirecting CIK cells with CD123 CAR should soon find a place in the plethora of novel alternative approaches used to treat AML, because the advantages in immune efficacy and in vivo persistence of CAR-redirected T-cells would represent a relevant beneficial effect [244]. CD123 based myeloablation may also be used as a novel conditioning therapy for HSCT [245]. Eventually anti-CD123 CAR-based strategy, coupled with a suicide gene system, could truly represent a major advancement in the field of AML therapeutics, providing a novel magic bullet for AML therapies, particularly for high-risk transplanted patients with MRD or as an alternative biological therapy for older patients in whom standard chemotherapeutic approaches are not applicable [246].

CD123 (IL-3-receptor α chain) has been identified as a potential immunotherapeutic target as it is overexpressed on AML LSCs and AML blasts rather than HSCs [247]. Two fusion proteins (anti-CD3 Fv-ΔIL3 and disulfide-stabilized anti-CD3 Fv-ΔIL3) display anti-leukemic activity against CD123-expressing cell lines and leukemic progenitors both in vitro and in vivo. Therefore, these 2 fusion proteins could be the promising candidates for future immunotherapy in AML [247].

11.6. Leukemia stem cells

Tumors possess a minor fraction of cancer stem cells (CSCs) which maintains the propagation of the malignancy [248]. In many cancers, it is difficult to completely eliminate the CSCs by chemotherapy or radiotherapy, thus recurrence or relapse of cancer usually occurs [248]. Perhaps the Holy Grail in cancer therapy today is CSCs or cancer initiating cells [248]. Despite the recent increase in understanding the pathogenesis of AML, the disease remains with poor outcome due to the overwhelming relapse rate [249]. Given the general lack of significant success in treating AML with conventional therapies, new approaches to treat the disease are warranted. The coming years will witness the performance of active clinical trials on targeted therapies against LSCs [249].

In 1994, CSCs were first described in AML cells by Dick and co-workers who dissociated LSCs from the bulk of AML cells [248,250]. The immature LSCs resided within the CD34 positive/CD38 negative subpopulation and they represented a small fraction of the total leukemic blasts [248]. The discovery of LSCs has important clinical implications [250]. LSCs are relatively insensitive to current therapies and they are considered amongst the leading causes of treatment failure and relapse in patients with AML [247,248,250]. Many of the critical biological properties of LSCs have been elucidated and these include the following: (1) distinct replicative properties, (2) cell surface phenotypes, (3) increased resistance to chemotherapy, and (4) involvement of growth-promoting chromosomal translocations [248]. In recent years, research has focused on the characterization of LSCs population which is the disease compartment most difficult to eliminate with conventional chemotherapy and the disease compartment most responsible for relapse [249].

LSCs represent a rare self-renewing cellular subpopulation in AML and their property of resistance to chemotherapy is associated with poor outcome. The characterization of genes which express surface markers of LSCs is likely to reveal novel targets that may improve therapeutic outcomes [251]. However, studies have shown that gene expression profiling of LSCs lacks reproducibility. Also, diverse signatures obtained from the analysis of LSC gene expression profiles confirm the heterogeneity of AML [251]. Analysis of gene sets that are essential for regulating LSC functions and improving the reproducibility and clinical characteristics of the relevant LSC signatures at gene levels are vital for biologic, therapeutic and prognostic levels in AML [251].

Although the field of specific therapeutic targeting of LSCs is still in its infancy as it is relatively new, it is a highly promising battleground that may reveal the Holy Grail of cancer therapy and may undoubtedly result in novel strategies to treat not only AML, but also leukemias in general [248]. Due to the unique features of LSCs, drugs are designed to target these cells and to eliminate them, but such drugs and therapies must be tested in the setting of clinical trials [249]. To be successful, novel therapeutic options in AML should aim at eradicating LSCs. Recently, the identification of targets on the cell surface of LSCs has been receiving particular attention [247]. Also, the tumor cell microenvironment or niche is an important therapeutic target, thus Rac inhibitors and various anti-integrin antibodies may be appropriate therapeutic modalities [248]. However, targeting LSCs can be achieved by: (1) targeting the key signal transduction pathways, namely: PI3K, Wnt and Rac, (2) targeting specific cell surface molecules such as CD33, CD44 and CD123 with effective cytotoxic monoclonal antibodies, (3) statins that have shown promising potential in targeting LSCs, and (4) inhibitors of ATP-binding cassette transporter proteins that are being extensively studied in combating drug resistance which is a frequent characteristic feature of LSCs [247,248].

11.7. Dendritic cells

The ability of DCs to activate T-cells is dependent upon their activation state [252]. Myeloid progenitors are prominent source of DCs under homeostatic conditions. LSCs and leukemic blasts can give rise to malignant DCs [253]. Immune tolerance to AML may be initiated at the level of the innate immune system. A specific subset of DCs, called CD8α^+DCs, may be responsible for mediating tolerance in AML, thus targeting the innate immune system may be beneficial in AML [252].

Leukemia-derived DCs can express leukemia antigens and may either induce anti-leukemic T cell responses or favor tolerance to the leukemia, depending on the co-stimulatory or inhibitory molecules or cytokines [253]. Active immunotherapy aimed at the generation of specific CTLs may represent a powerful approach to target LSCs in the setting of MRD [253]. To fully activate CTLs, leukemia antigens have to be successfully captured, processed and presented by mature DCs [253,254]. DC-based immunotherapy is a promising therapeutic strategy for the elimination of MRD in patients with AML [254]. Immunotherapy may be most effective in the setting of MRD after successful induction and PRT [253,254]. AML patients who are at high risk of relapse and who are not eligible for HSCT are particularly suited for such therapeutic approach [253,254].

Studies have shown that DC-vaccination has resulted in potent anti-leukemia CTL-responses and that DC-vaccination protocols remain a promising supplementary strategy in the treatment of leukemia [253]. The vaccination procedure includes: (1) the choice of LAAs, (2) the source of DCs, (3) the DC maturation protocol, and (4) the way the application has to be defined and standardized [253]. The timing and application of potential co-treatment including chemotherapy/HSCT or immunomodulatory therapies have to be considered carefully [253].

12. Personalized therapy for AML

Over the past 7 years, the application of advanced technology in genetic sequencing has revolutionized our understanding of AML biology [255]. Knowledge of somatic mutations in AML and their clinical relevance has increased our ability to determine prognosis depending on the pre-treatment risk stratification [125,255].

In many targeted agents, the initial response may be impressive, but ultimately the duration of response is often modest due to the evolution of drug-resistant malignant cell populations [125,255]. Additionally, the predominant clones at AML relapse may differ from the clones encountered at presentation prior to the administration of chemotherapy [255]. Therefore, repeat molecular profiling and drug susceptibility testing at relapse following targeted therapy allows the determination of the mechanisms of resistance and the potential use of combined targeted therapies to overcome drug resistance [125,255]. The ability to determine drug sensitivity in the laboratory prior to administration of specific therapy (an approach similar to antimicrobial susceptibility testing in microbiological disease) has long been an aspiration in AML management [255]. However, personalized therapy may be more appropriate for certain groups of patients such as older AML patients and those having relapsed disease [97,125,255].

13. Conclusions and future directions

AML is a heterogeneous disease, with multifactorial etiology, characterized by specific chromosomal abnormalities and genetic mutations. AML has numerous complications including: anemia, bleeding diathesis, venous thrombosis, extramedullary involvement, leukostasis, electrolytic disturbances and various infectious complications. Once the diagnosis of AML is established, the disease should be classified into the appropriate subtype according to the WHO and FAB classification systems, then patients should be thoroughly evaluated to determine their fitness for therapy.

The management of AML in older patients is a real therapeutic challenge. However, treatment of AML in older subjects should be tailored according to the circumstances of each patient taking into consideration the age, comorbidities, performance state and the risk category according to the cytogenetic and molecular profiles. Recently, several therapeutic options have been made available for older patients with AML. Interestingly, targeted therapies and monoclonal antibodies are more tolerable and more efficacious than the standard chemotherapies. Philadelphia chromosome positive de novo AML is extremely rare and has several distinguishing features. The available therapeutic options include: cytotoxic chemotherapy, TKIs and allogeneic HSCT. The prognosis of this type of AML is generally poor and the median survival is relatively short. Recently, the incidence of t-AML has been found to be increasing due to the longer survival of cancer patients and the wider utilization of chemotherapy, radiotherapy and immunosuppressive agents. This form of AML can be treated with chemotherapy, allogeneic HSC, investigational agents or the best supportive care.

The aims of induction therapy in patients with AML are induction of CR and restoration of normal BM function. Cytarabine and anthracyclines are still the backbone of the frontline therapy of AML. Response to the induction phase of chemotherapy is evaluated by BM examination, cytogenetic analysis, mutational studies and MRD by flow cytometry and PCR.

The evolution of new genetic mutations and MDR genes contribute to drug resistance that may be encountered during AML treatment. Drug resistance in AML can be treated with salvage chemotherapy and investigational therapies. For relapsed/refractory AML, the following treatment options are available: salvage chemotherapeutic regimens, allogeneic HSCT, immunotherapy with DLI, several novel and targeted therapies, appropriate clinical trials and the best supportive care. PRTs in patients with AML include: (1) consolidation cycles of chemotherapy, (2) autologous or allogeneic HSCT, and (3) maintenance therapy, in patients at high risk of relapse, with the recently introduced novel therapies that can be can administered even after successful HSCT.

The indications of allogeneic HSCT in patients with AML are: (1) AML refractory to induction therapy, (2) refractory AML in CR2, (3) intermediate- or high-risk cytogenetics, (4) AML with extramedullary disease, (5) AML secondary to MDS or chronic MPNs, and (6) t-AML not having favorable cytogenetics. Myeloablative allogeneic HSCT is usually performed in younger patients having good performance state and no major systemic dysfunction, while RIC-allogeneic HSCT is generally offered to older patients with AML and patients who are unfit to receive myeloablative-conditioning therapies. The antineoplastic potency of RIC-allogeneic HSCT relies mainly on the GVL effect of the allograft rather than the ablation of all residual leukemic cells. Currently, several myeloablative and non-myeloablative conditioning therapies are available for AML patients who are eligible for HSCT. Also, several donor or stem cell sources are being utilized such as MRD, MUD, and UCB as well as the haploidentical form of HSCT. In AML patients subjected to allogeneic HSCT, the following strategies to enhance immune reconstitution can be employed: DLI, in vitro T-cell depletion, rapamycin to promote expansion of T-regulatory cells and cyclophosphamide administered on day 3 post-allogeneic HSCT to reduce alloreactive lymphocytes. Autologous HSCT is indicated for older patients with comorbid medical conditions who are not candidates for allogeneic HSCT. Several lines of immunotherapy can be used for AML patients and these include: (1) allogeneic HSCT including RIC-allografts, (2) DLIs and GVL effect of RIC-allogeneic HSCT, (3) autologous anti-leukemic T-cell infusions, (4) adoptive transfer of T-cells and NK cells, (5) vaccination with tumor or leukemic cells and peptides, (6) immunomodulatory agents, (7) DCs and ILs, and (8) monoclonal antibodies and WT1 antigen targeting. Recently, several lines of novel and targeted therapies have been evolving in the management of AML and these include: FLT3 inhibitors, HSPs, HDAC inhibitors, purine analogs, CBF targeting agents, Bcl-2 inhibitors, CXCR4 antagonists and monoclonal antibodies.

The prognosis of AML is very variable and depends on the: age of the patient at diagnosis, comorbidity index, performance status and the specific karyotype. The incorporation of gene mutational analysis as well as gene expression and micro-RNA profiling in the diagnostics of AML is likely to enrich the risk stratification and consequently more targeted and novel therapeutics may be utilized in the frontline management of AML in the future. The recent advancements in the diagnostics and therapeutics have facilitated the introduction of personalized therapy in patients with AML. Regular evaluation of molecular profiling is essential in the modern management of AML. Drug susceptibility testing particularly at the time of relapse, resembling antimicrobial susceptibility testing in microbiology laboratories, may become a reality in the future.

Author details

Khalid Ahmed Al-Anazi*

Address all correspondence to: kaa_alanazi@yahoo.com

Department of Adult Hematology and Hematopoietic Stem Cell Transplantation, Cancer Center, King Fahad Specialist Hospital, Dammam, Saudi Arabia.

References

[1] Horton SJ, Huntly BJP. Recent advances in acute myeloid leukemia stem cell biology. Haematologica 2012; 97 (7): 966-974.

[2] Stock W, Thirman MJ. Pathogenesis of acute myeloid leukemia. UpToDate, 2014. Topic edited by Larson RA and Conner RF. Topic last updated: October, 28, 2014.

[3] Ayala F. Dewar R, Kieran M, Kalluri R. Contribution of bone microenvironment to leukemogenesis and leukemia progression. Leukemia 2009, 23: 2233-2241.

[4] Greim H, Kaden DA, Larson RA, Palermo CM, Rice JM, Ross D, et al. The bone marrow niche, stem cells, and leukemia: impact of drugs, chemicals and the environment. Ann N Y Acad Sci. 2014; 1310 (1): 7-31.

[5] El-Cheikh J, Crocchiolo R. Therapy of acute myeloid leukemia. Koschmieder S (ed.). In Tech 2012. ISBN: 978-953-307-886-1.

[6] Schiffer CA, Anastasi J. Clinical manifestations, pathologic features and diagnosis of acute myeloid leukemia. UpToDate 2014. Topic edited by Larson RA and Conner RF. Topic last updated: January, 14, 2014.

[7] Schiffer CA. Prognosis of acute myeloid leukemia. UpToDate 2014. Topic edited by Larson RA and Conner RF. Topic last updated: October, 28, 2014.

[8] Schiffer CA, Anastasi J. Classification of acute myeloid leukemia. UpToDate 2013. Topic edited by Larson RA and Conner RF. Topic last updated: October, 30, 2013.

[9] Larson RA, Induction therapy for acute myeloid leukemia in young adults. UpToDate 2014. Topic edited by Lowenberg B and Conner RF. Topic last updated: September, 04, 2014.

[10] Larson RA. Treatment of acute myeloid leukemia in older adults. UpToDate 2014. Topic edited by Lowenberg B, Schmader KE and Connor RF. Topic last updated: October, 08, 2014.

[11] Ossenkoppele G, Löwenberg B. How I treat the older patient with acute myeloid leukemia. Blood 2015; 125: 767-774.

[12] Schlenk RF. Post-remission therapy for acute myeloid leukemia. Haematologica 2014; 99 (11): 1663-1670.

[13] Alcalay M, Meani N, Gelmetti V, Fantozzi A, Fagioli M, Orleth A, et al. Acute myeloid leukemia fusion proteins deregulate genes involved in stem cell maintenance and DNA repair. J Clin Invest. 2003; 112: 1751-1761.

[14] Gulley ML, Shea TC, Fedoriw Y. Genetic tests to evaluate prognosis and predict therapeutic response in acute myeloid leukemia. J Mol Diagn. 2010; 12 (1): 3-16.

[15] Kumar CC. Genetic abnormalities and challenges in the treatment of acute myeloid leukemia. Gen Cancer 2011; 2 (2): 95-107.

[16] Walker A, Marcucci G. Molecular prognostic factors in ctogenetically normal acute myeloid leukemia. Expert Rev Hematol. 2012; 5 (5): 547-558.

[17] Pemmaraju N, Kantarjia H, Ravandi F, Cortes J. FLT3 inhibitors in the treatment of acute myeloid leukemia. Cancer 2011; 117 (15): 3293-3304.

[18] Ilyas AM, Ahmed S, Faheem M, Naseer MI, Kumosani T, Al-Qahtani MH, et al. Next generation sequencing of acute myeloid leukemia: influencing prognosis. BMC Genomics 2015; 16 (Suppl 1) S5.

[19] O'Brien EC, Prideaux S, Chevassut T. The epigenetic landscape of acute myeloid leukemia. Adv Hematol. 2014; Article ID 103175.

[20] Zaidi SZ, Owaidah T, Al Sharif F, Ahmed SA, Chaudhri N, Aljurf M. The challenge of risk stratification in acute myeloid leukemia with normal cytogenetics. Hematol Oncol Stem Cell Ther. 2008; 1 (3): 141-158.

[21] Filip AA, Libura M, Giebel S, Haus O. Genetic mechanisms and molecular markers of neoplastic transformation in acute myeloid leukemia. Witt M.,et al. (eds.), Molecular Aspects of Hematologic Malignancies, Principles and Practice, Springer-Verlag Berlin Heidelberg 2012. doi: 10.1007/978-3-642-29467-2_2

[22] Estey EH. Acute myeloid leukemia: 2014 update on risk-stratification and management. Am H Hematol. 2014; 89 (11): 1064-1081.

[23] Larson RA, Klepin HD. Pretreatment evaluation and prognosis of acute myeloid leukemia in older adults. UpToDate 2013. Topic edited by Lowenberg B and Conner RF. Topic last updated: December, 19, 2013.

[24] Tallman MS, Gilliland DG, Rowe JM. Drug therapy for acute myeloid leukemia. Blood 2005; 106 (4):1154-1163. Epub May 3, 2005.

[25] Schiffer CA. Overview of the complications of acute myeloid leukemia. UpToDate 2014. Topic edited by Larson RA and Connor RF. Topic last updated Jun. 25, 2014.

[26] Zuckerman T, Ganzel C, Tallman MS, Rowe JM. How I treat hematologic emergencies in adults with acute leukemia. Blood 2012; 120 (10): 1993-2002.

[27] Gorschlüter M, Mey U, Strehl J, Ziske C, Schepke M, Schmidtwolf IGH; et al. Neutropenic enterocolitis in adults: systematic analysis of evidence quality. Eur J Haematol. 2005; 75: 1-13.

[28] Schiffer CA. Hyperleukocytosis and leukostasis. UpToDate 2013. Topic edited by Larson RA and Connor RF. Topic last updated Nov. 21, 2013.

[29] Larson RA, Pui C-H. Tumor lysis syndrome: prevention and treatment. UpToDate 2015. Topic edited by Dews RE, Freedman AS, Poplack DG and Savarese DMF. Topic last updated Jan. 12, 2015.

[30] Howard SC, Jones DP, Pui C-H. The tumor lysis syndrome. New Engl J Med. 2011; 364 (19): 1844-1854.

[31] Chandran R, Hakki M, Spurgeon S. Infection in leukemia. Luciano Azevedo (ed.). Sepsis: an Ongoing and Significant Challenge. In Tech 2014, ISBN: 978-953-51-0780-4.

[32] Lech-Maranda E, Seweryn M, Giebel S, Holowiecki J, Piatkowska-Jakubas B, Wegrzyn J, et al. Infectious complications in patients with acute myeloid leukemia treated according to the protocol with daunorubicin and cytarabine with or without addition of cladrabine. A multicenter study by the Polish Adult Leukemia Group (PALG). Int J Infect Dis. 2010; 14: e132-e140.

[33] Malagola M, Peli A, Damiani D, Candoni A, Tiribelli M, Martinelli G, et al. Incidence of bacterial and fungal infections in newly diagnosed acute myeloid leukemia patients younger than 65 yr treated with induction regimens including fludarabine: retrospective analysis of 224 cases. Eur J Haematol. 2008; 81 (5): 354-363.

[34] Biswal S, Godnaik C. Incidence and management of infections in patients with acute leukemia following chemotherapy in general wards. eCancer 2013; 7: 310, 1-16.

[35] Gupta A, Singh M, Singh H, Kumar L, Sharma A, Bakhshi S, et al. Infections in acute myeloid leukemia: an analysis of 382 febrile episodes. Med Oncol. 2010; 27 (4): 1037-1045.

[36] Pea F, Viale P, Damiani D, Pavan F, Cristini F, Fanin R, et al. Ceftazidime in acute meyloid leukemia patients with febrile neutropenia: helpfulness of continuous intravenous infusion in maximizing pharmacodynamic exposure. Antimicrob Agents Chemother. 2005; 49 (8): 3550-3553.

[37] De Rosa FG, Motta I, Audisio E, Frairia C, Busca A, Di Perri G, et al. Epidemiology of bloodstream infections in patients with acute myeloid leukemia undergoing levofloxacin prophylaxis. BMC Infect Dis. 2013; 13: 563, 1-5.

[38] Lee DG, Choi SM, Choi JH, Yoo JH, Park YH, Kim YJ, et al. Selective bowel decontamination for the prevention of infection in acute myeloid leukemia: a prospective randomized trial. Korean J Inter Med 2002; 17(1): 38-44.

[39] Rybka J, Butrym A, Wröbel T, Jaźwiec B, Stefano E, Dobrzyńska O, et al. The expression of toll-like receptors and development of severe sepsis in patients with acute myeloid leukemia after induction chemotherapy. Med Oncol. 2014; 31: 319, 1-4.

[40] Sayed HA, El-Mahallawy HA, Kaddah AM, Ismael HT, Talaat SM. Profile of infections in newly diagnosed patients with acute myeloid leukemia during the induction phase of treatment. J Egyptian Nat Cancer Inst. 2009; 21 (4): 315-322.

[41] Madani TAS. Clinical infections and bloodstream isolates associated with fever in patients undergoing chemotherapy for acute myeloid leukemia. Infection 2000; 28 (6): 367-373.

[42] Cannas G, Pautas C, Raffoux E, Quesnel B, de Botton S, de Ravel T, et al. Infectious complications in adult acute myeloid leukemia: analysis of the Acute Leukemia

French Association-9802 prospective multicenter clinical trial. Leuk Lymphoma 2012; 53 (6): 1068-1076.

[43] Bhatt VR, Viola GM, Ferrajoli A. Invasive fungal infections in acute leukemia. Ther Adv Hematol. 2011; 2 (4): 231-247.

[44] Gomez MZR, Mulanovich VE, Jiang Y, Lewis RE, Kontoyiannis DP. Incidence density of invasive fungal infections during primary antifungal prophylaxis in newly diagnosed acute myeloid leukemia patients in a tertiary cancer center, 2009 to 2011. Antimicrob Agents Chemother. 2014; 58 (2): 865-873.

[45] Nucci M, Anaissie E. How we treat invasive fungal diseases in acute leukemia: the importance of an individualized approach. Blood 2014; 124 (26): 3858-3869.

[46] Safdar A. Difficulties with fungal infections in acute myelogenous leukemia patients: immune enhancement strategies. Oncologist 2007; 12 (Suppl 2): 2-6.

[47] Odabasi Z, Mattiuzzi G, Estey E, Kantarjian H, Saeki F, Ridge RJ, et al. B-D-Glucan as a diagnostic adjunct for invasive fungal infections: validation, cutoff development and performance in patients with acute myelogenous leukemia and myelodysplastic syndrome. Clin Infect Dis. 2004; 39: 198-205.

[48] Caira M, Candoni A, Verga L, Busca A, Delia M, Nosari A, et al. Pre-chemotherapy risk factors for invasive fungal diseases: prospective analysis of 1192 patients with newly diagnosed acute myeloid leukemia (SEIFEM 2010-a multicenter study). Haematologica 2015; 100 (2): 284-292.

[49] Rüping MJ, Vehreschild JJ, Cornely DA. Patients at high risk of invasive fungal infections: when and how to treat. Drugs 2008; 68 (14): 1941-1962.

[50] Laventakos K, Lewis RF, Kontoyiannis DP. Fungal infections in leukemia patients: how do we prevent and treat them? Clin Infect Dis. 2010; 50: 405-415.

[51] Vehreschild JJ, Böhme A, Buchheidt D, Arenz D, Harnischmacher U, Heussel CP, et al. A double-blind trial on prophylactic voriconazole (VRC) or placebo during induction chemotherapy for acute myelogenous leukemia (AML). J Infect 2007; 55 (5): 445-449.

[52] Heng S-C, Slavin MA, Al-Badriyeh D, Kirsa S, Seymour JF, Grigg A, et al. Pharmacoeconomic evaluation of fluconazole, posaconazole and voriconazole for antifungal prophylaxis in patients with acute myeloid leukemia undergoing first consolidation chemotherapy. J Antimicrob Chemother. 2013; 68: 1669-1678.

[53] Cattaneo C, Borlenghi E, Panzali A, Antoniazzi F, Petulla M, Schieppati F, et al. Impact of posaconazole prophylaxis on invasive fungal infection during acute myeloid leukemia induction therapy: correlation with posaconazole serum levels. Blood 2013; 122 (21).

[54] Gomez MZR, Jiang Y, Mulanovich VE, Lewis RE, Kontoyiannis DP. Effectiveness of primary anti-aspergillus prophylaxis during remission induction chemotherapy for acute myeloid leukemia. Antimicrob Agents Chemother. 2014; 58 (5): 2775-2780.

[55] Cornely OA, Böhme A, Schmitt-Hoffmann A, Ullmann AJ. Safety and pharmacokinetics of isavuconazole as antifungal prophylaxis in acute myeloid leukemia patients with neutropenia: results of a phase 2, dose escalation study. Antimicrob Agents Chemother. 2015; 1-37.

[56] Annino L, Chierichini A, Anaclerico B, Finolezzi E, Norata M, Cortese S, et al. Prospective phase II single-center study of the safety of a single very high dose of liposomal amphotericin B for antifungal prophylaxis in patients with acute myeloid leukemia. Antimicrob Agents Chemother. 2013; 57 (6): 2596-2602.

[57] Larson RA, Boogaerts M, Estey E, Karanes C, Stadtmauer EA, Sievers EL, et al. Antibody-targeted chemotherapy of older patients with acute myeloid leukemia in first relapse using myelotarg (gemtuzumab ozogamicin). Leukemia 2002; 16: 1627-1636.

[58] Baer MR, Gojo I. Novel agents for the treatment of acute myeloid leukemia in the older patient. J Natl Compr Canc Netw. 2011; 9 (3): 331-335.

[59] Juliusson G. Older patients with acute myeloid leukemia benefit from intensive chemotherapy: an update from the Swedish acute leukemia registry. Clin Lymphoma Myeloma Leuk. 2011; 11 (1): S54-S59.

[60] Juliusson G, Billström R, Gruber A, Hellström-Lindberg E, Höglund M, Karlsson K, et al. Attitude towards remission induction for elderly patients with acute myeloid leukemia influences survival. Leukemia 2006; 20: 42-47.

[61] Lowenberg B, Ossenkoppele GJ, van Putten W, Schouten HC, Graux C, Ferrant A, et al. High-dose daunorubicin in older patients with acute myeloid leukemia. N Engl J Med 2009; 361 (13): 1235-1248.

[62] Lübbert M, Rüter BH, Claus R, Schmoor C, Schmid M, Germing U, et al. A multicenter phase II trial of decitabine as first-line treatment for older patients with acute myeloid leukemia judged unfit for induction chemotherapy. Haematologica 2012; 97 (3): 393-401.

[63] Attar EC, Johnson JL, Amrein PC, Lozanski G, Wadleigh M, De Angelo DJ, et al. Bortezomib added to daunorubicin and cytarabine during induction therapy and to intermediate-dose cytarabine for consolidation in patients with previously untreated acute myeloid leukemia age 60 to 75 years: CALG B (Alliance) Study 10502. J Clin Oncol. 2012; 31 (7): 923-929.

[64] Brandwein JM, Lever BF, Howson-Jan K, Schimmer AD, Schuh AC, Gupta B, et al. A phase I study of tipifarnib combined with conventional induction and consolidation therapy for previously untreated patients with acute myeloid leukemia aged 60 years and over. Leukemia 2009; 23: 631-634.

[65] Tran H, Yang D. Clofarabine in the treatment of newly diagnosed acute myeloid leukemia in older adults. Ann Pharmacother. 2012; 46 (1): 89-96.

[66] Tiley S, Claxton D. Clofarabine in the treatment of acute myeloid leukemia in older adults. Ther Adv Hematol. 2013; 4 (1): 5-13.

[67] Burnett AK, Russel NH, Kell J, Dennis M, Miligan D, Paolini S, et al. European development of clofarabine as treatment for older patients with acute myeloid leukemia considered unsuitable for intensive chemotherapy. J Clin Oncol. 2010; 28 (14): 2389-2395.

[68] Burnett AK, Russel NH, Hunter AE, Milligan D, Knapper S, Wheatley K, et al. Clofarabine doubles the response rate in older patients with acute myeloid leukemia but does not improve survival. Blood 2013; 122: 1384-1394.

[69] Lim MY, Jamieson K. Profile of sapacitabine: potential for the treatment of newly diagnosed acute myeloid leukemia in elderly patients. Clin Interv Aging 2014; 9: 753-762.

[70] Chevallier P, Delaunay J, Turlure P, Pigneux A, Hunault M, Garand R, et al. Long-term disease-free survival after gemtazumab, intermediae-dose cytarabine and mitoxantrone in patients with CD33 (+) primary resistant or relapsed acute myeloid leukemia. J Clin Oncol. 2008; 26 (32): 5192-5197.

[71] Burnett AK, Russel NH, Hills RK, Kell J, Freeman S, Kjeldsen L, et al. Addition of gemtuzumab ozogamicin to induction chemotherapy improves survival in older patients with acute myeloid leukemia. J Clin Oncol. 2012; 30 (32): 3924-3931.

[72] Brunnberg U, Mohr M. Noppeney R, Dürk HA, Sauer land MC, Müller-Tidow C, et al. Induction therapy of AML with ara-C plus daunorubicin versus ara-c plus gemtuzumab ozogamicin: a randomized phase II trial in elderly patients. Ann Oncol. 2012; 23: 990-996.

[73] Candoni A, Martinelli G, Toffoletti E, Chiarvesico A, Tiribelli M, Malagola M, et al. Gemtuzumab-ozogamicin in combination with fludarabine, cytarabine, idarubicin (FLAI-GO) as induction therapy in CD33-positive AML patients younger than 65 years. Leuk Res. 2008; 32 (12): 1800-1808.

[74] Jentsch-Ullrich K, Pelz A-F, Braun H, Koenigsmann M, Mohren M, Wieacker P, et al. Complete molecular remission in a patient with Philadelphia-chromosome positive acute myeloid leukemia after conventional therapy and imatinib. Haematologica 2004; 89: 49-51.

[75] Jameel A. Philadelphia chromosome positive acute myeloid leukemia: a rare hematological disorder, a case report. J Postgrad Med Inst. 2012; 26 (1): 111-114.

[76] Reboursiere E, Chantepie S, Gac A-C, Reman O. Rare but authentic Philadelphia-positive acute myeloblastic leukemia: two case reports and a literature review of charac-

teristics, treatment and outcome. Hematol Oncol Stem Cell Ther. 2014; pii: S1658-3876(14)00079-X.

[77] Soupir CP, Vergilio J-A, Cin PD, Muzikansky A, Kantarjian H, Jones D, et al. A rare aggressive leukemia with clincopathologic features distinct from chronic myeloid leukemia in myeloid blast crisis. Am J Clin Pathol. 2007; 127: 642-650.

[78] Cuneo A, Ferrant A, Michaux J-L, Demuynck H, Boorgaerts M, Louwagie A, et al. Philadelphia chromosome-positive acute myeloid leukemia: cytoimmunologic and cytogenetic features. Haematologica 1996; 81: 423-427.

[79] Tirado CA, Valdez F, Klesse L, Karandikar NJ, Uddin N, Arbini A, et al. Acute myeloid leukemia with inv (16) with CBFB-MYH11, 3'CBFB deletion, variant t (9;22) with BCR-ABL1, and del (7) (q22q32) in a pediatric patient: case report and literature review. Cancer Genet Cytogenet. 2010; 200 (1): 54-59.

[80] Bhatt VR, Akhtari M, Bociek G, Sanmann JN, Yuan J, Dave BJ, et al. Allogeneic stem cell transplantation in Philadelphia chromosome-positive acute myeloid leukemia. J Natl Compr Canc Netw. 2014; 12 (7): 963-968.

[81] Yamaguchi H, Inokuchi K, Yokomizo E, Miyata J, Watanabe A, Inami M, et al. Philadelphia-chromosome positive acute myeloid leukemia with tetraploidy. Int J Hematol 2002; 75 (1): 63-66.

[82] Larson RA. Therapy-related myeloid neoplasms: acute myeloid leukemia and myelodysplastic syndrome. UpToDate 2014; Topic edited by Lowenberg B and Connor RF. Topic last updated: January 24, 2014.

[83] Guenova M, Balatzenko G, Mihaylov G. Therapy-related acute myeloid leukemia. In Tech 2013. http://dx.doi.org/ 10.5772/52459.

[84] Larson RA. Etiology and management of therapy-related myeloid leukemia. Hematology 2007; 453-459.

[85] Pedersen-Bjergaard J, Christiansen DH, Desta F, Andersen MK. Alternative genetic pathways and cooperating genetic abnormalities in the pathogenesis of therapy-related myelodysplasia and acute myeloid leukemia. Leukemia 2006; 20: 1943-1949.

[86] Mauritzson N, Albin M, Rylander L, Billström R, Ahlgren T, Mikoczy Z, et al. Pooled analysis of clinical and cytogenetic features in treatment-related and de novo adult acute myeloid leukemia and myelodysplastic syndromes based on a consecutive series of 761 patients analyzed 1976-1993 and on 5098 unselected cases reported in the literature 1974-2001. Leukemia 2002; 16: 2366-2378.

[87] Pedersen-Bjergaard J, Andersen MK, Andersen MT, Christiansen DH. Genetics of therapy-related myelodysplasia and acute myeloid leukemia. Leukemia 2008; 22: 240-248.

[88] Christiansen DH, Pedersen-Bjergaard J. Internal tandem duplications of the FLT3 and MLL genes are mainly observed in atypical cases of therapy-related acute mye-

loid leukemia with a normal karyotype and are unrelated to type of previous therapy. Leukemia 2001; 15: 1848-1851.

[89] Schoch C, Kern W, Schnittger S, Hiddemann W, Haferlach T. Karyotype is an independent prognostic parameter in therapy-related acute myeloid leukemia (t-AML): an analysis of 93 patients with t-AML in comparison to 1091 patients with de novo AML. Leukemia 2004; 18: 120-125.

[90] Larson RA. Should therapy-related myeloid leukemia be treated like de novo acute myeloid leukemia? Haematologica Rep. 2006; 2 (15): 66-70.

[91] Carney DA, Westerman DA, Tam CS, Milner A, Prince HM, Kenealy M, et al. Therapy-related myelodysplastic syndrome and acute myeloid leukemia following fludarabine combination chemotherapy. Leukemia 2010; 24: 2056-2062.

[92] Atlas M, Head D, Behm D, Schmidt E, Zeleznik-Le NJ, Roe BA, et al. Cloning and sequence analysis of four t(9,11) therapy-related leukemia breakpoints. Leukemia 1998; 12: 1895-1902.

[93] Jacoby MA, De Jesus Pizarro RE, Shao J, Koboldt DC, Fulton RS, Zhou G, et al. The DNA double-strand break response is abnormal in myeloblasts from patients with therapy-related acute myeloid leukemia. Leukemia 2014; 28: 1242-1251.

[94] Gustafson SA, Lin P, Chen SS, Chen L, Abruzzo LV, Luthra R, et al. Therapy-related acute myeloid leukemia with t(8,21) (q22, q22) shares many features with de novo acute myeloid leukemia with t(8,21) (q 22,q 22) but does not have a favorable outcome. Am J Clin Pathol. 2009; 131: 647-655.

[95] Larson RA. Remission criteria in acute myeloid leukemia and monitoring of residual disease. UpToDate 2014. Topic edited by Lowenberg B and Conner RF. Topic last updated: September 14, 2014.

[96] Tefferi A, Letendre L. Going beyond 7+3 regimens in the treatment of adult acute myeloid leukemia. J Clin Oncol. 2012; 30 (20): 2425-2428.

[97] Burnett AK. Treatment of acute myeloid leukemia: are we making progress? Hematology 2012; 1-6.

[98] Gardin C, Chevret S, Pautas C, Turlure P, Raffoux E, Thomas X, et al. Superior long-term outcome with idarubicin compared with high-dose daunorubicin in patients with acute myeloid leukemia age 50 years and older. J Clin Oncol. 2013; 31 (3): 321-327.

[99] Estey E. Recent developments in management of older patients with acute myeloid leukemia. Ther Adv Hematol. 2012; 3 (2): 89-96.

[100] Willemze R, Suciu S, Meloni G, Labar B, Marie JP, Halkes CJ, et al. High-dose cytarabine in induction treatment improves the outcome of adult patients younger than age

46 years with acute myeloid leukemia: results of the EORTEC-GIMEMA AML-12 trial. J Clin Oncol. 2014; 32 (3): 219-228.

[101] Döhner H, Lübbert M, Fiedler W, Fouillard L, Haaland A, Brandwein JM, et al. Randomized phase II trial of low-dose cytarabine with or without volasertib in AML patients not suitable for induction therapy. Blood 2014; 124: 1426-1433.

[102] Hourigan CS, Karp JE. Minimal residual disease in acute myeloid leukemia. Nat Rev Clin Oncol. 2013; 10 (8): 460-471.

[103] Köhnke T, Sauter D, Ringel K, Hoster E, Laubender RP, Hubmann M, et al. Early assessment of minimal residual disease in AML by flow cytometry during aplasia identifies patients at increased risk of relapse. Leukemia 2015; 29: 377-386.

[104] Bacher U, Haferlach T, Fehse B, Schnittger S, Kroger N. Minimal residual disease diagnostics and chimerism in the post-transplant period in acute myeloid leukemia. Sci Word J. 2011; 11: 310-319.

[105] Walter RB, Buckley SA, Pagel JM, Wood BL, Storer BE, Sandmaier BM, et al. Significance of minimal residual disease before myeloablative hematopoietic cell transplantation for AML in first and second complete remission. Blood 2013, 122: 1813-1821.

[106] Kern W, Haferlach T, Schoch C, Löffler H, Gassmann W, Heinecke A, et al. Early blast clearance by remission induction therapy is a major independent prognostic factor for both achievement of complete remission and long-term outcome in acute myeloid leukemia: data from the German AML-Cooperative Group (AMLCG) 1992 Trial. Blood 2003; 101 (1): 64-70.

[107] Estey EH. How to manage high-risk acute myeloid leukemia. Leukemia 2012; 26: 861-869.

[108] Fiegl M, Unterhalt M, Kern W, Braess J, Spiekermann K, Staib P, et al. Chemomodulation of sequential high-dose cytarabine by fludarabine in relapsed or refractory acute myeloid leukemia: a randomized trial of the AMLCG. Leukemia 2014; 28: 1001-1007.

[109] Walter RB, Othus M, Burnett AK, Löwenberg B, Kantarjian HM, Ossenkoppele GJ, et al. Resistance prediction in AML: analysis of 4601 patients from MRC/NCRI, HOVON/SAKK, SWOG and MD Anderson Cancer Center. Leukemia 2015; 29: 312-320.

[110] Visani G, Miligan D, Leoni F, Chang J, Keley S, Marcus R, et al. Combined action of PSC 833 (valspodar), a novel MDR reversing agent, with mitoxantrone, etoposide and cytarabine in poor-prognosis acute myeloid leukemia. Leukemia 2001; 15: 761-771.

[111] Holowiecki J, Grosicki S, Robak T, Kyrcz-Krzemien S, Gieble S, Hellmann A, et al. Addition of cladrabine to daunorubicin and cytarabine increases complete remission rate after a single course of induction treatment in acute myeloid leukemia. Multicenter, Phase III study. Leukemia 2004; 18: 989-997.

[112] Platzbecker U, Germing U. Combination of azacitidine and lenalidomide in myelodysplastic syndromes or acute myeloid leukemia - a wise liaison? Leukemia 2013; 27: 1813-1819.

[113] Lokody I. Overcoming resistance in acute myeloid leukemia treatment. Nature Rev Cancer 2014; 14: 452-453.

[114] Cornelissen JJ, Versluis J, Passweg JR, van Putten WLJ, Manz MG, Maertens J, Beverloo HB, et al. Comparative therapeutic value of post-remission approaches in patients with acute myeloid leukemia aged 40-60 years. Leukemia 2014; 29: 1041-1050.

[115] Larson RA. Post-remission therapy for acute myeloid leukemia in younger adults. UpToDate 2015. Edited by Lowenberg B and Connor RF. Topic last updated: February 18, 2015.

[116] Hourigan Cs, McCarthy P, de Lima M. Back to the future! The evolving role of maintenance therapy after hematopoietic stem cell transplantation. Biol Blood Marrow Transplant. 2014; 20: 154-163.

[117] Pusic I,Choi J, Bernabe N, Abboud CN, Westervelt P, Vij R, Cashen AF, et al. Maintenance therapy with decitabine after allogeneic hematopoietic stem cell transplantation for acute myeloid leukemia and high risk myelodysplastic syndrome. Blood 2013; 122 (21): 4638 – 4638.

[118] Lin TR, Levy MY. Acute myeloid leukemia: focus on novel therapeutic strategies. Clin Med Insights Oncol. 2012; 6: 205-217.

[119] Seval GC, Ozcan M. Treatment of acute myeloid leukemia in adolescent and young adult patients. J Clin Med. 2015; 4: 441-459.

[120] Ravandi F. Relapsed acute myeloid leukemia: why is there no standard of care? Best Pract Res Clin Haematol. 2013; 26 (3): 253-259.

[121] Othus M, Appelbaum FR, Petersdorf SH, Kopecky KJ, Slovak M, Nevill T, et al. Fate of patients with newly diagnosed acute myeloid leukemia who fail primary induction therapy. Biol Blood Marrow Transplant. 2015; 21 (3): 559-564.

[122] Szer J. The prevalent predicament of relapsed acute myeloid leukemia. Hematology 2012; 43-48.

[123] Larson RA. Treatment of relapsed or refractory acute myeloid leukemia. UpToDate 2014. Topic edited by Loweberg B and Connor RF. Topic last updated: June 19, 2014.

[124] Choi S-J, Lee J-H, Lee J-H, Kim S, Seol M, Lee Y-S, et al. Treatment of relapsed acute myeloid leukemia after allogeneic bone marrow transplantation with chemotherapy followed by G-CSF primed donor leukocyte infusion: a high incidence of isolated extramedullary relapse. Leukemia 2004, 18: 1789-1797.

[125] Ofran Y, Rowe JM. Treatment of relapsed acute myeloid leukemia: what is new? Curr Opin Hematol. 2012; 19: 89-94.

[126] Blum W, Klisovic RB, Becker H, Yang X, Rozewski DM, Phelps MA, et al. Dose escalation of lenalidomide in relapsed or refractory acute leukemia. J Clin Oncol 2010; 28 (33): 4919-4925.

[127] Kanate As, Pasquini MC, Hari PN, Hamadani M. Allogeneic hematopoietic cell transplant for acute myeloid leukemia: current state in 2013 and future directions. World J Stem Cells 2014; 6 (2): 69-81.

[128] Hamilton BK, Coplan EA. Concise review: the role of hematopoietic stem cell transplantation in the treatment of acute myeloid leukemia. Stem Cells 2012; 30: 1581-1586.

[129] Magenau J, Couriel DR. Hematopoietic stem cell transplantation for acute myeloid leukemia: to whom, when and how. Curr Oncol Rep. 2013; 15: 436-444.

[130] Vyas P, Appelbaum FR, Craddock C. Allogeneic hematopoietic cell transplantation for acute myeloid leukemia. Biol Blood Marrow Transplant. 2015; 21: 8-15.

[131] Martin-Antonia B, Suarez-Lledo M, Arroyes M, Fernandez-Aviles, Martinez C, Rovira M, et al. A variant in IRF3 impacts on the clinical outcome of AML patients submitted to allo-SCT. Bone marrow Transplant. 2013; 48: 1205-1211.

[132] Ayuk F, Zabelina T, Wortmann F, Alchalby H, Wolschke C, Lellek H, et al. Donor choice according to age for allo-SCT for AML in complete remission. Bone Marrow Transplant. 2013; 48: 1028-1032.

[133] Gupta V, Tallman MS, Weisdorf DJ. Allogeneic hematopoietic cell transplantation for adults with acute myeloid leukemia; myths, controversies and unknowns. Blood 2011; 117: 2307-2318.

[134] Cornelissen JJ, Löwenberg B. Role of allogeneic stem cell transplantation in current treatment of acute myeloid leukemia. Hematology 2005; 151-155.

[135] Appelbaum FR. Indications for allogeneic hematopoietic cell transplantation for acute myeloid leukemia in the genomic era. Am Soc Clin Oncol Educ Book 2014, e327-e333.

[136] Peccaroti J, Ciceri F. Allogeneic stem cell transplantation for acute myeloid leukemia. Hematologica 2010; 95 (6): 857-859.

[137] Aoki J, Ishiyama K, Taniguchi S, Fukuda T, Ohashi K, Ogawa H, et al. Outcome of allogeneic hematopoietic stem cell transplantation for acute myeloid leukemia patients with central nervous system involvement. Biol Blood Marrow Transplant. 2014; 20: 2029-2033.

[138] Lazarus HM, Rowe JM. Reduced-intensity conditioning for acute myeloid leukemia: is this strategy correct. Leukemia 2006, 20: 1673-1682.

[139] Koreth J, Schlenk R, Kopecky KJ, Honda S, Sierra J, Djulhegovich BJ, et al. Allogeneic stem cell transplantation for acute myeloid leukemia in first complete remission. J Am Med Assoc 2009, 301 (22): 2349-2361.

[140] Walter RB, Sandmaier BM, Storer BF, Godwin CD, Buckley SA, Page JM, et al. Number of courses of induction therapy independently predicts outcome after allogeneic transplantation for acute myeloid leukemia in first morphological remission. Biol Blood Marrow Transplant. 2015; 21 (2): 373-8. doi: 10.1016/j.bbmt. 2014. 09.022. Epub September 30, 2014.

[141] Cornelissen JJ, Breems D, van Putten WJJ, Gratwohl AA, Passweg JR, Pubst T, et al. Comparative analysis of the value of allogeneic hematopoietic stem cell transplantation in acute myeloid leukemia with monosomal karyotype versus other cytogenetic risk categories. J. Clin Oncol. 2012; 30 (17): 2140-2146.

[142] Middeke JM, Beelen D, Stadler M, Göhring G, Schlegelberger B, Baurmann H, et al. Outcome of high-risk acute myeloid leukemia after allogeneic hematopoietic cell transplantation: negative impact of abnl (17p) and -5/5q-. Blood 2012; 120: 2512-2528.

[143] Grunwald MR, Tseng L-H, Lin M-T, Pratz KW, Eshleman JR, Levis MJ, et al. Improved FLT3 internal tandem duplication PCR assay predicts outcome after allogeneic transplant for acute myeloid leukemia. Biol Blood Marrow Transplant. 2014; 20: 1989-1995.

[144] Chen Y-B, Li S, Lane AA, Connolly C, Del Rio C, Valles B, et al. Phase I trial of maintenance sorafenib after allogeneic hematopoietic stem cell transplantation for Fms-like tyrosine kinase 3 internal tandem duplication acute myeloid leukemia. Biol Blood Marrow Transplant 2014; 20: 2042-2048.

[145] Ustun C, Lazarus HM, Weisdorf D. To transplant or not: a dilemma for treatment of elderly AML patients in the twenty-first century. Bone Marrow Transplant. 2013; 48: 1497-1505.

[146] Sorror ML, Appelbaum FR. Risk assessment before allogeneic hematopoietic cell transplantation for older adults with acute myeloid leukemia. Expert Rev Hematol. 2013; 6 (5): 1-26.

[147] Takami A, Yano S, Yokoyama H, Kuwatsuka Y, Yamaguchi T, Kanda Y, et al. Donor lymphocyte infusion for the treatment of relapsed acute myeloid leukemia after allogeneic hematopoietic stem cell transplantation: a retrospective analysis by the adult Acute Myeloid Leukemia Working Group of the Japan Society of Hematopoietic Cell Transplantation. Biol Blood Marrow Transplant. 2014; 20: 1785-1790.

[148] Bejanyan N, WeisdorF DJ, Logan BR, Wang H-L Devine SM, de Lima M, et al. Survival of patients with acute myeloid leukemia relapsing after allogeneic hematopoietic cell transplantaion: a Center for International Blood and Marrow Transplant Research Study. Biol Blood Marrow Transplant 2015; 21 (3): 454-459.

[149] Kongtim P, Di Stasi A, Roudon G, Chen J, Adekola K, Ropat U, et al, Can a female donor for a male recipient decrease the relapse rate of patients with acute myeloid leukemia treated with allogeneic hematopoietic stem cell transplantation. Biol Blood Marrow transplant. 2015; 21: 713-719.

[150] Warklick ED, de Latour RP, Shanley R, Robin M, Bejanyan N, Xhaard A, et al. Allogeneic hematopoietic cell transplantation outcomes in acute myeloid leukemia: similar outcomes regardless of donor type. Biol Blood Marrow Transplant. 2015; 21: 357-363.

[151] Schlenk RF, Döhner K, Mack S, Stoppel M, Kiraly F, Götze K, et al. Prospective evaluation of allogeneic hematopoietic stem-cell transplantation from matched related and matched unrelated donors in younger adults with high-risk acute myeloid leukemia: German- Austrian Trial AMLHD 98A. J Clin Oncol. 2010; 28 (30): 4642-4648.

[152] Foran JM, Pavletic SZ, Logan BR, Agovi-Johnson MA, Perez WS, Bolwell BJ, et al. Unrelated donor allogeneic transplantation after failure of autologous transplantation for acute myeloid leukemia: a study from the CIBMTR. Biol Blood Marrow Transplant. 2013; 19 (7): 1102-1108.

[153] Gorin N-C, Labopin M, Piemontese S, Arcese W, Santarone S, Huang H, et al. T-cell-replete haploidentical versus autologous stem cell transplantation in adult acute leukemia: a matched pair analysis. Haematologica 2015; 100: 558-564; doi:10.3324/haematol.2014. 111450.

[154] Devillier R, Harbi S, Fürst S, Crocchiolo R, El-Chiekh J, Castagna L, et al. Poor outcome with nonmyeloablative conditioning regimen before cord blood transplantation for patients with high-risk acute myeloid leukemia compared to matched related or unrelated donor transplantation. Biol Blood Marrow Transplant. 2014; 20: 1560-1565.

[155] Mo X-D, Kong J, Zhao T, Xu L-P, Zhang X-H, Liu D-H, et al. Extramedullary relapse of acute leukemia after haploidentical hematopoietic stem cell transplantation: incidence, risk factors, treatment and clinical outcomes. Biol Blood Marrow Transplant. 2014; 20: 2023-2028.

[156] Di Stasi A, Milton DR, Poon LM, Hamdi A, Rondon G, Chen J, et al. Similar transplantation outcome for acute myeloid leukemia and myelodysplastic syndrome patients with haploidentical versus 10/10 human leukocyte antigen-matched unrelated and related donors. Biol Blood Marrow Transplant. 2014; 20: 1975-1981.

[157] Raj K. Haploidentical versus matched donor stem cell transplantation for acute myeloid leukemia/ myelodysplastic syndrome patients. Biol Blood Marrow Transplant. 2014; 20: 1873-1876.

[158] Gao L, Wen Q, Chen X, Liu Y, Zhang C, Gao L, et al. Effects of priming with recombinant human granulocyte colony-stimulating factor on conditioning regimen for high-risk acute myeloid leukemia patients undergoing human leukocyte antigen-

haploidentical hematopoietic stem cell transplantation: a multicenter randomized controlled study in Southwest China. Biol Blood Marrow Transplant. 2014; 20: 1932-1939.

[159] Yahng S-A, Kim J-H, Jeon Y-W, Yoon J-H, shin S-H, Lee S-F, et al. A well-tolerated regimen of 800 c Gy TBI-fludarabine-busulfan-ATG for reliable engraftment after unmanipulated haploidentical peripheral blood stem cell transplantation in adult patients with acute myeloid leukemia. Biol Blood Marrow Transplant. 2015; 21: 119-129.

[160] Abboud CN, Granulocyte colony-stimulating factor priming improves haploidentical stem cell transplantation in high-risk acute myeloid leukemia subsets: a new role for an old work horse. Biol Blood Marrow Transplant. 2014; 20: 1873-1876.

[161] Ustun C, Wiseman AC, DeFor TE, Yohe S, Linden MA, Oran B, et al. Acheiving stringent CR is essential before reduced-intensity conditioning allogeneic hematopoietic cell transplantation in AML. Bone Marrow Transplant. 2013; 48: 1415-1420.

[162] Ho AYL, Pagliuca A, Kenyon M, Parker JE, Mijovic A, Devereux S, et al. Reduced-intensity allogeneic hematopoietic stem cell transplantation for myelodysplastic syndrome and acute myeloid leukemia with multilineage dysplasia using fludarabine, busulphan and alemtuzumab (FBC) conditioning. Blood 2004; 104: 1616-1623.

[163] Valcarcel D, Martino R, Caballero D, Martin J, Ferra C, Nieto JB, et al. Sustained remissions of high-risk acute myeloid leukemia and myelodysplastic syndrome after reduced-intensity conditioning allogeneic hematopoietic transplantation: chronic graft-versus-host disease is the strongest factor improving survival, J Clin Oncol. 2008; 26 (4): 577-584.

[164] Gyurkocza B, Storb R, Storer BE, Chauncey TR, Lange T, Shizuru JA, et al. Nonmyeloablative allogeneic hematopoietic cell transplantation in patients with acute myeloid leukemia. J Clin Oncol 2010; 28 (17): 2859-2867.

[165] de Lima M, Anagnostopoulos A, Munsell M, Shahjahan M, Ueno N, Ippoliti C, et al. Nonablative versus reduced- intensity conditioning regimens in the treatment of acute myeloid leukemia and high-risk myelodysplastic syndrome: dose is relevant for long-term disease control after allogeneic hematopoietic stem cell transplantation. Blood 2004; 104: 865-872.

[166] Andersson BS, Valdez BC de Lima M, Wang X, Thall PF, Worth LL, et al. Clofarabine ± fludarabine with once daily IV busulfan as pretransplant conditioning therapy for advanced myeloid leukemia and MDS. Biol Blood Marrow Transplant. 2011; 17 (6): 893-900.

[167] Kröger N, Shimoni A, Zabelina T, Schieder H, Panse J, Ayuk F, et al. Reduced-toxicity conditioning with treosulfan, fludarabine and ATG as preparative regimen for allogeneic stem cell transplantation (alloSCT) in elderly patients with secondary acute myeloid leukemia (sAML) or myelodysplastic syndrome (MDS). Bone Marrow Transplant. 2006; 37: 339-344.

[168] Martins C, Lacerda JF, Lourenco F, Carmo JA, Lacerda JMF. Autologous stem cell transplantation in acute myeloid leukemia: factors influencing outcome. A 13 year single institution experience. Acta Med Port. 2005; 18: 329-338.

[169] Kakucs E, Benede KI, Benedek E, Köpoczi JB, Tunyogi A, Istrati M. Autologous stem cell transplantation in patients with acute myeloid leukemia: a single-center experience. Acta Med Marisiensis 2013; 59 (2): 91-93.

[170] Nagler A, Labopin M, Gorin N-C, Ferrara F, Sanz MA, Wu D, et al. Intravenous busulfan for autologous stem cell transplantation in adult patients with acute myeloid leukemia: a survey of 952 patients on behalf of the Acute Leukemia Working Party of the European Group of Blood and Marrow Transplantation. Haematologica 2014; 99 (8): 1380-1386.

[171] Vellenga E, van Putten W, Ossenkoppele GJ, Verdonck LF, Theobald M, Cornelissen JJ, et al. Autologous peripheral blood stem cell transplantation for acute myeloid leukemia. Blood 2011; 118: 6037-6042.

[172] Hengeveld H, Suciu S, Chelgoum Y, Marie J-P, Muus P, Lefrère F, et al. High numbers of mobilized CD34 + cells collected in AML in first remission are associated with high relapse rate irrespective of treatment with autologous peripheral blood SCT or autologous BMT. Bone Marrow Transplant. 2015; 50: 341-347.

[173] Breems DA, Löwenberg B, Acute myeloid leukemia and the position of autologous stem cell transplantation. Semin Hematol 2007; 44 (4): 259-266.

[174] Linker CA. Autologous stem cell transplantation for acute myeloid leukemia. Bone Marrow Transplant. 2003; 31: 731-738.

[175] Piccalaga PP, Paolini S, Meloni G, Visani G, Ferrara F. Autologous stem cell transplantation for acute myloid leukemia. In-Tech 2013.

[176] Thomas X, Suciu S, Rio B, Leone G, Broccia G, Fillet G, et al. Autologous stem cell transplantation after complete remission and consolidation in acute myeloid leukemia patients aged 61-70 years: results of the prospective EORTC-GIMEMA AML-13 study. Haematologica 2007; 92 (03): 389-396.

[177] Ossenkopple GJ, Janssen JJWM, Huijgens PC. Autologous stem cell transplantation in elder acute myeloid leukemia. Mediterr J Hematol Infect Dis. 2013; 5 (1): e20130218.

[178] Oriol A, Ribera J-M, Esteve J, Guardia R, Brunet S, Bueno J, et al. Feasibility and results of autologous stem cell transplantation in de novo acute myeloid leukemia in patients over 60 years old. Results of the CETLAM AML-99 protocol. Haematologica, 2004; 89 (7): 791-800.

[179] Wetzel D, Mueller BU, Mansouri Taleghani B, Baerlocher GM, Seipel K, Leibundgut K, et al. Delayed hematological recovery after autologous stem cell transplantation is

associated with favourable outcome in acute myeloid leukemia. Br J Haematol.2015; 168 (2): 268-273.

[180] Linker CA, Ries CA, Damon LE, Sayre P, Navarro W, Rugo HS, et al. Autologous stem cell transplantation for acute myeloid leukemia in first remission. Biol Blood Marrow Transplant. 2000; 6 (1): 50-57.

[181] el-Shami K, Smith BD. Immunotherapy for myeloid leukemias: current status and future directions. Leukemia 2008; 22: 1658-1664.

[182] Barrettt AJ, Le Blanc K. Immunotherapy prospects for acute myeloid leukemia. Clin Exper Immunol 2010; 161: 223-232.

[183] Frankel AE, Baer MR, Hogge DE, Stuart RK. Immunotherapy of acute myeloid leukemia. Curr Pharmaceutical Biotechnol. 2001; 2 (3): 209-215(7).

[184] Kadowaki N, Kitawaki T. Recent advances in antigen-specific immunotherapy for acute myeloid leukemia. Clin Dev Immunol 2011; 104926: 1-7.

[185] Smits ELJM, Berneman ZN, van Tendeloo VFI. Immunotherapy of acute myeloid leukemia: current approaches. Oncologist 2009; 14: 240-252.

[186] Vasu S, Blum W. Emerging immunotherapies in older adults with acute myeloid leukemia. Curr Opin Hematol. 2013; 20 (2): 107-114.

[187] Schürch CM, Riether C, Ochsenbein AF. Dendritic cell-based immunotherapy for myeloid leukemias. Front Immunol. 2013; 4: 496, 1-16.

[188] Bar M. Adoptive immunotherapy for acute myeloid leukemia: from allogeneic hematopoietic cell transplantation to CAR T cells. Leukemia 2014; 2, 134.

[189] Anguille S, van Tendeloo VF, Berneman ZN. Leukemia-associated antigens and their relevance to the immunotherapy for acute myeloid leukemia. Leukemia 2012; 26: 2186-2196.

[190] Walter RB, Appelbaum FR, Estey E, Bernstein ID. Acute myeloid leukemia stem cells and CD33-targeted immunotherapy. Blood 2012; 119: 6198-6208.

[191] Jurcic JG, Immunotherapy for acuter myeloid leukemia. Curr Oncol Rep. 2005; 7: 339-346.

[192] Jurcic JG, Rosenblat TL.Targeted alpha-particle immmunotherapy for acute myeloid leukemia. Am SocClinOncolEduc Book 2014; e126-e131.

[193] Powles RL, Crowther D, Bateman CJT, Beard MEJ, Mc Elwain TJ, Russel J, et al. Immunotherapy for acute myelogenous leukemia. Br J Cancer 1973; 28: 365-376.

[194] Foon KA, Smalley RV, Riggs CW, Gale RP. The role of immunotherapy in acute myelogenous leukemia. Arch Intern Med 1983; 143: 1726-1731.

[195] Snauwaert S, Vandekerckhove B, Kerre T. Can immunotheraphy specifically target acute myeloid leukemia stem cells? Oncoimmunology 2013; 2: 2, e 22943.

[196] Goswani M, Hensel N, Smith BD, Prince GT, Qin L, Levitsky HI, et al. Expression of putative targets of immunotherapy in acute myeloid leukemia and healthy issues. Leukemia 2014; 28: 1167-1170.

[197] Smith CC, Wang Q, Shin C-S, Salerno S, Damon LE, Levis MJ, et al. Validation of ITD mutations in FLT3 as a therapeutic target in human acute myeloid leukemia. Nature 2012, 485 (7397): 260-263.

[198] Lin TL, Levy MY. Acute myeloid leukemia: focus on novel therapeutic strategies. Clin Med Insights Oncol. 2012; 6: 205-217.

[199] Foran JM. Targeted therapy of acute myeloid leukemia in 2012: towards individualized therapy. Hematology; Suppl 1: S137-140.

[200] Daver N, Cortes J. Molecular targeted therapy in acute myeloid leukemia. Hematology 2012; Suppl 1: S59-S62.

[201] Larkin K, Blum W. Novel therapies in AML: reason for hope or just hype? Am Soc Clin Ooncol Educ Book 2014; e341-e351.

[202] Tallman MS. New strategies for the treatment of acute myeloid leukemia including antibodies and other novel agents. Hematology 2005; 143-150.

[203] Baker SD, Zimmerman EI, Wang Y-D, Orwick S, Zatechka DS, Buaboonnam J, et al. Emergence of polyclonal FLT3 tyrosine kinase domain mutation during sequential therapy with sorafenib and sunitinib in FLT3-ITD-positive acute myeloid leukemia. Clin Cancer Res. 2013; 19 (20): 5758-5768.

[204] Wander SA, Levis MJ, Fathi AT. The evolving role of FLT3 inhibitors in acute myeloid leukemia: quizartinib and beyond. Ther Adv Hematol. 2014; 5 (3): 65-77.

[205] Alvarado Y, Kantarjian HM, Luthra R, Ravandi F, Borthakar G, Garcia-Manero G, et al. Treatment with FLT3 inhibitor in patients with FLT3-mutated acute myeloid leukemia is associated with development of secondary FLT3-tyrosine kinase domain mutations. Cancer 2014; 120 (14): 2142-4149.

[206] Moore AS, Faisal A, de Castro DG, Bavetsias V, Sun C, Atrash B, et al. Selective FLT3 inhibition of FLT3-ITD^{+} acute myeloid leukemia resulting in secondary D 835 Y mutation: a model for emerging clinical resistance patterns. Leukemia 2012; 26: 1462-1470.

[207] Swords R, Freeman C, Giles F. Targeting the FMS-like tyrosine kinase 3 in acute myeloid leukemia. Leukemia 2012; 26: 2176-2185.

[208] Cortes J, Kantarjian H, Foran JM, Ghirdaladze D, Zodelava M, Borthakur G, et al. Phase I study of quizartinib administered daily to patients with relapsed or refracto-

ry acute myeloid leukemia irrespective of FMS-like tyrosine kinase 3- internal tandem duplication status. J Clin Oncol. 2013; 31 (9): 3681-3687.

[209] Ostronoff F, Estey E. The role of quizartinib in the treatment of acute myeloid leukemia. Expert Opin Investing Drugs 2013; 22 (12): 1659-1669.

[210] Smith CC, Lasater EA, Zhu X, Lin KC, Stewart WK, Damon LE, et al. Activity of ponatinib against clinically-relevant AC220-resitant kinase domain mutants of FLT3-ITD. Blood 2013; 121: 3166-3171.

[211] Zimmerman EI, Turner DC, Buaboonnam J, Hu S, Orwick S, Roberts MS, et al. Crenolanib is active against models of drug-resistant FLT3-ITD-positive acute myeloid leukemia. Blood 2013; 122 (22): 3607-3615.

[212] Jagtap AD, Chang PT Liu JR, Wang HC, Kondekar NB, Shen LT, et al. Novel acylureidoindolin-2-one derivatives as dual Aurora BlFLT3 inhibitors for the treatment of acute myeloid leukemia. Eur J Med Chem. 2014; 85: 268-288.

[213] Al-Hussaini M, Di Persio JF. Small molecule inhibitors in acute myeloid leukemia: from the bench to the clinic. Expert Rev Hematol. 2014; 7 (4): 439-464.

[214] Liu S, Klisovic RB, Vukosavljevic T, Yu J, Paschka P, Huynh L, et al. Targeting AML1/ETO-histone deacetylase receptor complex: a novel mechanism for valproic acid-mediated gene expression and cellular differentiation in AML1/ETO-positive acute myeloid leukemia cells. J Pharmacol Exper Therap. 2007; 321 (3): 953-960.

[215] Odenike OM, Alkan S, Sher D, Godwin JE, Huo D, Brandt SJ, et al. Histone deacetylase inhibitor romidepsin has differential activity in core binding factor acute myeloid leukemia. Clin Cancer Res. 2008; 14: 7095-7101.

[216] Fredly H, Gjertsen B, Bruserud Ø. Histone deacetylase inhibition in the treatment of acute myeloid leukemia: the effects of valproic acid on leukemia cells, and the clinical and experimental evidence for combining valproic acid with other antileukemic agents. Clin Epigenetics 2013; 5:12.

[217] Botts M, Verbrugge I, Martin BP, Salmon JM, Ghisi M, Baker A, et al. Differentiation therapy for the treatment of t(8,21) acute myeloid leukemia using histone deacetylase inhibitors. Blood 2014; 123: 1341-1352.

[218] Bruserud Ø, Stapnes C, Tronstad KJ, Ryningen A, Anensen N, Gjertsen BT. Protein lysine acetylation in normal and leukemic hematopoiesis: HDACs as possible therapeutic targets in adult AML. Expert Opin Ther Targets 2006; 10 (1): 51-66.

[219] Torgersen ML, Engedal N, Bøe S-O, Hokland P, Simonsen A. Targeting autophagy potentiates the apoptotic effect of histone deacetylase inhibitors in t(8,21) AML cells. Blood 2013; 122: 2467-2476.

[220] Reikvam H, Ersvaer E, Bruserud Ø. Heat shock protein 90- a potential target in the treatment of human acute myeloid leukemia. Curr Cancer Drug Tartgets 2009; 9 (6): 761-776.

[221] Boissel N, Renneville A, Leguay T, Cornillet-Lefebvre P, Recher C, Lecerf T, et al. Dasatinib in high-risk core binding factor acute myeloid leukemia in first complete remission - a French Acute Myeloid Leukemia Intergroup Trial. Haematologica 2015, Epub ahead of print.

[222] Lech-Maranda E, Korycka A, Robok T. Clofarabine as a novel nucleoside analogue approved to treatment patients with haematological malignancies: mechanism of action and clinical activity. Mini Rev Med Chem 2009; 9 (7): 805-812.

[223] Larson ML, Venugopal P. Clofarabine: a new treatment option for patients with acute myeloid leukemia. Expert Opin Pharmacother. 2009; 10 (8): 1653-1357.

[224] Nazha A, Ravandi F, Kantarjian H, Huang X, Choi S, Garcia-Manero G, et al. Clofarabine, idarubicin, cytarabine (CIA) as front line therapy for patients ≤ 60 years with newly diagnosed acute myeloid leukemia (AML). Am J Hematol. 2013; 88 (1): 961-966.

[225] Willemze R, Suciu S, Muus P, Halkes CJ, Meloni G, Meert L, et al. Clofarabine in combination with a standard remission induction regimen (cytosine arabinoside and idarubicin) in patients with previously untreated intermediate and bad-risk acute myelogenous leukemia (AML) or high-risk myelodysplastic syndrome (HR-MDS): phase I results of an ongoing phase I/II study of the leukemia groups of EORTC and GIMEMA (EORTC GIMEMA 06061/AML-14A trial). Ann Hematol. 2014; 93 (6): 965-975.

[226] Yamauchi T, Uzui K, Nishi R, Shigemi H, Ueda T. Cytarabine-resistant leukemia cells are moderately sensitive to clofarabine in vitro. Anticancer Res. 2014; 34 (4): 1657-1662.

[227] Steensma DP, Stone RM. Lenalidomide in AML: del (5q) or who? Blood 2011; 118: 481-482.

[228] Xie C, Edwards H, Caldwell JT, Taub JW, Ge Y. Obatoclax potentiates the cytotoxic effect of cytarabine on acute myeloid leukemia cells by enhancing DNA damage. Mol Oncol. 2014; S 1574-7891 (14) 00232-4.

[229] Thomas S, Schelker R, Klobuch S, Zaiss S, Troppmann M, Rehli M, et al. Bimodulatory therapy induces complete molecular remission in chemorefractory acute myeloid leukemia. Haematologica 2014; 1-10.

[230] Tavernier E, Aanei C, Solly F, Flandrin-Gresta P, Campos L, Guyotat D. $CXCR_4$: a new therapeutic target of the leukemic cell? Role of the SDF-1/$CXCR_4$ axis in acute myeloid leukemia. Bull Cancer 2014; 101 (6): 593-604.

[231] Peled A, Tavor S. Role of $CXCR_4$ in the pathogenesis of acute myeloid leukemia. Theranostics 2013; 3 (1): 34-39.

[232] Tavor S, Petit I. Can inhibition of the SDF-1/$CXCR_4$ axis eradicate acute leukemia? Semin Cancer Biol. 2010; 20 (3): 178-185.

[233] Zeng Z, Shi YX, Samudio IJ, Wang R-Y, Ling X, Frolova O, et al. Targeting the leukemia microenvironment by CXCR4 inhibition overcomes resistance to kinase inhibitors and chemotherapy in AML. Blood 2009; 113: 6215-6224.

[234] Ehninger A, Kramer M, Röllig C, Thiede C, Bornhäuser M, von Bonin M, et al. Distribution and levels of cell surface expression of CD33 and CD123 in acute myeloid leukemia. Blood Cancer J. 2014; 4: e 218.

[235] Giles F, Estey E, O'Brien S. Gemtuzumab ozogamicin in the treatment of acute myeloid leukemia. Cancer 2003, 98 (10): 2095-2104.

[236] Bross BF, Beitz J, Chen G, Chen XH, Duffy E, Kieffer L, et al. Approval summary: gemtuzumab ozogamicin in relapsed acute myeloid leukemia. Clin Cancer Res. 2001; 1490 (7): 1490-1496.

[237] Stasi R, Gemtuzumab ozogamicin: an anti-CD33 immuno-conjugate for the treatment of acute myeloid leukemia. Expert Opin Biol Ther. 2008; 8 (4): 527-540.

[238] Molnär I, Powell BL. What role does gemtuzumab ozogamicin have in the treatment of acute myelogenous leukemia. Curr Hematol Malig Rep. 2007; 2 (2): 104-110.

[239] Kharfan-Dabaja MA, Hamadani M, Reljic T, Pyngolil R, Komrokji RS, Lancet JE, et al. Gemtuzumab ozogamicin for treatment of newly diagnosed acute myeloid leukemia: a systemic review and meta-analysis. Br J Haematol. 2013; 163 (3): 315-325.

[240] Castaigne S, Pautas C, Terré C, Raffoux E, Bordessoule B, Bastie JN, et al. Effect of gemtuzumab ozogamicin on survival of adult patients with de novo acute myeloid leukemia (ALFA-0701): a randomised, open-label phase 3 study. Lancet 2012; 379 (9825): 1508-1516.

[241] Di Rocco A, Finolezzi E, Anaclerico B, Calabrese E, Levi A, Trasartis, et al. Therapeutic advances in neoplastic hematology: target therapy anti-CD33. Clin Ter. 2005, 156 (4): 183-186.

[242] Madiros A, Dos Santos C, Mc Donald T, Brown CE, Wang X, Elizabeth Budde L, et al. T cells expressing CD123-specific chimeric antigen receptors exhibit specific cytolytic effector functions and antitumor effects against human acute myeloid leukemia. Blood 2013; 122: 3138-3148.

[243] Tettamanti S, Marin V, Pizzitola I, Magnani CF, Giordano-Attianese GM, Cribioli E, et al. Targeting of acute myeloid leukemia by cytokine-induced killer cells redirected with a novel CD123-specific chimeric antigen receptor. Br J Haematol. 2013; 161 (3): 389-401.

[244] Pizzitola I, Anjos-Afonso F, Rouault-Pierre K, Lassailly F, Tettamanti S, Spinelli O, et al. Chimeric antigen receptors against CD33/CD123 antigens efficiently target primary acute myeloid leukemia cells in vitro. Leukemia 2014; 28: 1596-1605.

[245] Gill S, Tasian SK, Ruella M, Shestova O, Li Y, Porter DL, et al. Preclinical targeting of human acute myeloid leukemia and myeloablation using chimeric antigen receptor-modified T cells. Blood 2014; 123 (15): 2343-2354.

[246] Tettamanti S, Biondi A, Biagi E, Bonnet D. CD123 AML targeting by chimeric antigen receptors. Oncoimmunology 2014; 3: e28835-1.

[247] Fan D, Li Z, Zhang X, Yang Y, Yuan X, Zhang X, et al. AntiCD3Fv fused to human interleukin-3 deletion variant redirected T cells against human acute myeloid leukemia stem cells. J Hematol Oncol. 2015; 8: 18.

[248] Misaghian N, Ligresti G, Steelman LS, Bertrand FE, Bäsecke J, Libra M, et al. Targeting the leukemic stem cell: the holy grail of leukemia therapy. Leukemia 2009, 23: 25-42.

[249] Pollyea DA, Gutman JA, Gore L, Smith CA, Jordan CT. Targeting acute myeloid leukemia stem cells: a review and principles for the development of clinical trials. Haematologica 2014; 99 (8): 1277-1284.

[250] Chan WI, Huntly BJ. Leukemia stem cells in acute myeloid leukemia. Semin Oncol. 2008; 35(4): 326-135.

[251] Yang XH, Li M, Wang B, Zhu W, Desgardin A, Onel K, et al. Systematic computation with functional gene-sets among leukemic and hematopoietic stem cells reveals a favorable prognostic signature for acute myeloid leukemia. BMC Bioinformatics 2015; 16: 97.

[252] Curran E, Corrales L, Kline J. Targeting the innate immune system as immunotherapy for acute myeloid leukemia. Fron Oncol. 2015; 5 (83): 1-9.

[253] Schürch CM, Riether C, Ochsenbein AF. Dendritic cell-based immunotherapy for myeloid leukemias. Front Immunol. 2013; 4: 496.

[254] Subklewe M, Geiger C, Lichtenegger FS, Javorovic M, Kvalheim G, Schendel DJ, et al. New generation dendritic cell vaccine for immunotherapy of acute myeloid leukemia. Cancer Immunol Immunother. 2014; 63: 1093-1103.

[255] Hourigan CS, Karp JE. Personalized therapy for acute myeloid leukemia. Cancer Discov. 2013; 3 (12): 1-4.

Chapter 6

Clofarabine and Adult Acute Myeloid Leukemia

Branimir Spassov, Gueorgui Balatzenko, Georgi Mihaylov and Margarita Guenova

Additional information is available at the end of the chapter

http://dx.doi.org/10.5772/61435

Abstract

Acute myeloid leukemia (AML) is a clonal, malignant disease of hematopoietic tissues that is characterized by accumulation of abnormal blast cells, principally in the marrow and impaired production of normal blood cells. The unsatisfactory clinical outcomes of AML patients urged the development of new therapy strategies, one of which includes the implementation of new nucleoside analogs. Clofarabine has offered new promising perspectives within induction and consolidation therapies. This chapter will evaluate the efficacy and tolerability of clofarabine as a single agent and in combination therapy, including hematopoietic stem cell transplantation, for AML patients.

Keywords: Clofarabine, adult acute myeloid leukemia

1. Introduction

Acute myeloid leukemia (AML) is defined as a clonal disorder characterized by the uncontrolled proliferation and survival of immature myeloid progenitors that undergo a differentiation block at various maturation steps, leading to accumulation of leukemic cells in bone marrow and inhibition of normal hematopoiesis [1].

The treatment of AML patients includes both induction and consolidation chemotherapy. The overall goal of induction is to provide complete remission (CR) – <5% blast cells in the bone marrow, absolute neutrophils count >1,000/μl and platelet count >100,000/μl. Consolidation or post-remission chemotherapy, with or without hematopoietic stem cell transplantation (HSCT), further improves the outcome by decreasing relapses.

Unfortunately, the therapy of AML patients has shown only partial progress over the past 20 years. For many years, the conventional induction chemotherapy for AML patients has consisted of cytarabine plus an anthracycline (7+3 regimen; i.e., 7 days of treatment with cytarabine and 3 days of treatment with an anthracycline) [2]. Although the overall response rate (ORR) to this combination is 70–80%, only 30–50% of them remains alive for more than 5 years since most patients will relapse and die from their disease or associated complications [3]. Numerous modifications of this combination (using different anthracylines, adding a third agent such as mitoxantrone or etoposide, extending the number of days of cytarabine, priming of leukemia blasts with hematopoietic growth factors) failed to improve response rates and overall survival (OS) [4–8].

Some 15–25% de novo AML patients fail to achieve CR because of resistance to treatment and 40% of CR patients will relapse within 2 years. Although several different salvage chemotherapy combinations have been administered to patients with refractory/relapsed AML, the prognosis in this subset of patients is very poor, with a CR rate ranging from 30 to 50% [9]. The goal of salvage chemotherapy is to provide a bridge to HSCT aimed at prolonged OS.

Older AML patients do very poorly [10]. Standard induction therapy with 7+3 in older patients has resulted in CR rates ranging from 30 to 50% and induction mortality rates of 10–35% [11,12]. Remissions are usually transient and rarely last more than 12 months. The median OS is 5–10 months, with less than 10% of patients remaining in remission at 3 years [13].

The unsatisfactory clinical outcomes of patients with AML urged the development of new nucleoside analogs. Over the past years, a series of deoxyadenosine analogs have been synthesized with the aim to improve drug efficacy [14]. Several of these compounds, such as fludarabine, cladribine, nelarabine, or gemcitabine, have been introduced into the clinical practice for hematological malignancies. Clofarabine has progressively gained some attention as a possible new weapon available for patients with AML [15] since this drug could be implemented in induction and consolidation therapy including HSCT.

2. Clofarabine pharmacology

Clofarabine (2-chloro-20-fluoro-deoxy-9-b-D-arabinofuranosyladenine) is a second-generation nucleoside analog synthesized in the 1990s. The rationale behind its design was to combine the most favorable pharmacokinetic properties of fludarabine and cladribine. Like cladribine and fludarabine, clofarabine is toxic to both non-proliferating human lymphocytes and rapidly proliferating cells. Clofarabine is believed to enter cells by both facilitated and active nucleoside transport mechanisms as well as, at higher concentrations and upon longer exposure, by passive diffusion across lipid membranes [16]. Once inside the cell, clofarabine is phosphorylated to its active triphosphate form by cellular enzymes, including deoxycytidine and deoxyguanosine kinases [17]. Clofarabine metabolites are retained by cells to a greater extent than are the metabolites of cladribine. This could lead to more pronounced anti-tumoral effect and higher hematological toxicity of the former [18]. The anti-cancer activity of clofarabine involves three major mechanisms: inhibition of deoxyribonucleic acid (DNA) synthesis, inhibition of ribonucleotide reductase, and direct induction of apoptosis [19,20]. Clonogenicity assays showed a strong inverse correlation between cell survival and incorporation of clofarabine monophosphate into DNA, thus suggesting this latter mechanism as a critical step for the cytotoxic potential of this drug [18].

http://dx.doi.org/10.5772/61435

Given its mechanisms of action, clofarabine was predicted to work separately or synergistically with other chemotherapeutic agents such as other purine nucleoside analogs and DNA-damaging or cross-linking agents such as anthracyclines and platinum agents [21]. Therefore, it is not a big surprise that clofarabine has gained so much interest in the past years. A lot of clinical trials had been performed and relevant English language studies are summarized in Table 1.

Reference	Study phase	AML study population	Patients, N	Median age	ORR %	CR %	Median OS (weeks)	Induction mortality %
			Combination with cytarabine					
Faderl et al. [27]	2	Untreated	60	61	60	52	41	7
Becker et al. [28]	2	Untreated	50	53	82	76	97	2
Faderl et al. [30]	3	Untreated	70	71	67	63	46	16
Faderl et al. [32]	2	Untreated	60	70	66	58	51	7
Martínez-Cuadrón et al. [31]	2	Untreated	11	74	27	27	Not reported	73
Becker et al. [40]	1–2	Relapsed/refractory	46	53	61	46	36	11
Tse et al. [42]	2	Relapsed/refractory	21	45		43	Not reported	9.5
Scappini et al. [43]	2	Relapsed/refractory	47	50.5	61.5	51	28	13
Faderl et al. [38]	2	Relapsed/refractory	25	63	40	28	23	3
Faderl et al. [39]	3	Relapsed/refractory	163	67	47	35	26	16
			Combination with idarubicin and cytarabine					
Willemze et al. [23]	1	Untreated	25	55.9	84	76	Not reported	16
Selleslag et al. [24]	1/2	Untreated	62	50	84	74	74% at 1 year	
Nazha et al. [29]	2	Untreated	59	48	79	74	Not reached	4
			Combination with daunorubicin					
Vigil et al. [34]	2	Untreated	21	69	38	28.6	45	14
			Monotherapy					
Kantarjian et al. [35]	2	Untreated	112	71	46	38	41	16
Burnett et al. [36]	2	Untreated	106	71	48	32	19	18
Burnett et al. [37]	3	Untreated	203	74	38	22	13% at 2 years	32
Kantarjian et al. [26]	2	Relapsed/refractory	31	54	55	42	Not reported	5

List of abbreviations:

AML – acute myeloid leukemia; ORR – overall response rate; CR – complete remission; OS – overall survival

Table 1. Studies evaluating clinical responses of patients with acute myeloid leukemia to clofarabine combination and monotherapy

According to data from phase 1 trial, the maximum tolerated dose (MTD) of clofarabine, given as 1-h infusion daily for 5 days in patients with hematological malignancies, was determined to be 40 mg/m^2/day. The dose-limiting toxicity (DLT) was hepatotoxicity. Among 16 AML patients 16% ORR was registered, as two of them achieved CR and three had CR with incomplete platelet recovery (CRi) [22].

In order to determine the MTD of clofarabine combined with 3 + 10 induction regimen (idarubicin + cytarabine) in adults with untreated intermediate and unfavorable risk AML or high-risk myelodysplastic syndrome (MDS), a phase 1 of the EORTC/Gimema AML-14A study was carried out [23]. The study included 25 patients with median age of 55.9 years that received clofarabine 1-h infusion (arm A) or push injection (arm B) for 5 days at the dose level of 5 × 10 mg/m^2/day or 5 × 15 mg/m^2/day in an algorithmic dose escalation 3 + 3 design. Patients in CR were planned to receive a consolidation course (intermediate dose cytarabine, idarubicin). Primary endpoint was safety and tolerance as measured by dose-limiting toxicity (DLT). The clofarabine dose of 5 × 15 mg/m^2/day resulted in four DLTs and three patients' withdrawals due to adverse events not classified as DLT while clofarabine dose of 5 × 10 mg/m^2/day was associated with one DLT and no treatment withdrawals. The latter clofarabine dose was considered by the authors as MTD. CR and CRi were achieved in 21 patients (11/12 (92%) receiving clofarabine 10 mg/m^2/day; 10/13 (77%) receiving clofarabine 15 mg/m^2/day).

Selleslag et al. reported the final results of the combined phase 1 and 2 parts of the EORTC/Gimema AML-14A study that explored the antitumor activity of clofarabine containing induction combination regimens at the aforementioned phase 1 selected dosage schedules [24]. Patients 18–60 years old (n = 57) with previously untreated intermediate- and bad risk AML or high risk MDS (n = 5) were included in the study. Clofarabine was administered as 1-h infusion (Arm A) or push injection (Arm B) at 10 mg/m^2 on days 2, 4, 6, 8, and 10 in combination with cytarabine (100 mg/m^2/day on days 1–10) and idarubicin (10 mg/m^2/day, on days 1, 3, and 5). One cycle of consolidation including cytarabine (500 mg/m^2 every 12 h on days 1–6) and idarubicin (10 mg/m^2/day on days 4, 5, and 6) was administered in patients who achieved a CR/CRi. The two tested clofarabine (5x10 mg/m^2) containing regimens yielded an impressive (84%) CR/CRi rate, whereas OS of both regimens was 74% at 1 year.

2.1. Clofarabine in AML induction therapy

2.1.1. Newly diagnosed AML patients

2.1.1.1. Clofarabine combination therapy

The benefit of combining clofarabine with cytarabine, was hypothesized given in vitro data showing increased conversion of cytarabine to its active triphosphate form (ara-CTP) via deoxycytidine kinase when cytarabine was given after clofarabine, and this drug combination produced synergistic killing of myeloid leukemia cells [25]. The infusion of cytarabine was begun 4 h after starting clofarabine as previous studies demonstrated that this was the time of maximum clofarabine triphosphate accumulation in leukemia blasts [26].

The combination of clofarabine and cytarabine was studied as an induction therapy by Faderl and colleagues [27]. They had enrolled 60 patients with newly diagnosed AML or high-risk

MDS patients. The median age of the study group was 61 years (range, 50–74 years). The induction therapy consisted of intravenous clofarabine 40 mg/m^2 for 5 days (days 2 to 6) followed 4 h later by intravenous cytarabine 1 g/m^2 on days 1 to 5. On day 1, only cytarabine was administered; on day 6, only clofarabine was administered. This cytarabine infusion rate generated cytarabine concentrations in plasma that maximize the rate of ara-CTP accumulation in leukemic blasts. Cycles were repeated every 4 to 6 weeks depending on leukemia response, recovery of normal hematopoiesis, or occurrence of treatment-related toxicities. Patients were allowed to receive a maximum of three induction cycles or until a CR, CRi or partial response (PR) was achieved. The maintenance therapy given as a consolidation in responding patients consisted of up to six additional courses with clofarabine 40 mg/m^2 daily followed 4 h later by cytarabine 1 g/m^2 daily for three consecutive days. Of 60 patients, 48% had secondary AML, 50% had abnormal karyotypes, and 21% showed *FLT3* gene abnormalities. The ORR was 60% with 52% of CR and 8% of CRi. Induction death was observed in 7% of the patients. Despite the good CR rate, OS did not appear to be improved compared with other induction regimens.

In order to improve the clinical outcomes of previously untreated AML patients, combination therapy of clofarabine and cytarabine was tested with granulocyte colony-stimulating factor (G-CSF) priming [28]. This therapy regimen was named GCLAC and 50 newly diagnosed patients with AML or advanced MDS or advanced myeloproliferative neoplasm (MPN) were included in the study. The median age was 53 years (range, 22–64 years). The treatment consisted of intravenous clofarabine (30 mg/m^2/day) followed 4 h later by intravenous cytarabine (2 g/m^2/day) for five consecutive days. Patients received daily subcutaneous G-CSF priming from the day before chemotherapy until neutrophil recovery. A second induction cycle was administered if a patient had >5% marrow blasts 21 days post induction. Patients in remission received up to three post remission cycles with reduced dosages. Twenty-six percent of the patients had unfavorable, 64% intermediate, and 8% favorable cytogenetics. The ORR was 82% with 76% of CR and 6% of CRi. For patients with an antecedent hematologic disorder (AHD), the CR rate was 65%, compared to 85% for those without an AHD. Seventy percent of AML patients with the internal tandem duplication of fms-like tyrosine 3 (*FLT3*-ITD) achieved CR after treatment with GCLAC without the inclusion of a *FLT3* inhibitor. The 60-day mortality was 2%. Median overall survival was 24.3 months and at a median follow-up of 15 months, 32 patients were alive of whom 21 were in remission. The authors concluded that front-line GCLAC is a well-tolerated, effective induction regimen for AML and advanced myelodysplastic or myeloproliferative disorders although GCLAC was not compared with other induction regimens.

The combination of clofarabine, cytarabine, and idarubicine was applied in phase 2 study with newly diagnosed AML patients less than 60-years-old. The study included 59 patients with median age of 48 years (range, 19–60 years). The therapy consisted of clofarabine (20 mg/m^2) and cytarabine (1 g/m^2) both for 5 days and idarubicin (10 mg/m^2) for 3 days, followed in patients in remission by up to six consolidation cycles with reduced dosages. The ORR was 79%. With a median follow-up of 10.9 months, the median OS was not reached and the median event-free survival (EFS) was 13.5 months. Four-week and eight-week mortality were 2% and 4%, respectively. Forty-two percent of the patients proceeded with allogeneic SCT in first remission. The authors performed a retrospective comparison with patients treated with idarubicine and cytarabine, and concluded that the addition of clofarabine showed an apparent improvement in both OS and EFS. According to authors, patients ≤40 years and those with unfavorable karyotype benefited most of triple combination therapy [29].

Several different clofarabine combinations were tested in previously untreated older AML patients to find more effective and less toxic treatments.

The combination of clofarabine and low-dose cytarabine (LDAC) was tested as front-line therapy in previously untreated older AML patients aged 60 years and older. The study included 70 patients with newly diagnosed AML and median age was 71 years (range, 60–83 years). The patients were randomized to treatment with clofarabine alone versus clofarabine plus LDAC [30]. Fifty percent of the patients had secondary AML/MDS, 50% had abnormal karyotypes, and 11% showed *FLT3* abnormalities. Clofarabine (30 mg/m^2/day) was given intravenously over 1 h (days 1 through 5) and in combination arm cytarabine was added (20 mg/m^2/day) given by subcutaneous injection daily for 14 days (days 1 through 14), but beginning 4 h after the start of clofarabine. On days 1 to 5, administration of clofarabine preceded the injection of cytarabine by approximately 4 h. A second induction cycle was permitted for stable disease, partial response, or hematologic improvement after the first induction cycle. Patients with at least a CRi could receive up to 12 consolidation cycles. During the consolidation, clofarabine (30 mg/m^2/day) was given on days 1 through 3 with or without 7 days of cytarabine. Overall, 56% achieved CR and CR rate was significantly higher with the combination. Induction mortality was not significantly different in both treatment arms (19% with the combination versus 31% with clofarabine alone). The combination showed better EFS but not OS.

Similar clinical study was performed on much smaller group of patients [31]. The study included 11 patients with median age of 74 years (range, 63–87 years). Clofarabine (20 mg/m^2/day) was given intravenously over 1 h (days 1 through 5) in combination with LDAC (20 mg/m^2/day) given by subcutaneous injection daily for 14 days (days 1 through 14). Patients in CR could receive a maximum of 10 consolidation courses with intravenous clofarabine (15 mg/m^2/day) during five consecutive days and subcutaneous cytarabine (20 mg/m^2/day) during seven consecutive days. CR was achieved in 27%. The mortality rates at 4 and 8 weeks were 46% and 73%, respectively. Due to this unacceptable early mortality rate, the study was prematurely discontinued. High mortality rate could be in part explained by inadequate supportive care of the patients. The authors concluded that tight patients' clinical monitoring, follow-up, and intensive supportive care seem crucial to achieve at least acceptable clinical outcomes in elderly AML patients receiving clofarabine plus LDAC.

The combination of clofarabine and LDAC was evaluated as an induction and consolidation therapy, latter alternating with decitabine [32]. Decitabine is an important drug in induction of global and gene-specific DNA hypomethylation [33]. Sixty patients with a median age of 70 years (range, 60–81 years) with newly diagnosed AML were included in the study. Induction therapy consisted of clofarabine 20 mg/m^2 by intravenous infusion daily (days 1 through 5) plus cytarabine 20 mg subcutaneously twice daily (days 1 through 10). On days 1 through 5, clofarabine preceded the cytarabine injections by about 3 to 4 h. Patients who did not achieve a CR could receive one reinduction cycle at the same dose and schedule. In the case of persistent disease after reinduction, patients could proceed with decitabine 20 mg/m^2 as a 1- to 2-h intravenous infusion daily for five consecutive days. Responding patients received consolidation therapy consisting of same clofarabine and cytarabine scheme alternating with decitabine 20 mg/m^2 for 5 days up to 17 cycles. Overall, 66% achieved CR and CRi. Notably, all of the seven patients with an FLT3-ITD responded, which included CR in six of them (86%). Induction mortality was low (7% at 8 weeks) and toxicities manageable. Among the 40 patients who have achieved CR/CRi, the median relapse-free survival (RFS) and OS were 14.1 and 24.2 months, respectively. The median OS of all patients was 12.7 months. However, compared with a historical group of patients who received clofarabine plus low-dose cytarabine with a shorter consolidation, RFS was not statistically different.

The combination of clofarabine and daunorubicin was tested as a first-line therapy in previously untreated older AML patients aged 60 years and older [34]. The median age of the 21 patients was 69 years (range, 60–85 years). Fourteen patients (67%) had unfavorable risk features. Induction mortality was 14%. CR was registered in 28.6% of the patients and the median OS was 11.2 months.

2.1.1.2. Clofarabine monotherapy

Clofarabine monotherapy was tested as an induction therapy predominantly in newly diagnosed older AML patients.

A phase 2 study assessed the efficacy of clofarabine monotherapy in older adults with untreated AML and at least one unfavorable baseline prognostic factor [35]. The study included 112 patients with median age of 71 years (range, 60–88 years). Sixty two percent of patients were ≥70 years old, 41% had intermediate, and 55% had unfavorable cytogenetics. Clofarabine was administered intravenously daily at 30 mg/m^2/d during induction (days 1 through 5) and 20 mg/m^2/d during reinduction/consolidation (six cycles maximum). The median duration of remission was 56 weeks. The ORR was 46% and according to authors it did not seem to be affected by the presence of multiple unfavorable prognostic factors. Noteworthy, five patients in remission proceeded to HSCT. The all-cause 30-day mortality rate was 9.8% and the all-cause 60-day mortality rate was 16%. Median OS was 41 weeks for all patients, 59 weeks for patients who achieved CR or CRi, and 72 weeks for patients who achieved a CR.

Another two consecutive phase 2 studies (UWCM-001 and BIOV-121) assessed the efficacy of clofarabine monotherapy in older adults with untreated AML [36]. UWCM-001 patients were either older than 70 years or 60–69 years of age with cardiac comorbidity or poor performance status (WHO >2) whereas BIOV-121 patients were at least 65 years of age and considered not eligible for intensive chemotherapy. The studies enrolled 106 patients. Clofarabine was administered intravenously daily at 30 mg/m^2/d for 5 days and the patients could receive up to four or six courses of this drug. CR+CRi were achieved in 48% of the patients and induction death within 30 days was 18%. Interestingly, response and overall survival were not inferior in the adverse cytogenetic risk group. The authors performed a retrospective comparison with patients treated with LDAC and showed that the rate of CR/CRi with clofarabine was significantly superior (48% vs 17%). They had also demonstrated that OS with clofarabine was significantly superior to LDAC and non-significantly inferior to intensive chemotherapy.

To confirm survival benefit of clofarabine, a randomized comparison of LDAC vs clofarabine was performed in 406 untreated older patients with AML and high-risk MDS [37]. The median age of the patients was 74 years (range, 51–90 years). LDAC was given as a twice-daily 20-mg subcutaneous injection (days 1 through 10) with the aim of delivering four courses at approximately 6-week intervals and clofarabine was given as 20 mg/m^2 daily (days 1 through 5) by intravenous infusion for four courses approximately 4 to 6 weeks apart. Patients who were considered to be benefiting (CR or stable disease) were permitted to receive additional courses of treatment. The ORR (CR + CRi) was significantly improved in the clofarabine arm (38% vs 19%). However, there was no OS difference between the treatment arms. The authors explained the lack of clofarabine survival benefit by the superior survival of LDAC patients who failed to enter CR or who relapsed from CR.

2.1.2. *Refractory or relapsed AML patients*

2.1.2.1. *Clofarabine combination therapy*

Several clinical trials proved the clinical activity of clofarabine combination therapy in refractory or relapsed AML patients. Although many clofarabine combinations had been tested, the combination of clofarabine and cytarabine was largely applied in these patients.

Faderl and colleagues published a phase 2 study of clofarabine in combination with cytarabine to treat patients with relapsed AML [38]. The trial was conducted in 32 patients with relapsed acute leukemia, 25 of which are with AML. The median age of the whole study population was 59 years (range, 18 to 84 years). Clofarabine 40 mg/m^2 was administered as a 1-h intravenous infusion daily (days 2 through 6) followed 4 h later by an intermediate dose of cytarabine (1 g/m^2 as a 2-h constant-rate intravenous infusion) once daily (days 1 through 5). On day 1, only cytarabine was administered; on day 6, only clofarabine was administered. Patients were allowed to receive a maximum of two cycles of induction therapy and responding patients could receive up to six additional cycles of maintenance therapy at 75% of the induction doses of both clofarabine and cytarabine. ORR among AML patients was 40%. Only one patient died during induction (within 4 weeks of therapy start), constituting an induction mortality of 3%. The authors demonstrated that the combination of clofarabine with cytarabine is safe and active.

Given the encouraging clinical results of the previous study, a phase 3, randomized, double-blind, placebo-controlled trial based on the administration of clofarabine 40 mg/m^2 or placebo followed by cytarabine 1 g/m^2 for five consecutive days was carried out in relapsed or refractory AML patients [39]. The primary end point of the trial was OS. The median age was 67 years and 320 patients were included in the trial. Although OS did not differ between the treatment arms, it was clearly demonstrated that the combination of clofarabine and cytarabine significantly improved response rates and EFS.

The combination regimen of clofarabine and high-dose cytarabine with G-CSF priming (GCLAC) was tested in a phase 1–2 study in patients with relapsed or refractory AML [40]. The median age of the patients was 53 years. Most patients were treated at the maximum dose of clofarabine 25 mg/m^2 per day and cytarabine 2 g/m^2 beginning 4 h after the start of clofarabine for 5 days. G-CSF 5 μg/kg was given from the day before chemotherapy until neutrophil recovery. The 30-day mortality for GCLAC was 0%. CRs were seen in 21 of the 46 evaluable patients (46%) and the ORR was 61%. The authors demonstrated that CR rates were considerably higher among relapsed patients whose first CR durations had exceeded 6 months. Median survival for all 50 patients was 9 months with 17 patients remaining alive after a median follow up of 1.9 years since beginning GCLAC. Thirteen of these 17 received HSCT after treatment with GCLAC. The authors showed that GCLAC is highly active in relapsed and refractory AML.

Given the positive clinical activity of GCLAC in relapsed or refractory AML, this regimen was retrospectively compared to fludarabine at 30 mg/m^2 and cytarabine 2 g/m^2 both daily for 5 days with (FLAG) or without (FA) G-CSF priming [41]. It was shown that after accounting for the duration of first complete remission, salvage number, age, and cytogenetics, GCLAC was associated with a higher CR rate and longer OS. Despite the retrospective nature of the analyses, the authors concluded that GCLAC may be superior to FA/FLAG, particularly in patients with short duration of first complete remission or unfavorable cytogenetics.

The combination of clofarabine and high-dose cytarabine was evaluated in 21 AML patients with refractory or relapsed disease [42]. The median age of the patients was 45 years (range, 22–62 years). The treatment comprised intravenous clofarabine (40 mg/m^2/day) and intravenous cytarabine (1–2 g/m^2/day) starting 4 h after clofarabine infusion for five consecutive days. Patients in CR could receive further consolidation chemotherapy with clofarabine + cytarabine, high-dose cytarabine, or allogeneic HSCT. CR was achieved in 42.9% of the patients. The authors demonstrated that although the small number of the cases, CR could be achieved only in relapsed or refractory AML receiving clofarabine in combination of cytarabine at 2 g/m^2/day.

Another dose combination of clofarabine and cytarabine was tested in high-risk AML patients who relapsed or failed to respond to at least two induction therapies [43]. The study was conducted on 47 patients with median age of 50.5 years (range, 21–71 years). The therapy consisted of clofarabine 22.5 mg/m^2 given i.v., followed after 3 h by intravenous cytarabine at 1 g/m^2 daily for five consecutive days. Patients achieving CR or partial response (PR) were slated to receive a further consolidation cycle with clofarabine at 22.5 mg/m^2 and cytarabine at 1 g/m^2 on days 1 through 4. Induction mortality was 13%. Among all patients, ORR was 61.5% – 24 (51%) achieved a CR and another five patients (10.5%) had a PR. Notably, among the 24 patients, 13 patients underwent allogeneic HSCT. Given the poor prognosis of these patients, combination therapy of clofarabine and cytarabine definitely represented a "bridge" to transplantation.

The combination of clofarabine and high-dose cytarabine was tested in 35 refractory or relapsed AML patients, at a median age of 39.4 years (range, 21–60 years), treated in our institution [44]. Clofarabine was given 40 mg/m^2 daily i.v. for five consecutive days (days 2–6) followed 4 h later by cytarabine 1 or 2 g/m^2 administered i.v. for five consecutive days (days 1–5). Eighteen patients (51.4%) achieved CR, whereas thirteen patients (37.1%) had resistant disease, and four (11.4%) died during induction. In patients with CR, 55.6% (10/18) were able to proceed to allogeneic HSCT. The 24-month OS for the whole patients' cohort was 28.8%. We concluded that clofarabine in combination with cytarabine is effective in refractory and relapsed AML patients, and it represents a useful remission induction strategy to serve as a bridge to transplantation in these patients.

2.1.2.2. Clofarabine monotherapy

A phase 2 clinical and pharmacologic study of clofarabine in patients with refractory or relapsed acute leukemia was performed [22]. The study included 62 patients of which 50% had AML. Clofarabine was administered intravenously at 40 mg/m^2 over 1 h daily for 5 days every 3 to 6 weeks. CR was achieved in 42% of the patients whereas ORR (CR+CRi) was 55%. Response rates were higher in patients with longer first CR durations.

2.2. Clofarabine and hematopoietic stem cell transplantation

Over the past few years, the potential role of clofarabine has been studied also as a cytoreduction therapy for patients candidate to transplant and within different conditioning regimens.

2.2.1. Clofarabine as a cytoreductive agent for patients candidate to transplant

The feasibility of a cytoreductive strategy based on clofarabine before allogeneic SCT for refractory AML was specifically explored [45]. Clofarabine 30–40 mg/m^2 i.v. daily for 5 days was administered in 17 patients with plans to initiate conditioning during the nadir, 14 days later. Bone marrow biopsy 12 days after clofarabine showed effective cytoreduction in 59% of the patients which correlated with higher progression-free survival (PFS) and OS. The toxicity of the regimen was acceptable. Sixteen patients received their hematopoietic stem cell infusion at a median of 22 days after starting clofarabine. Transplant-related mortality at day 100 and 2-year was 6 and 36% respectively, while 1 year PFS and OS were 25 and 38%, respectively. These results showed that clofarabine cytoreduction followed by immediate HSCT is feasible with acceptable toxicity and transplantation-related mortality (TRM).

A retrospective analysis was performed in order to evaluate the antileukemic efficacy and toxicity of clofarabine-based chemotherapy followed by reduced-intensity conditioning (RIC) and allogeneic SCT for high-risk, relapsed, or refractory AML or MDS [46]. A total of 27 patients underwent allogeneic SCT after treatment with clofarabine and cytarabine for 5 days and RIC based on 4 Gy total body irradiation, cyclophosphamide, and anti-thymocyte globulin (ATG). Prophylaxis of graft-versus-host disease (GvHD) consisted of cyclosporine and mycophenolate mofetil. Most transplants were performed from peripheral blood stem cells and unrelated donors. The rates of OS and RFS were 56 and 52% at 2 years, respectively. Clofarabine-based chemotherapy followed by RIC showed good antileukemic efficacy even in patients with high-risk AML or MDS, with engraftment and GvHD-incidence comparable to other RIC regimens.

A retrospective study was performed to evaluate the feasibility and anti-leukemic activity of a sequential therapy using clofarabine for cytoreduction followed by conditioning for haploidentical HSCT in patients with non-remission acute leukemia [47]. Patients received clofarabine (5 × 30mg/m^2 i.v.) followed by a T cell replete haploidentical transplantation for AML (n = 15) or ALL (n = 3). Conditioning consisted of fludarabine, cyclophosphamide plus either melphalan, total body irradiation or treosulfan/etoposide. High-dose cyclophosphamide was administered for post-grafting immunosuppression. Neutrophil engraftment was achieved in

83% and complete remission in 78% at day +30. The toxicity of the regimen was acceptable and the non-relapse mortality (NRM) at 1 year was 23%. The estimated OS and RFS at 1 year from haploidentical HSCT were 56 and 39%, respectively. The concept of a sequential therapy using clofarabine for cytoreduction followed by haploidentical HSCT proved to be feasible and allows successful engraftment, while providing an acceptable toxicity profile and anti-leukemic efficacy in patients with advanced acute leukemia.

Very recently, the combination of clofarabine 30 mg/m^2 and cytarabine 1 g/m^2 on days 1–5 (CLARA) was tested on 84 patients with relapsed or refractory AML with median age of 61 years (range, 40–75) [48]. Patients with a donor received HSCT in aplasia after first CLARA. In case of a prolonged donor search, HSCT was performed as soon as possible. The conditioning regimen consisted of clofarabine 30 mg/m^2, day -6 to -3, and melphalan 140 mg/m^2 on day -2. In patients with partially matched unrelated donors, ATG at a cumulative dose of 4.5 mg/kg was recommended. GvHD prophylaxis consisted of cyclosporine and mycophenolate mofetil. Donors were HLA-identical siblings in eight cases (14%), HLA-compatible unrelated donors in 30 cases (55%), and unrelated donors with one mismatch in 17 cases (31%). ORR assessed at day 15 after start of CLARA was 80% while 31% of patients having less than 5% BM blasts at that time. Treatment success was achieved in 61% of the patients. With a median follow-up of 25 months, OS and leukemia-free survival (LFS) for all enrolled patients at 2 years was 42 and 52%, respectively. At the time of enrollment, 14% of patients had a related donor and 33% had an unrelated donor available. In 46% of the patients, donor search was initiated at the time of enrollment. The OS at 2 years for patients with a related or an unrelated donor available was 75 and 47%, respectively, while it was 29% for patients for whom donor search was initiated at the time of enrollment.

2.2.1.1. Clofarabine in different conditioning regimens

Given the evidence of clinical activity of clofarabine and cytarabine in induction therapy of AML patients, a RIC regimen containing both drugs was explored in AML and MDS patients [49]. Seven patients were enrolled. Their median age was 54 years; three were with MDS and four with AML. The treatment plan consisted of clofarabine 40 mg/m^2 i.v. and cytarabine 1 g/m^2 i.v. both on days –6 to –2 and ATG 1 mg/kg on day –4 and 2.5 mg/kg on days –3 and –2. The median duration of neutropenia was 14 days and that of thrombocytopenia was 22 days. No acute GVHD was observed. Enrollment to the trial was halted due to unacceptable high mortality. The high mortality rate was caused by the insufficiently immunosuppressive activity of the regimen to ensure engraftment.

In order to improve the immunosuppressive activity of clofarabine and cytarabine combination as a conditioning regimen, the addition of cyclophosphamide, busulfan, and ATG was performed [50]. A phase 2 prospective multicenter trial aimed to assess the efficacy and safety of a sequential conditioning regimen was conducted. Twenty-seven AML patients in primary induction failure were included. The treatment consisted of clofarabine 30 mg/m^2/d for 5 days, cytarabine 1g/m^2/d for 5 days, and after a 3 days rest, cyclophosphamide 60 mg/kg/d for 1 day, IV busulfan 3.2 mg/kg/d for 2 days, and ATG 2.5 mg/kg/d for 2 days. For GVHD prophylaxis, patients received cyclosporine alone in case of a family donor, and cyclosporine + mycophenolate mofetil in case of an HLA-matched unrelated donor. The cumulative incidence of disease progression and NRM at 1 and 2 years were 46, 59, 8, and 13%, respectively. The OS and LFS at 1 and 2 years were 54, 37, 46, and 28%, respectively.

Clofarabine had been tested in many other combination therapies in the context of conditioning regimens. A phase 1 trial was conducted to determine the MTD of clofarabine with high-dose busulfan followed by allogeneic SCT in patients with high-risk and refractory acute leukemia, most of which are with AML [51]. A total of 15 patients, median age 48 (30–58) years were included in the study. Patients received intravenous busulfan 0.8 mg/kg every 6 h on days −6 to −3 and clofarabine 30–60 mg/m^2 per day on days −6 to −2. Graft-versus-host disease prophylaxis included sirolimus plus tacrolimus. All the patients engrafted, and the MTD was not reached. One-year EFS and OS were 53 and 60%, respectively.

Very recently, clofarabine busulfan 4 (Clo/Bu4) conditioning regimen was compared in AML patients with active disease with standard conditioning regimens (cytoxan/total body irradiation (Cy/TBI) or fludarabine/busulfan (Flu/Bu). The study included 16 patients whose outcomes were compared to those of 16 historical controls. RFS at 1 year for the Clo/Bu4 and control patients was 79 and 19%, respectively. OS in the Clo/Bu4 and control groups is 81 and 25%, respectively [52]. While more than half of the patients experienced some level of GvHD, most cases remained mild to moderate in both acute and chronic presentations.

The addition of clofarabine to combination of fludarabine and busulfan was tested as pretrnsplant conditioning for advanced AML and MDS [53]. Patients were randomized between four different arms combining different dosages of nucleoside analogs followed on each day by busulfan infused to a specific pharmacokinetically targeted daily area under the curve. Fifty-one patients with a median age of 45 years have been enrolled with a minimum follow-up exceeding 100 days. The prophylaxis of GvHD consisted of tacrolimus and mini-methotrexate (MTX) ± low-dose rabbit-ATG. All patients engrafted and despite that forty-one patients had active leukemia at the time of transplant, CR was achieved in 85%. The projected median OS was 23 months.

A phase 1 study combining escalating doses of clofarabine with high-dose melphalan as RIC for allogeneic SCT was conducted in adult AML patients [54]. Sixteen patients with median age of 63 years were included in the study. Two patients died during dose escalation. All other patients demonstrated complete engraftment by day 30 with a median time to absolute neutrophil and platelet count recovery of 14 and 16 days, respectively. Only two patients relapsed and four patients died with a median follow-up of 17 months.

The combination of clofarabine–melphalan–alemtuzumab had been tested as a conditioning regimen for patients with advanced hematologic malignancies phase 1–2 study [55]. No DLT was observed in the phase 1 study and clofarabine 40 mg/m^2 for 5 days, melphalan 140 mg/m^2 for 1 day, and alemtuzumab 20 mg for 5 days were adopted for the phase 2 study. Seventy two patients with a median age of 54 years were included in the study of which 44 had AML or MDS. All evaluable patients engrafted. Median neutrophil and platelet recovery time was 10 and 18 days, respectively. At 1 year, the cumulative incidence of TRM, cumulative incidence of relapse, OS, and PFS were 26, 29, 59, and 45%, respectively. The main toxicity in the phase 2 study was rapid-onset renal, which was observed more frequently in older patients and those with baseline decrease in glomerular filtration rate. In 21% of the patients treated at the phase 2 doses was observed grade 3–5 renal toxicity.

http://dx.doi.org/10.5772/61435

3. Conclusion

Clofarabine exhibits efficacy in AML patients as a single agent and in combination with other cytotoxic drugs. Regarding older AML patients, first-line clofarabine monotherapy is associated with similar efficacy and potentially lower induction mortality compared with intensive chemotherapy regimens. Therefore, it may be an appropriate alternative treatment option for older patients with decreased PS or those who are unable to tolerate an anthracycline.

Clofarabine combinations with cytarabine and idarubicine provided encouraging results in untreated younger AML patients. Clofarabine containing induction regimens yielded an impressive CR/CRi rate, low mortality rate, and high OS at 1 year [23,24].

Combinations of clofarabine and cytarabine as a second-line therapy have offered promising results showing ORR ranging between 47% in elderly subjects and 61% in younger patients [32,40,43].

Another important aspect of clofarabine implementation is the transplantation strategy – as a cytoreductive agent for patients candidates to transplant and within conditioning regimens [45–50,52]. Considering that in most studies clofarabine has shown a possible impact on response rates and DFS but not on OS, one of the best possible achievements offered by this drug could be the opportunity to bring more patients to SCT with a good disease control, especially in subjects treated in second line [15].

These data confirm that clofarabine could be a useful option in the induction, reinduction, and transplantation therapy of AML patients.

Author details

Branimir Spassov[1,4*], Gueorgui Balatzenko[2,4], Georgi Mihaylov[1,4] and Margarita Guenova[3,4]

*Address all correspondence to: branispassov@gmail.com

1 National Specialized Hospital for Active Treatment of Hematological Diseases, Department of Clinical Hematology, Sofia, Bulgaria

2 National Specialized Hospital for Active Treatment of Hematological Diseases, Laboratory of Cytogenetics and Molecular Biology, Sofia, Bulgaria

3 National Specialized Hospital for Active Treatment of Hematological Diseases, Laboratory of Hematopathology and Immunology, Sofia, Bulgaria

4 Center of Excellence – Translational Research in Haematology, National Specialized Hospital for Active Treatment of Haematological Diseases, Sofia, Bulgaria

References

[1] Jan M, Majeti R. Clonal evolution of acute leukemia genomes. Oncogene 2013;10;32(2):135–40.

[2] O'Donnell MR, Abboud CN, Altman J, et al. Acute myeloid leukemia. J Natl Compr Canc Netw 2011;9:280–317.

[3] Fernandez HF, Sun Z, Yao X, et al. Anthracycline dose intensification in acute myeloid leukemia. N Engl J Med 2009;361:1249–59.

[4] Mandelli F, Vignetti M, Suciu S, et al. Daunorubicin versus mitoxantrone versus idarubicin as induction and consolidation chemotherapy for adults with acute myeloid leukemia: The EORTC and GIMEMA Groups Study AML-10. J Clin Oncol 2009;27:5397–403.

[5] Burnett AK, Hills RK, Milligan DW, et al. Attempts to optimize induction and consolidation treatment in acute myeloid leukemia: results of the MRC AML12 trial. J Clin Oncol 2010;28:586–95.

[6] Holowiecki J, Grosicki S, Robak T, et al. Addition of cladribine to daunorubicin and cytarabine increases complete remission rate after a single course of induction treatment in acute myeloid leukemia. Multicenter, phase III study. Leukemia 2004;18:989–97.

[7] Ohtake S, Miyawaki S, Fujita H, et al. Randomized study of induction therapy comparing standard-dose idarubicin with high-dose daunorubicin in adult patients with previously untreated acute myeloid leukemia: the JALSG AML201 study. Blood 2011;117:2358–65.

[8] Lowenberg B, van Putten W, Theobald M, et al. Effect of priming with granulocyte colony-stimulating factor on the outcome of chemotherapy for acute myeloid leukemia. N Engl J Med 2003;349:743–52.

[9] Pastore D, Specchia G, Carluccio P, Liso A, Mestice A, Rizzi R, Greco G, Buquicchio C, Liso V. FLAG-IDA in the treatment of refractory/relapsed acute myeloid leukemia: single-center experience. Ann Hematol 2003 Apr;82(4):231–5.

[10] Tallman MS, Gilliland DG, Rowe JM: Drug therapy for acute myeloid leukemia. Blood 2005;106:1154–63.

[11] Büchner T, Berdel WE, Haferlach C, et al. Age-related risk profile and chemotherapy dose response in acute myeloid leukemia: a study by the German Acute Myeloid Leukemia Cooperative Group. J Clin Oncol 2009;27:61–9.

[12] Estey E. Acute myeloid leukemia and myelodysplastic syndromes in older patients. J Clin Oncol 2007;25:1908–15.

[13] Roboz GJ. Treatment of acute myeloid leukemia in older patients. Expert Rev Anticancer Ther 2007;7:285–95.

[14] Montgomery JA, Shortnacy-Fowler AT, Clayton SD, Riordan JM, et al. Synthesis and biologic activity of 20-fluoro-2-halo derivatives of 9-b-D-arabinofuranosyladenine. J Med Chem 1992;35:397–401.

[15] Fozza C. The role of Clofarabine in the treatment of adults with acute myeloid leukemia. Crit Rev Oncol Hematol 2015Mar;93(3):237–45.

[16] King KM, Damaraju VL, Vickers MF, Yao SY, Lang T, Tackaberry TE, et al. A comparison of the transportability, and its role in cytotoxicity, of clofarabine, cladribine, and fludarabine by recombinant human nucleoside transporters produced in three model expression systems. Mol Pharmacol 2006;69:346–53.

[17] Sjoberg AH, Wang L, Eriksson S. Substrate specificity of human recombinant mitochondrial deoxyguanosine kinase with cytostatic and antiviral purine and pyrimidine analogs. Mol Pharmacol 1998;53:270–3.

[18] Xie C, Plunkett W. Metabolism and actions of 2-chloro-9-(2-deoxy-2-fluoro-beta-D-arabinofuranosyl)-adenine in human lymphoblastoid cells. Cancer Res 1995;55:2847–52.

[19] Zhenchuk A, Lotfi K, Juliusson G, Albertioni F. Mechanisms of anti-cancer action and pharmacology of clofarabine. Biochem Pharmacol. 2009 Dec 1;78(11):1351–9.

[20] Tran H, Yang D. Clofarabine in the treatment of newly diagnosed acute myeloid leukemia in older adults. Ann Pharmacother 2012 Jan;46(1):89–96.

[21] Tiley S, Claxton D. Clofarabine in the treatment of acute myeloid leukemia in older adults. Ther Adv Hematol 2013 Feb;4(1):5–13.

[22] Kantarjian HM, Gandhi V, Kozuch P, Faderl S, Giles F, Cortes J, et al. Phase I clinical and pharmacology study of clofarabine in patients with solid and hematologic cancers. J Clin Oncol 2003;21:1167–73.

[23] Willemze R, Suciu S, Muus P, et al. Clofarabine in combination with a standard remission induction regimen (cytosine arabinoside and idarubicin) in patients with previously untreated intermediate and bad-risk acute myelogenous leukemia (AML) or high-risk myelodysplastic syndrome (HR-MDS): phase I results of an ongoing phase I/II study of the leukemia groups of EORTC and GIMEMA (EORTC GIMEMA06061/AML-14A trial). Ann Hematol 2014;93:965–75.

[24] Selleslag D, Suciu S, Meloni G, Muus P, Halkes C, Venditti A, Ramadan S, Pruijt H, Meert L, Vignetti M, Marie J-P, Bron D, MD, de Witte T12, Amadori S, Willemze R, Frederic Baron F. Clofarabine in Combination with a Standard Remission Induction Regimen in Patients 18-60 Years Old with Previously Untreated Intermediate and Bad Risk Acute Myelogenous Leukemia (AML) or High Risk Myelodysplasia (MDS):

Combined Phase I/II Results of the EORTC/Gimema AML-14A Trial. (Abstract 3675;56th congress of ASH; December 6–9, 2014).

[25] Cooper T, Ayres M, Nowak B, et al. Biochemical modulation of cytarabine triphosphate by clofarabine. Cancer Chemother Pharmacol 2005;55:361–8.

[26] Kantarjian H, Gandhi V, Cortes J, et al. Phase 2 clinical and pharmacologic study of clofarabine in patients with refractory or relapsed acute leukemia. Blood 2003;102:2379–86.

[27] Faderl S, Verstovsek S, Cortes J, et al. Clofarabine and cytarabine combination as induction therapy for acute myeloid leukemia (AML) in patients 50 years of age or older. Blood 2006;108:45–51.

[28] Becker PS, Medeiros BC, Stein AS, Othus M, Appelbaum FR, Forman SJ, Scott BL, Hendrie PC, Gardner KM, Pagel JM, Walter RB, Parks C, Wood BL, Abkowitz JL, Estey EH. Am J Hematol 2014 Dec 24. doi: 10.1002/ajh.23927. [Epub ahead of print].

[29] Nazha A, Kantarjian H, Ravandi F, et al. Clofarabine, idarubicin, and cytarabine (CIA) as frontline therapy for patients≤60 years with newly diagnosed acute myeloid leukemia. Am J Hematol 2013;88:961–6.

[30] Faderl S, Ravandi F, Huang X, et al. A randomized study of clofarabine versus clofarabine plus low-dose cytarabine as front-line therapy for patients aged 60 years and older with acute myeloid leukemia and high-risk myelodysplastic syndrome. Blood 2008;112:1638–45.

[31] , Montesinos P, Oriol A, Salamero O, Vidriales B, Bergua J, Herrera P, Vives S, Sanz J, Carpio C, Rodríguez-Veiga R, Moscardó F, Sanz MA. Phase II trial to assess the safety and efficacy of clofarabine in combination with low-dose cytarabine in elderly patients with acute myeloid leukemia. Ann Hematol 2014 Jan;93(1):43–6.

[32] Faderl S, Ravandi F, Huang X, et al. Clofarabine plus low-dose cytarabine followed by clofarabine plus low-dose cytarabine alternating with decitabine in acute myeloid leukemia frontline therapy for older patients. Cancer 2012;118:4471–7.

[33] Daskalakis M, Nguyen TT, Nguyen C, et al. Demethylation of a hypermethylated P15/INK4B gene in patients with myelodysplastic syndrome by 5-Aza-2_-deoxycytidine (decitabine) treatment. Blood 2002;100:2957–64.

[34] Vigil CE, Tan W, Deeb G, et al. Phase II trial of clofarabine and daunorubicin as induction therapy for acute myeloid leukemia patients greater than or equal to 60 years of age. Leuk Res 2013;37:1468–71.

[35] Kantarjian HM, Erba HP, Claxton D, et al. Phase II study of clofarabine monotherapy in previously untreated older adults with acute myeloid leukemia and unfavorable prognostic factors. J ClinOncol 2010;28:549–55.

[36] Burnett AK, Russell NH, Kell J, et al. European development of clofarabine as treatment for older patients with acute myeloid leukemia considered unsuitable for intensive chemotherapy. J Clin Oncol 2010;28:2389–95.

[37] Burnett AK, Russell NH, Hunter AE, et al. Clofarabine doubles the response rate in older patients with acute myeloid leukemia but does not improve survival. Blood 2013;122:1384–94.

[38] Faderl S, Gandhi V, O'Brien S, et al. Results of a phase 1–2 study of clofarabine in combination with cytarabine (ara-C) in relapsed and refractory acute leukemias. Blood 2005;105:940–7.

[39] Faderl S, Wetzler M, Rizzieri D, et al. Clofarabine plus cytarabine com-pared with cytarabine alone in older patients with relapsed or refractory acute myelogenous leukemia: results from the CLASSIC I Trial. J Clin Oncol 2012;30:2492–9.

[40] Becker PS, Kantarjian HM, Appelbaum FR, et al. Clofarabine with high dose cytarabine and granulocyte colony-stimulating factor (G-CSF) priming for relapsed and refractory acute myeloid leukaemia. Br J Haematol 2011;155:182–9.

[41] Becker PS, Kantarjian HM, Appelbaum FR, et al. Retrospective comparison of clofarabine versus fludarabine in combination with high-dose cytarabine with or without granulocyte colony-stimulating factor as salvage therapies for acute myeloid leukemia. Haematologica 2013;98:114–8.

[42] Tse E, Leung AY, Sim J, et al. Clofarabine and high-dose cytosine arabinoside in the treatment of refractory or relapsed acute myeloid leukaemia. Ann Hematol 2011;90:1277–81.

[43] Scappini B, Gianfaldoni G, Caracciolo F, et al. Cytarabine and clofarabine after high-dose cytarabine in relapsed or refractory AML patients. Am J Hematol 2012;87:1047–51.

[44] Spassov B, Balatzenko G, Angelova S, Toshkov S, Guenova M, Arnaudov G, Mihaylov G. Combination of clofarabine and cytarabine in the treatment of refractory or relapsed acute myeloid leukemia. (Abstract E943;20th congress of EHA; June 11–14, 2015).

[45] Locke FL, Artz A, Rich E, et al. Feasibility of clofarabine cytoreduction before allogeneic transplant conditioning for refractory AML. Bone Marrow Transplant 2010;45:1692–8.

[46] Buchholz S, Dammann E, Stadler M, et al. Cytoreductive treatment with clofarabine/ara-C combined with reduced-intensity conditioning and allogeneic stem cell transplantation in patients with high-risk, relapsed or refractory acute myeloid leukemia and advanced myelodysplastic syndrome. Eur J Haematol 2012;88:52–60.

[47] Tischer J, Stemmler HJ, Engel N, et al. Feasibility of clofarabine cytoreduction followed by haploidentical hematopoietic stem cell trans-plantation in patients with relapsed or refractory advanced acute leukemia. Ann Hematol 2013;92:1379–88.

[48] Middeke J, Herbst R, Parmentier S, Bug G, Hänel M, Stuhler G, Kerstin Schäfer-Eckart, Rösler W, Klein S, Bethge W, Bitz U, Alakel N, Schaich M, Morgner A, Kramer M, Platzbecker U, Röllig C, Thiede C, Ehninger G, Bornhäuser M, Schetelig J. Updated Results from the Bridge Trial: Long-Term Survival and Impact of Donor Availability – Clofarabine Salvage Therapy Prior to Allogeneic Hematopoietic Stem Cell Transplantation in Patients with Relapsed or Refractory AML. (Abstract 1204;56thcongress of ASH; December 6–9, 2014).

[49] Martin MG, Uy GL, Procknow E, et al. Allo-SCT conditioning for myelodysplastic syndrome and acute myeloid leukemia with clofarabine, cytarabine and ATG. Bone Marrow Transplant 2009;44:13–7.

[50] Mohty M, Malard F, Blaise D, Milpied N, Socie G, Huynh A, Oumedaly R, Yakoub-Agha I, Furst S, Guillaume Th, Tabrizi R, Delaunay J, Moreau P, Labopin M, Chevallier P. Sequential Regimen of Clofarabine, Cytarabine and Reduced Intensity Conditioning (RIC) Prior to Allogeneic Stem Cell Transplantation (allo-SCT) for Acute Myeloid Leukemia (AML) in Primary Treatment Failure (Abstract 1228;56thcongress of ASH; December 6–9, 2014).

[51] Farag SS, Wood LL, Schwartz JE, et al. Phase I trial and pharmacokinetic study of high-dose clofarabine and busulfan and allogeneic stem cell transplantation in adults with high-risk and refractory acute leukemia. Leukemia 2011;25:599–605.

[52] Zebrowski A, Hanlon A, Mangan J, Martin J, Luger S, Loren A, Hexner E, Reshef R, Gill S, Smith J, Stadtmauer E, Porter D and Frey N. Clofarabine Busulfan Conditioning Improves Outcomes in Patients with Active Acute Myelogenous Leukemia Undergoing Allogeneic Stem Cell Transplant.(Abstract 1239;56thcongress of ASH; December 6–9, 2014).

[53] Andersson BS, Valdez BC, de Lima M, et al. Clofarabine± fludarabine with once daily i.v. busulfan as pretransplant conditioning therapy for advanced myeloid leukemia and MDS. Biol Blood Marrow Transplant 2011;17:893–900.

[54] Kirschbaum MH, Stein AS, Popplewell L, et al. A phase I study in adults of clofarabine combined with high-dose melphalan as reduced-intensity conditioning for allogeneic transplantation. Biol Blood Marrow Transplant 2012;18:432–40.

[55] van Besien K, Stock W, Rich E, et al. Phase I–II study of clofarabine-melphalan-alemtuzumab conditioning for allogeneic hematopoietic cell transplantation. Biol Blood Marrow Transplant 2012;18:913–21.

Chapter 7

Perspective on Therapeutic Strategies of Leukemia Treatment — Focus on Arsenic Compounds

Bo Yuan, Noriyoshi Iriyama, Xiao-Mei Hu,
Toshihiko Hirano, Hiroo Toyoda and Norio Takagi

Additional information is available at the end of the chapter

http://dx.doi.org/10.5772/60786

Abstract

Leukemia is a type of cancer of the body's blood-forming tissues, including the bone marrow and the lymphatic system. Treatments for leukemia are complex, depending upon the type of leukemia and other factors. Acute promyelocytic leukemia (APL) is a distinct subtype of acute myeloid leukemia (AML) and accounts for approximately 10-15% of all cases of AML in adults. Arsenic and its compounds are widely distributed in the environment and have been used medicinally for over 2,000 years. In fact, investigators from China and the USA have demonstrated that treatment with ATO (As_2O_3, As^{III}) results in complete remission in 90% of relapsed APL patients since mid-1990s. Moreover, As_2S_2 or As_4S_4, also known as realgar, has been gaining increasing attention and is traditionally used to treat certain types of hematological disorders including chronic myeloid leukemia (CML), AML, myelodysplastic syndrome (MDS) and MDS/AML in China. In this chapter, we first highlight the pharmacokinetics of ATO and realgar in leukemia patients and/or healthy volunteer. We will further summarize the detailed mechanisms underlying the cytocidal effects of these arsenic compounds. We also provide detailed insight into potential future clinical application of those promising candidates endowed with potent antitumor activities in view of combination with arsenic compounds.

Keywords: leukemia, arsenic trioxide, realgar, combination therapy, naturally derived substances

1. Introduction

Leukemia is a type of cancer of the body's blood-forming tissues, including the bone marrow (BM) and the lymphatic system. Treatments for leukemia are complex, depending on the type of leukemia and other factors. At present, treatment may include some combination of chemotherapy, radiation therapy, targeted therapy, and hematopoietic stem cell transplantation, in addition to supportive care and palliative care as needed.

Acute promyelocytic leukemia (APL) is a distinct subtype of acute myeloid leukemia (AML) and accounts for approximately 10–15% of all cases of AML in adults. Morphologically, it is identified as AML–M3 by the French–American–British classification. Cytogenetically, APL is characterized by a balanced reciprocal translocation between chromosomes 15 and 17, generating a promyelocytic leukemia (PML)/retinoic acid receptor α (RARα) fusion gene, which is thought to play a central role in the initiation of leukemogenesis [1–4]. The oncogenic fusion protein PML-RARα has been demonstrated to recruit corepressor (CoR) complexes containing nuclear receptor CoRs, histone deacetylases (HDACs), resulting in myeloid differentiation arrest observed in APL [5, 6]. An introduction of all-*trans* retinoic acid (ATRA) since 1986 has dramatically improved the outcome of treatment of this disease [5]. It has been reported that ATRA induces differentiation of APL cells through not only dissociating CoRs from the PML-RARα oncoprotein but also recruiting coactivators that possess histone acetylase activity [5–7]. For detailed mechanisms underlying the efficacy of ATRA, please refer to some excellent research and review articles [6, 8–11]. In fact, in 90% of *de novo* APL patients, administration of ATRA induces differentiation of leukemic blasts and clinical remission, and 70% of them have been cured by ATRA administration in combination with chemotherapy [4, 6, 12]. Due to its good clinical outcomes, ATRA is used as a first-line administration for *de novo* APL patients. Nevertheless, the remaining 30% of patients relapse and often become resistant to this conventional treatment [4, 6, 12].

Arsenic and its compounds are widely distributed in the environment and exist in organic and inorganic forms. There are three inorganic forms of arsenic: yellow arsenic (As_2S_3, also known as orpiment and Cihuang "female yellow" in China); red arsenic (As_2S_2 or As_4S_4, also known as realgar and Xionghuang"male yellow" in China); and white arsenic or ATO (As_2O_3, As^{III}), which is made by burning realgar or orpiment [6]. Although a well-known poison, arsenic has been used medicinally for over 2 000 years. Since the mid-1990s, investigators from China and the USA have demonstrated that treatment with ATO results in complete remission in 90% of relapsed APL patients [4, 13–15]. From then on, a dramatic clinical efficacy of ATO-based regimens against APL has been reported around the world. An impressive drug efficacy against APL led to its approval in the USA and in Europe under the brand name Trisenox for "the induction of remission and consolidation in patients with APL whose conditions are refractory to, or who have relapsed from retinoid and anthracycline chemotherapy, and whose APL is characterized by the presence of the t(15:17) translocation or PML-RARα gene expression" [13]. Moreover, As_2S_2 as another important arsenic compound has been gaining increasing attention and traditionally used to treat certain types of hematological disorders, including chronic myeloid leukemia (CML), AML, myelodysplastic syndrome (MDS) and MDS/AML in

China [16–18]. Although realgar has not yet been approved by the U.S. Food and Drug Administration (FDA) and other major countries for clinical use, it has become another research for focus following ATO due to its good therapeutic efficacy and perceived low toxicity [19, 20].

In this chapter, we first highlight the pharmacokinetics of ATO and realgar in leukemia patients and/or a healthy volunteer. We will further summarize the detailed mechanisms underlying the cytocidal effects of these arsenic compounds. We also provide detailed insight into potential future clinical applications of those promising candidates endowed with potent antitumor activities in view of combination with arsenic compounds.

2. Pharmacokinetics of arsenic compounds in leukemia patients

2.1. Pharmacokinetic studies of ATO in Peripheral Blood (PB)

It has been established that biomethylation, which primarily occurred in the liver [21, 22], is a major metabolic pathway for inorganic arsenic in human and many animal species [23], by which arsenic undergoes metabolic conversion by the reduction of As^{V} to As^{III} with subsequent methylation, yielding monomethylated and dimethylated metabolites [24, 25]. A postulated metabolic pathway is as follows: As^{V} → As^{III} → methylarsonic acid (MAs^{V}) → methylarsonous acid (MAs^{III}) → dimethylarsinic acid ($DMAs^{V}$) → dimethylarsinous acid ($DMAs^{III}$) (Figure 1). It has been demonstrated that, following arsenic exposure, 40–60% of arsenic intake is eliminated through urine. The standard profile of urinary arsenic in human is comprised of 10–30% inorganic arsenic, 10–20% monomethylated arsenic (MAs: MA^{III} + MA^{V}), and 60–80% dimethylated arsenic (DMAs: DMA^{III} + DMA^{V}) [26, 27].

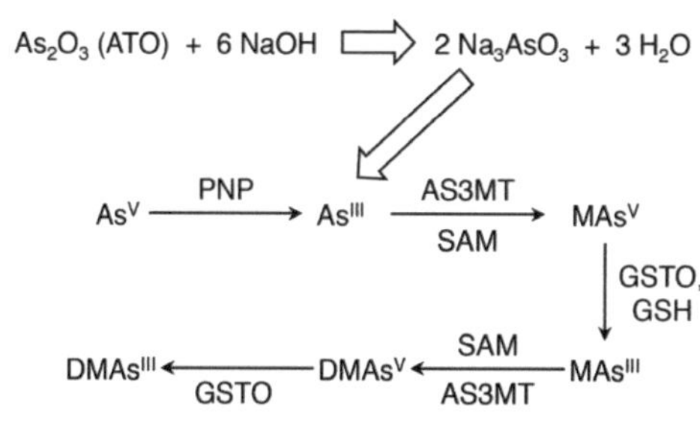

Figure 1. Postulated pathways of the biotransformation of arsenic in mammalian systems. Biomethylation, which primarily occurs in the liver, is a major metabolic pathway for inorganic arsenic in human and many animal species. In human, dimethylarsinous acid ($DMAs^{III}$) and dimethylarsinic acid ($DMAs^{V}$) appear to be the end products of this pathway [133]. In the pathway, arsenate reductases, such as the omega isoform of glutathione S-transferase (GSTO) and purine nucleoside phosphorylase (PNP), catalyse the reduction of arsenate species [4, 22]. Human arsenic (+ 3 oxidation state) methyltransferase (AS3MT) catalyse the methylation of arsenite [4, 22]. S-adenosylmethionine (SAM) is the methyl donor [4, 22].

In order to provide an effective treatment protocol for individual APL patients, detailed studies have been conducted on the pharmacokinetics of As^{III} in APL patients using biological samples such as peripheral blood (PB), cerebrospinal fluid (CSF), BM, and urine [14, 28–31]. Compared with a limited understanding of metabolic profiles of realgar and its pharmacokinetics, many detailed systematic analyses of the metabolites of ATO in blood cells and plasma of APL patients have been performed. In this regard, by using high-performance liquid chromatography (HPLC)/inductively coupled plasma mass spectrometry (ICP-MS), we have conducted studies on the total arsenic and speciation of ATO metabolites in an APL patient when 0.15 mg/kg/day was infused. Blood samples were obtained from the patient at various time points after remission induction therapy and during consolidation therapy [31]. Of note, biological samples, such as blood and urine, contain much higher concentrations of chloride ion, which interferes with arsenic detection at *m*/*z* 75 due to the formation of argon chloride ($^{40}Ar^{35}Cl^{+}$: *m*/*z* 75) in argon plasma [28, 32]. Therefore, arsenic was detected as the adduct ion of $^{75}As^{16}O^{+}$ (*m*/*z* 91), which is produced by the oxidization of arsenic in the oxygen atmosphere with the dynamic reaction cell techniques [31].

We first demonstrated that, in all blood samples collected either after the remission induction therapy or during the consolidation therapy, approximately 80–90% of the total arsenic in the blood samples was observed in the blood cells, suggesting that most of the blood arsenic is bound to hemoglobin [31]. These results are in good agreement with a previous report showing that 90% of blood arsenic is bound to hemoglobin [33]. These findings suggest that careful attention should be paid to profiles of total arsenic in blood cells and consequently provide valuable insight into clinical applications of As^{III}. We further clarified that, during the drug withdraw period, the amount of As^{V} in plasma was more readily eliminated among all arsenic metabolites [31], as reported by other groups [32, 34]. We also demonstrated that As^{III} concentrations in plasma initially declined more quickly than those of MAs^{V} and $DMAs^{V}$ [31]. These results suggest that methylated metabolites (MAs^{V} and $DMAs^{V}$) are major metabolites in plasma and are similar to those reported by other groups [23–25]. Furthermore, we demonstrated that the concentrations of methylated metabolites (MAs^{V} and $DMAs^{V}$) as well as inorganic arsenic (As^{III} and As^{V}) in plasma increased with multiple administration during the consolidation therapy period [31]. In comparison, Fujisawa et al. demonstrated no increase in the maximum concentrations of inorganic arsenic (As^{III} and As^{V}) despite multiple administrations, suggesting that inorganic arsenic plasma may reach a steady state after multiple administration [28]. It is noteworthy that only one of the 14 patients enrolled in the study of Fujisawa et al. was in the first relapse, and the remaining patients were in the second to fifth relapse [28]. In contrast, the patient in our study was in the first relapse [31]. Although the exact reason for the above-mentioned apparent differences in the profiles of the concentrations of inorganic arsenic (As^{III} and As^{V}) in the plasma of APL patients is not clear, the differences in patient characteristics may explain the discrepancy in the concentrations of inorganic arsenic. These results also suggest that understanding the differences in metabolism among patients is very useful for providing an effective treatment protocol for individual patients with leukemia.

2.2. Pharmacokinetic studies of ATO in the CSF

Although the central nervous system (CNS) relapse of APL occurs in 1–5% of patients, the optimal therapy for this case remains unclear [35, 36]. Fortunately, several clinical data have demonstrated that ATO seems to be capable of crossing the blood–brain barrier in humans and can be considered as an effective treatment strategy for the CNS relapse of APL [37–40]. We have recently determined the total arsenic and speciation of ATO metabolites in the CSF and PB plasma samples from three patients with APL who were treated with intravenous ATO as salvage therapy [0.15 mg/kg/day ATO + intrathecal chemotherapy (methotrexate + cytosine arabinoside + prednisolone)] [29]. In this study, PB was collected before and after the infusion, and the CSF was collected after the infusion, respectively. Furthermore, in order to prepare samples for arsenic speciation, the PB plasma was ultrafiltered with a 10-kDa molecular mass cutoff. The filtrates were thus defined as low-molecular-weight fraction (LMW-F) and subjected to arsenic speciation analysis. The remains trapped in filters were defined as high-molecular-weight fraction (HMW-F) and subjected to total arsenic determination [29]. We first demonstrated that not only inorganic arsenic (As^{III} and As^{V}) but also methylated arsenic metabolites (MAs^{V} and $DMAs^{V}$) existed in the CSF and that the total CSF arsenic concentrations ranged from 148 nM to 250 nM (mean: 199 nM) [29]. It has been demonstrated that ATO exerts a dual effect on APL cells; that is, ATO induces apoptosis at relatively high concentrations, ranging from 1 μM to 2 μM, whereas trends to promote differentiation of APL cells at low concentrations range from 0.1 μM to 0.5 μM [4, 6, 41]. Therefore, the beneficial effects of arsenic on the CNS relapse of APL patients might be attributed to its differentiation induction, rather than apoptosis induction. Furthermore, we found that the total PB plasma arsenic concentration is about twice of the sum of the amount of each arsenic metabolite present in LMW-F [29]. We also demonstrated that the total arsenic concentration in HMW-F accounted for approximately 50% of the total PB plasma arsenic concentration, suggesting that considerable amounts of arsenic species exist in clinical samples as a protein-bound complex.

Similar to previous reports showing that arsenic concentrations in the CSF were about 10% of those in whole blood or plasma [38, 40], we also demonstrated that the arsenic concentrations of the CSF were 8–17% of the plasma levels [29]. Taken together, it is possible to use a combination of arsenic with other chemotherapeutics to achieve a favorable clinical outcome in APL patients with CNS relapse, although a further larger scale randomized study must be conducted to reach a firm conclusion. It is noteworthy that Meng et al. have developed a non-invasive method via a concomitant with 20% mannitol intravenous bolus injection to help ATO enter into the CNS [42]. Their regimens include 125 ml of 20% mannitol bolus through the medial cubital vein at the rate of 12 ± 30 ml/min, followed with 250 ml of mixed solution (including 20% mannitol and ATO 0.08 mg/kg/day) through intravenous infusion at the rate of 6 ml/min, followed by ATO 0.08 mg/kg/day + 5% glucose 250-ml infusion at the rate of 0.5 ml/min in the total dosage of ATO (0.16 mg/kg/day) [42]. Compared with the general ATO intravenous infusion, the mannitol-assisted ATO penetration followed by the slow-speed continuous ATO intravenous infusion can not only increase the elemental arsenic concentration in the CNS but also keep the plasma arsenic at prolonged effective therapeutic levels without remarkable plasma arsenic peak. Therefore, the non-invasive method was supposed to be more beneficial to the CNS relapse of APL and increase the prevention and treatment efficiency of APL marrow relapse, as well as less side effects to normal tissues [42]. The same group has recently extended the application of the non-invasive method to additional patients [43]. They demonstrated that, in 16 of the 17 patients examined, abnormal blasts/promyelocytes from the CSF were eliminated in 18 to 32 days (median: 24 days) after the start of induction treatment and that all the patients tolerated the induction well. Importantly, there were no complaints of side effects associated with the use of mannitol [43]. Of note, over the course of the entire induction treatment process, the concentrations of arsenic in the blood and CSF were fairly stable in each patient. For each individual, the arsenic level in the CSF was ~99.7% of those in the paired blood samples, although the arsenic levels in different individuals were highly variable in the blood and CSF [43].

2.3. Pharmacokinetic studies of ATO in the BM

Although an initial report demonstrated that the total arsenic concentrations in the plasma of a BM sample from five relapsed APL patients were close to levels for differentiation induction, the analysis was conducted for the BM sample collected at only one collection time point [44]. Moreover, despite the fact that BM is a vital site for regulating the production of blood cells, no speciation analysis of arsenicals in the BM from APL patients undergoing long-term administration of ATO has been done before. In this regard, in order to gain more detailed information on the distribution of arsenic, we have recently investigated, for the first time, the arsenic speciation in the plasma of the BM and compared the arsenic speciation profiles between the PB and BM collected before and after the start of administration of 0.15-mg/kg/day ATO [30]. In this study, we first demonstrated a time-dependent increase of the total arsenic concentrations in the BM plasma, which was similar to that in the PB plasma. Furthermore, the total arsenic concentration levels tended to be higher in the BM plasma than those in the PB plasma, raising clinical concerns and inspiring us to unravel the detailed information on the distribution of arsenic as well as its speciation in these biological samples [30]. In this study, the concentrations of MAs^{V} and $DMAs^{V}$ substantially increased after the start of administration, whereas those of As^{III} were still kept at a low level until day 10, followed by a substantial increase from day 14 after the start of administration. As mentioned in Section 2.1, we have previously demonstrated that the PB plasma concentrations of both methylated arsenic metabolites (MAs^{V} and $DMAs^{V}$) and inorganic arsenic (As^{III} and As^{V}) remarkably increased after the start of administration in a Japanese APL patient undergoing consolidation therapy [31]. Compared with the APL patient in our previous study [31], the patient enrolled in this study appeared to have relatively higher metabolic efficiency, probably due to her relatively young age or without clinical complications. Collectively, our findings suggest that the efficiency of drug metabolism is obviously different in individual patients with different backgrounds, such as age range, with or without organ failure or disseminated intravascular coagulation (DIC), which, in turn, affect clinical outcomes and appearance of side effects. Of note, a close similarity of the arsenic speciation profiles between the PB and BM plasma was observed throughout the remission induction therapy, suggesting for the first time that the arsenic speciation analysis of the PB plasma could be predicative for BM speciation without applying BM aspiration [30]. Investigation of the total amount of arsenic in HMW-F trapped in a 10-kDa molecular mass cutoff filters further demonstrated that arsenic concentrations were much higher in the BM plasma than those in the PB plasma. One important biological effect of arsenic has been suggested to be mediated by reaction with closely spaced cysteine residues on a critical cell protein [45]. Several proteins such as tubulin, thioredoxin reductase, human arsenic methyltransferase (AS3MT, responsible for arsenic methylation) with a high cysteine content, and accessible thiol group are candidates for interactions with arsenic [4, 46]. In fact, arsenic bound to high molecular weight proteins (MW > 10-kDa) has been detected in livers and kidneys in rats after an intravenous injection of arsenite [47]. In view of the vital role of the BM microenvironment in maintaining the homeostasis of hematopoietic system, we assumed that a higher amount of proteins (MW > 10-KDa)-bound arsenic complex contributes to the protection effect from the attack of free arsenic species. Likewise, patients with low-proteinemia besides liver and/or renal dysfunctions might frequently develop arsenic-mediated side effects. Understandably, further investigation of the detailed information about these proteins is needed.

2.4. Pharmacokinetic studies of ATO in urine

The pharmacokinetic studies in APL patients have been well discussed by using urine samples [14, 28, 32, 48]. Previous studies on urinary arsenic excretion profiles demonstrated that there are large variations among individual patients with regard to the arsenic metabolic profiles and excretion patterns. For instance, an initial study demonstrated that urinary arsenic contents slightly increased during drug administration and the total amounts of arsenic excreted daily into the urine accounted for approximately 1–8% of the daily dose [14]. However, a previous report revealed that the mean total arsenic excretion rate including inorganic arsenic and methylated arsenic was about 20% of the daily dose on day 1 and remained at about 60% of the daily dose during subsequent weeks [28]. A clinical pharmacokinetic study performed in an APL patient showed that, in the urine sample collected for 24 h after administration of ATO, the total amount of inorganic arsenic and the methylated metabolites was almost 30% more of the daily dose [32]. Furthermore, Wang et al. [48] have demonstrated that there is an interindividual difference in excretion profiles and the relative concentrations of major arsenic species in the urine among four Chinese APL patients undergoing ATO treatment. In addition, other pathways of excretion, such as through the bile, have also been suggested to play a partial role in the elimination of arsenic [14, 48]. Therefore, systematic monitoring of the speciation of arsenic compounds in not only urine samples but also other biological samples such as the PB plasma has important implications for achieving favorable outcomes and minimizing side effects in leukemia patients treated with arsenic-based regimens.

2.5. Pharmacokinetic studies of realgar in leukemia patients as well as a healthy volunteer

Realgar has been widely used clinically in China [17, 18]. Moreover, an As_2S_2-containing formula, Qinghuang powder (QHP), was used as a folk medicine recorded in a famous traditional Chinese medicine (TCM) book, Shi Yi De Xiao Fang, published in 1345. Despite this, the systematic study on metabolic profiles of realgar and its pharmacokinetics have not yet been fully investigated. Compared with intravenous administration of ATO, oral administration of realgar is advantageous and would be more suitable for consolidation and maintenance therapy and consequently make better patient compliance and quality of life [16]. In this regard, Lu and colleagues designed a pilot study in which 129 APL patients with different disease stages were enrolled and received oral administration of highly purified crystalline realgar (As_4S_4) [19]. In this pilot study, encouraging responses such as high complete remission rate, long disease-free survival period, and tolerable side effects after oral administration of realgar alone were observed [19]. Furthermore, clinical pharmacokinetic studies on seven volunteers with APL and hematologic complete remission (HCR) by using 60 mg/kg oral As_4S_4 in a single dose demonstrated that arsenic could be detected in the blood 30 min after oral administration of As_4S_4. The peak time (T_{peak}) was 3.4 ± 1.4 h, and the maximum concentration (C_{max}) was 24.9 ± 8.0 μg/l. As expected, there was a wide interpatient variation in area under the concentration–time curve ($AUC_{0\text{-infinity}}$) (899.01 ± 705.64 μg/h per liter) and elimination half-life ($t_{1/2}$) (30.1 ± 11.1 h). These pharmacokinetic data revealed that rapid absorption of arsenic occurred after oral administration of As_4S_4 [19]. In addition, most urinary arsenic excretion occurred within the first 24 h. Measurement of blood arsenic levels in eight patients who were given oral As_4S_4 at a dosage of 50 mg/kg/day for 2 weeks followed by a break of 2 weeks during the first year of treatment demonstrated that blood arsenic levels declined during the drug withdraw period [19]. Arsenic concentrations in plasma and red cells were also measured in five patients with newly diagnosed APL and showed that the red-cell arsenic level was approximately two times higher than the plasma level, similar to the findings observed in an APL patient treated with ATO. Similar to the behavior of blood arsenic levels, urinary arsenic levels also quickly declined after discontinuation of As_4S_4. Of note, the arsenic level in the CSF in nine patients on the 10th day of treatment was 5.6–14.6 μg/l, a level similar to that in plasma, indicated that oral As_4S_4 is capable of penetrating into the CSF, suggesting the usefulness of As_4S_4 for the CNS relapse of APL [19]. These previous findings suggested that As_4S_4 treatment alone is highly effective and safe in both remission induction and maintenance therapy in patients with APL, regardless of disease stage.

Recently, the therapeutic effects of QHP have been evaluated in MDS patients with different karyotypes, including normal karyotype, trisomy 8 karyotype, and other cytogenetic abnormalities after receiving one to two 3-month courses of oral administration of QHP (containing realgar 0.16 g/capsule/day). Furthermore, the PB samples were collected 10–12 h after ingestion, and the total arsenic concentrations in the PB or PB plasma were determined using HPLC/ICP-MS. A positive correlation was found between the efficacy of QHP and total arsenic concentrations in the PB, but not in the PB plasma. Compared with patients with other cytogenetic abnormalities, much better clinical efficacy was observed in patients with normal or trisomy 8 karyotype, in agreement with our previous findings [49]. Surprisingly, no significant difference in the total arsenic concentrations in the PB was observed between the high-efficacy groups (patients with normal or trisomy 8 karyotype) and low-efficacy groups (patients with other cytogenetic abnormalities). Furthermore, no correlation between total arsenic concentrations in the PB or PB plasma and administration period was found in the study, suggesting that realgar might have a relatively low absorption/accumulation rate. Interestingly, compared with patients who did not receive oral administration of QHP, no apparent alteration in the mitochondria membrane potential ($\Delta\Psi m$) was found in primary blasts from the BM in patients treated with QHP. Moreover, among 28 patients treated with QHP, no correlation between $\Delta\Psi m$ and total arsenic concentrations in the PB was observed, suggesting that the mitochondria might not be the main target for QHP, although further detailed studies are obviously needed.

Currently, as much as 49 items among approximately 500 TCMs contain realgar [16]. Furthermore, there are 22 registered oral formulae containing realgar in the *Chinese Pharmacopoeia 2010*, which account for nearly 50% of the 49 realgar-containing formulae listed in the Pharmacopoeia [16]. Since TCM has been evolved and developed through long-term historical clinical practice, many TCMs are available over the counter. However, the lack of scientific evidence, especially in pharmacokinetics, results in a difficulty in its clinical application. In this regard, Koch and colleagues investigated the bioaccessibility (a surrogate measurement for bioavailability) and excretion of *Niu Huang Jie Du Pain* (translated as cow bezoar detoxifying pills), one of the most commonly used over-the-counter TCMs containing about 7% of arsenic in the form of realgar [50]. Analysis of the amount of arsenic available for absorption using three different bioaccessibility methods demonstrated that, although the total arsenic exist as high as 28 mg in a single pill, only 4% of it was available for absorption into the bloodstream (1 mg of arsenic per pill), suggesting that the bioaccessibility of realgar is very poor [50]. In fact, the poor bioaccessibility and/or bioavailability of realgar has also been reported by other researchers [51, 52]. Therefore, these observations raise the possibility that mild toxicity of the clinical application of realgar reported might be attributed to poor bioaccessibility and/or bioavailability, rather than its low toxic nature. Obviously, in order to draw a firm conclusion, more detailed studies are needed.

Koch and colleagues also evaluated arsenic concentrations and their speciation in urinary samples collected from a volunteer aged 70 years before and after ingestion of one pill of *Niu Huang Jie Du Pain*. [50]. The maximum value of the total arsenic species excreted after the ingestion of the one pill appeared approximately 14 h after ingestion, and methylated arsenic metabolites (MAs^{V} and $DMAs^{V}$) were the predominant species. The proportion of methylated arsenic metabolites in all arsenical species are in total agreement with previous arsenic metabolic profiles observed in other clinical samples, including the PB plasma, the CSF, and BM obtained from APL patients undergoing ATO treatment [4, 29–31], and healthy individuals who have drunk water containing inorganic arsenic [26, 27], reconfirming that biomethylation is a major detoxification pathway for inorganic arsenicals, regardless of different forms of arsenic. Interestingly, compared with previous findings showing that MAs^{III} and $DMAs^{III}$ have been detected in the urine of APL patients undergoing ATO treatment [48] and healthy individuals who have drunk water containing inorganic arsenic [25, 53], no traces of MAs^{III} and $DMAs^{III}$ were detected in the urine collected at any time after ingestion of one pill of *Niu Huang Jie Du Pain*, although two different HPLC/ICP-MS conditions, which were certified as the optimal condition for distinguishing MAs^{III} and $DMAs^{III}$ from other arsenic species, were used [50]. It is important to note that there should be some differences in metabolic profiles between taking a single dose or multiple doses. Since the aforementioned sampling of the urine was from a single individual who just took only one dose of *Niu Huang Jie Du Pain*, further research is desirable to study the more realistic exposure of multiple chronic doses, as well as to include more individuals to gain more statistical strength for populations consuming these medicines [50].

Due to the poor bioaccessibility and/or bioavailability of realgar mentioned above, realgar nanoparticles (NPs) were designed to improve its pharmacological and toxicological profiles [16]. It has been demonstrated that, compared with commercially used coarse realgar powder, realgar NPs with a size less than 200 nm prepared even by different methods show much higher efficiency in cytotoxicity associated with apoptosis induction and differentiation induction in leukemic cells such as HL-60 and U937 [54–57]. Although the detailed pharmacokinetic studies on realgar NPs have not yet been investigated in human beings, an *in vivo* bioavailability of realgar NPs prepared by cryo-grinding with polyvinylpyrrolidone (PVP) and/or SDS was evaluated in rats [58]. In this study, a remarkable increase in the urinary recovery of arsenic was observed in rats after a single oral administration of the cryo-ground realgar particle suspension. A range of 58.5–69.6% of the administered dose of arsenic was recovered in urine in the first 48 h from the PVP and/or SDS co-ground preparations; whereas the original realgar powder gave a urinary recovery of only 24.9%, suggesting that size reduction of realgar particles to nano levels could substantially enhance their bioavailability [58]. Furthermore, the cytotoxicity of the realgar NPs to human gynecological cell lines such as GI80-13S, Hela cells was comparable with the ATO observed previously [58]. Interestingly, realgar NPs were also found to be successfully delivered by transdermal administration, which gave more therapeutic efficiency than intraperitoneal administration in a model of treating melanoma skin tumor-bearing C57BL/6 mice, raising the possibility of its new clinical use [59].

It is well known that, besides administration of arsenic to patients in clinical practice, arsenic can also enter the body through food chains. The most common exposure to high levels of arsenic in food is through marine products in the form of arsenobetaine or plant products in the form of various arsenosugars [4]. Arsenobetaine, a trimethylarsenic compound, is one of the major organic arsenic in seafood and is not produced by the metabolism of As^{III} in human [34, 60]. Once arsenobetaine is ingested during periods of arsenic-based therapy, it will be excreted from the body in the same form and consequently interrupt the accuracy of evaluation of the pharmacokinetics of arsenic species. Therefore, controlling the daily diet, in particular seafood, during the periods of remission induction therapy and/or consolidation therapy is very important to accurately monitor the metabolic profiles of arsenic.

3. Mechanisms underlying the cytocidal effects of arsenic compounds

3.1. Involvement of oxidative stress in arsenic-mediated apoptosis induction

The remarkable clinical results achieved with ATO and realgar in relapsed as well as newly diagnosed APL patients have promoted investigations to determine the mechanisms underlying their activity. Accumulating evidence has shown that ATO exerts dose-dependent dual effects in APL cells such as NB4, with preferential apoptosis at relatively high concentrations ranging from 0.5 μM to 2.0 μM and partial differentiation at relatively low concentrations ranging from 0.1 to 0.5 μM [4, 61, 62]. The apoptosis-inducing effect is primarily associated with the mitochondrial-mediated intrinsic apoptotic pathway, whereas the extrinsic pathway through death receptors, such as the tumor necrosis factor receptor (TNFR) and Fas, have also been reported to be implicated in ATO-induced apoptosis in human leukemia, lymphoma, as well as glioma cell lines [63–65]. Moreover, a third pathway involving endoplasmic reticulum and caspase-12 has been reported to associate with ATO-mediated apoptosis in the chronic myeloid leukemia cell line K562 [66].

It has become clear that oxidative damage is one of the main mechanisms by which arsenic induces apoptosis [4, 6, 55, 61, 62, 67]. This idea is consistent with the binding capacity of arsenite to adjacent sulfhydryl (SH) groups present in many vital biomolecules [4, 6, 61, 62, 67] and also strongly supported by clinical data that levels of 8-hydroxy-2′-deoxyguanosine (8-OH-dGuo), one of the most abundant oxidative products of DNA, are increased in plasma from APL patients after remission induction and consolidation therapy with ATO [68]. Similar to ATO, realgar NPs also caused elevated urinary 8-OH-dGuo excretion in rats from day 1 after oral administration [69]. ATO has been demonstrated to disrupt mitochondrial respiration through blockading of electron flow at complex III and IV to elevate the generation of oxygen free radicals [70]. It has also been reported that reduced nicotinamide adenine dinucleotide phosphate (NADPH) oxidase-derived reactive oxygen species (ROS) are responsible for the susceptibility to arsenic cytotoxicity in leukemia cells [71, 72]. Furthermore, downregulation of the ROS elimination system, comprising glutathione (GSH), thioredoxin, and anti-oxidative enzymes including superoxide dismutase (SOD), catalase, as well as glutathione peroxidase (GPx), has been reported to be involved in cytocidal effects of arsenic compounds [73–78]. In line with these findings, GPx inhibitors such as mercaptosuccinic acid [79], catalase inhibitors such as 3-amino-1,2,4-trizaole [79], and SOD inhibitors such as 2-methoxyestradiol have been reported to potentiate the apoptosis-inducing activity of arsenic in NB4 cells as well as primary leukemia cells from patients with chronic lymphocytic leukemia [70, 73, 80]. Collectively, through not only enhancing the ROS production system but also impairing the ROS elimination system, arsenic compounds are able to induce intracellular ROS accumulation, which, in turn, activates apoptotic pathways in hematological cell lines including the APL cell line [41, 73, 74, 81–84].

3.2. Differentiation induction

In vitro and *in vivo* studies have demonstrated that a low-dose of ATO (0.1 ~ 0.5 μM) induces differentiation of NB4, a human APL cell line with t(15;17), as well as fresh APL cells [15, 81, 85]. Morphological changes such as condensation of chromatin, lobulation of nuclei, and the expression profiling of surface markers have been used as markers of the differentiation of APL cells [15, 81, 85]. Consistent with previous findings, we have recently demonstrated that 0.125 μM ATO also induced differentiation in HT93A cells, another t(15;17)-positive APL cell line established from the peripheral blood of a patient with APL [86], as evidenced by the appearance of jelly-bean-shaped nuclei in almost all cells, accompanied by a significant increase in CD11c and CD15 expression [87]. Furthermore, we demonstrated that As_2S_2 induced granulocyte differentiation in HL-60 cells, as evidenced by the increment in CD11b expression, in which oxidative stress associated with GSH depletion and p38 mitogen-activated protein kinase (MAPK) activation was involved [77, 84]. More interestingly, we have recently found that treatment with As_2S_2 induced erythroid differentiation in F36p, derived from MDS/AML, and HL-60 cells, as evidenced by a dose-dependent increase in the expression level of CD235a, a marker for the detection of the erythroid cell lineage [88, 89]. We further demonstrated that, although the alteration in the expression level of phosphorylated and total p38 MAPK was observed to some extent in parallel with As_2S_2-induced erythroid differentiation, no alteration was observed in the expression level of CD235a, regardless of the presence or absence of SB203580, a specific inhibitor for p38 MAPK, suggesting that p38 MAPK plays a small role in As_2S_2-induced erythroid differentiation in HL-60 cells [89]. Therefore, our findings suggest that p38 MAPK plays a critical role in As_2S_2-induced differentiation into granulocytes, rather than erythroid differentiation.

It has been demonstrated that higher DNA methylation levels at a few CpG sites in some erythroid specific genes correlated with a decreased erythroid differentiation capacity of K562 cells, which has been proposed as a very useful *in vitro* model system for studying erythroid differentiation [90, 91]. We have recently evaluate the effects of the As_2S_2-containing Chinese herbal formula QHP on the genomic methylation level in primarily diagnosed MDS patients [49], since MDS patients, especially those with high-risk MDS, have been reported to possess abnormal hypermethylation in tumor suppressor genes [92]. In this study, global DNA methylation detection (ChIP-on-chip assays) demonstrated that the number of hypermethylated genes decreased from 1,063 to 75 and that the methylated genes involved in multicellular organismal development, signal transduction, and apoptosis were demethylated after treatment with QHP [49]. We thus suggest that demethylation status, which might be resulted from As_2S_2 treatment, attributed to the above-mentioned erythroid differentiation of F36 and HL-60 cells, although further investigation of a correlation between erythroid differentiation and As_2S_2-triggered demethylation in these cells is needed to draw a more conclusive idea. Collectively, our findings provide a conceptual basis for the establishment of clinical protocols of As_2S_2 for the treatment of hematological disorders, in particular MDS and MDS/AML.

3.3. Degradation of PML-RARα

It is no doubt that PML-RARα plays a central role in the initiation of leukemogenesis, although there is evidence to suggest that the fusion gene expression is not the sole genetic event required for the development of APL [4–6]. It has been clarified that arsenic-mediated modulation/degradation of the PML-RARα oncoprotein is one of the major mechanisms responsible for the efficacy of arsenic compounds in APL [4–6, 93]. Furthermore, the PML moiety, but not the RARα moiety, of the PML-RARα chimera represents the target for arsenic treatment [6, 61]. It has been clarified that both PML and PML-RARα form high-molecular-weight conjugates with a small ubiquitin-related modifier (SUMO)-1 and are recruited from the nucleoplasm to the nuclear body (NB), followed by ubiquitin-mediated proteolysis [94–96]. Degradation of PML-RARα is closely associated with differentiation, growth inhibition associated with the induction of apoptosis, as well as cell cycle arrest in APL cells treated with arsenic compounds [4–6, 93]. In addition, degradation of the PML-RARα protein associated with its redistribution was also reported in fresh APL cells obtained from the PB and BM of APL patients after treatment with As_4S_4 [97]. More intriguingly, Tian and colleagues have recently investigated the effects of As_4S_4 on RA-resistant human APL NB4-R1 cells and found that treatment with As_4S_4 induced apoptosis in cells through the downregulation of expression of the SET gene, which is a natural inhibitor for protein phosphatase 2 (PP2A), a pro-apoptotic protein [93]. They further demonstrated that the addition of As_4S_4 strengthened the SET RNAi-induced upregulation of PP2A and the downregulation of PML-RARα, suggesting that As_4S_4 induces apoptosis through the downregulation of the SET protein expression, which, in turn, increases PP2A expression and reduces PML-RARα expression, consequently leading to the apoptosis of NB4-R1 cells [93].

4. Potential combination therapies with arsenic compounds

An extensive body of literature has clearly demonstrated superiority in treating APL simultaneously with ATO and ATRA [4–6, 61, 98]. It has been demonstrated that ATRA synergizes ATO activity to provide superior efficacy of combination therapy in patients by promoting the effects of ATO on several signaling pathways such as apoptosis induction, differentiation, as well as the degradation of PML-RARα [4–6]. In this regard, we have recently investigated the effects of ATO, ATRA, and the granulocyte colony-stimulating factor (G-CSF), alone or in combination, on the APL cell line HT93A by focusing on differentiation, growth inhibition, as well as arsenic uptake [87]. Our experimental data demonstrated that ATRA induced greater differentiation in cells than ATO and that G-CSF promoted differentiation-inducing activities of both ATO and ATRA [87]. Similar to a previous report showing that ATRA induced aquaporin-9 (AQP-9), which is a member of the aquaporin superfamily and proposed to be responsible for arsenic uptake [99–101], in HL-60 cells, we also demonstrated that ATRA induced AQP9 expression in a time- and dose-dependent manner in HT93A cells [87]. However, probably due to its cytotoxicity, treatment with 1 μM ATRA decreased arsenic uptake compared with the control subject. Interestingly, the addition of G-CSF recovered the reduced arsenic uptake to the same level as that in controls by increasing the number of viable cells, although G-CSF itself did not affect the expression levels of AQP9 [87]. Collectively, our results indicate that G-CSF not only promotes differentiation-inducing activities of both ATRA and ATO but also makes APL cells vulnerable to increased arsenic uptake, providing new insight into combination therapy using these three agents for the treatment of APL.

Since HDACs play a key role in the transcriptional regulation and pathogenesis of cancer [102, 103], its inhibitors (HDACi) are currently being developed for the therapy of several types of cancer, including leukemia [104]. Furthermore, aberrant recruitment of HDACs through the expression of PML-RARα has been implicated as an initiating tumorigenic event in APL [5–7]. Based on these previous findings, we hypothesized that treatment with ATRA in combination with HDACi could provide therapeutic benefit for patients with APL. In this regard, we investigated the effects of ATRA and valproic acid (VPA), alone and in combination, on the NB4 cells in view of differentiation induction and growth inhibition [105], since VPA is a member of class I HDACi and has shown potential anti-leukemic activities either alone or in combination with other anti-leukemic agents [102, 103, 106, 107]. In this study, we demonstrated that not only ATRA but also VPA induced differentiation in NB4 cells, and their combination further augmented the differentiation activity [105]. We further demonstrated that the upregulation of transcription factors, including CCAAT/enhancer-binding proteins (CEBPα, β, ε) and PU.1, which are known to be critical factors for normal myelopoiesis, granulocytic maturation, and being repressed in APL, concurred with the differentiation induction [105]. Given the importance of CEBPs and PU.1 in myeloid development, our results thus suggest that restoration of the normal function of the myeloid cell transcriptional machinery is a major molecular mechanism underlying the differentiation induction in NB4 cells [105]. It has been suggested that ATO/ATRA degrades the PML-RARα oncoprotein, resulting in the eradication of leukemia-initiating cells [108, 109]. Therefore, as a new therapeutic approach, a multi-target therapy based on a combination of ATRA, ATO, and VPA would be useful and worth evaluating further for its beneficial clinical effects.

Although advances in science and technology have replaced raw herbs and/or herbal compounds with powerful synthetic drugs, including molecular target-based drugs, in cancer therapy, the issue of concern is still resistance, disease relapse, and side effects of drugs in a clinical setting. In the case of arsenic compounds, side effects such as white blood cell count, QT prolongation, as well as liver dysfunction are still a serious concern and limit further clinical application, although the remarkable clinical efficacy of arsenic compound-based regimens against APL has been reported [4, 16]. Therefore, application of new arsenic-based therapies may require the generation of sensitizing strategies for improving the efficacy of arsenic compounds as well as minimizing their side effects. In order to optimize and/or maximize future clinical applications of arsenic compounds in patients with leukemia or even other malignancies, including solid tumors, combination therapy has attracted considerable interest as new therapeutic strategies. In this regard, we have been interested in the effects of naturally derived substances such as flavonoids on different kinds of cancerous cells, including leukemic cells [110–115]. Of these, Vitex, an extract from the ripe fruit of Vitex agnus-castus, has attracted great attention [112, 113, 115, 116]. We have investigated the effects of Vitex and its major component, casticin (Figure 2), on leukemia cell lines, HL-60 and U-937, and found that HL-60 cells were more sensitive to the cytotoxicity of Vitex/casticin compared with U-937 cells [112]. Furthermore, compared with unstimulated HL-60 cells, phorbol 12-myristate 13-acetate (PMA)- and 1,25-dihydroxyvitamin D3 (VD3)-differentiated HL-60 cells acquired resistance to Vitex/casticin. Based on the observation that the HL-60 cell line is more immature than the U-937 cell line, our results suggest that the levels of cytotoxicity of Vitex/casticin were largely attributed to the degree of differentiation of leukemia cells; that is, cell lines with less differentiated phenotype were more susceptible than the differentiated ones [112]. More importantly, much less cytotoxicity was observed in peripheral blood mononuclear cells (PBMNCs) from healthy volunteers when treated with concentrations of Vitex/casticin showing significant cytotoxicity in both leukemic cell lines [112]. Since recent studies have demonstrated that less differentiated cancer cells, referred to as leukemia stem cells (LSCs), acquired limitless self-renewal through oncogenic transformation and that the incomplete eradication of primary LSCs is closely linked to chemotherapy resistance and consequently contribute to eventual disease relapse [117], our findings thus provide fundamental insight into the clinical application of Vitex/casticin for hematopoietic malignancy in combination with arsenic compounds. We further demonstrated [113, 114] that Vitex/casticin-triggered cytotoxicity in HL-60 cells was implicated in histone H3 phosphorylation through the activation of the p38 MAPK pathway, which is a common signaling pathway involved in the mechanism underlying the cytocidal effects of arsenic compounds [4, 6, 16]. These findings suggest that Vitex/casticin could be promising candidates of adjunct therapeutic reagents for leukemia patients.

Delphinidin (Figure 2), a major anthocyanidin known to be present in pigmented fruits and vegetables, such as pomegranate, berries, dark grapes, eggplant, and red onion, is a diphenylpropane-based polyphenolic ring structure that carries a positive charge in its central ring [118]. Delphinidin has been gaining considerable attention, as it appears to possess a strong antioxidant/oxidant property as well as other potentially beneficial traits, such as anti-inflammatory, antimutagenesis, and antiangiogenesis activities [119, 120]. Furthermore, delphinidin and its glycosides have been demonstrated to trigger apoptosis in HL-60 cells

http://dx.doi.org/10.5772/60786

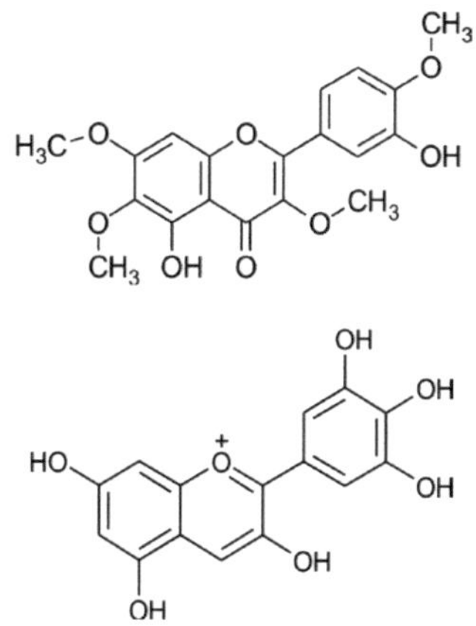

Figure 2. Chemical structures of casticin and delphinidin.

through a ROS/JNK-mediated mitochondrial death pathway [121, 122]. We have recently demonstrated that delphinidin exhibited a dose- and time-dependent cytotoxic effect against NB4 cells, in which intrinsic/extrinsic pathway-mediated apoptosis, but not cell cycle arrest, was involved (Yuan et al, submitted). We further demonstrated that delphinidin exerted more potent cytotoxicity against NB4 cells than normal PBMNCs and that delphinidin in combination with arsenite achieved an enhanced cytocidal effect against NB4 cells, but lesser on PBMNCs (Yuan et al, submitted). These results suggest that delphinidin selectively sensitizes NB4 cells to arsenite, resulting in an enhancement of arsenite cytotoxicity by strengthening intrinsic/extrinsic pathway-mediated apoptosis induction. Our observations may offer a rationale for the use of delphinidin to improve the clinical efficacy of arsenite.

Intriguingly, it has been revealed that flavonoids can inhibit the function of ATP-binding cassette transporters such as multidrug-resistance-associated proteins (MRPs) as well as P-glycoprotein (P-gp) [123, 124], which are known to be responsible for the efflux of arsenic and may consequently contribute to resistance to arsenic therapy [4, 125, 126]. In addition, we have recently demonstrated [101] that MRP2 and AQP9, which belongs to the aquaporin superfamily and is closely associated with arsenic uptake, contribute to the differential sensitivity of primary human-derived normal cells to arsenite using a unique *in vitro* primary cell culture system [79, 127, 128]. Therefore, the influence of naturally derived substances on the expression of transporters associated with intracellular arsenic accumulation should be taken into account during treatment in combination with arsenic compounds. More recently, by using human embryonic kidney epithelial (HEK) 293 cells overexpressing MRP4 cells, we have demonstrated (Yuan et al., manuscript in preparation) that MRP4, another member of ABC transporters, could be one of the major contributors to arsenic resistance, although further investigation into the correlation between the expression status of MRP4 and the treatment outcome of leukemia patients treated with arsenic-based regimens is needed.

In traditional medicines, including TCM, formulae consisting of more than one active ingredients are actually much more frequently used, aiming to act on more than one pharmacological targets and thus exerting synergistic therapeutic effects. One of the most successful models is the realgar–indigo naturalis formula (RIF), in which arsenic sulfide (A), indirubin (I), and tanshinone IIA (T) are three major components, and has been found effective against APL in China [16]. In this regard, Wang and colleagues performed the dissection of mechanisms of RIF using an APL murine model and APL cells, including NB4, NB4-R2 (ATRA-resistant NB4-derived cell lines), and primary leukemic cells from APL patients [129]. Their results not only indicated the functions of each component, e.g., A acted as a principal component, whereas I and T served as adjuvant ones, but also demonstrated the generation of expected synergistic effects in view of prolongation of the life span of treated mice, the efficiency of terminal differentiation induction, and the upregulation of APQ9 expression associated with increment in intracellular arsenic accumulation, without apparent severe side effects [129]. This study provides new insight into exploring the value of traditional formulae on a larger scale and helping to bridge Western and Eastern medicines in the era of systems biology. Besides, we also focused on the effects of products derived from the human body, such as progesterone (Pg), and demonstrated that Pg induced a dose- and time-dependent cell growth inhibition in A3 and I9.2 cells, both of which are subclones of a T-cell-derived leukemic Jurkat cell line [130]. We further suggested that growth suppression accompanied with the induction of apoptosis by Pg in these cells was mediated through the mitochondrial membrane disruption, followed by the activation of the caspase cascade [130]. These results provide a novel insight into Pg actions toward its use for clinical application in patients with lymphocytic T-cell leukemia and raise the possibility of combination with arsenic compounds.

5. Conclusions

A striking global *in vivo* and *in vitro* study on the treatment with arsenic compounds, alone or in combination, is being explored to understand detailed mechanisms underlying their efficiency in not only APL but also many other malignancies, including arsenic-resistant hematopoietic cancer or even solid tumors. Due to the higher reactivity and instability of trivalent methyl arsenic metabolites such as MAs^{III} and $DMAs^{III}$, a more accurate assessment of these metabolites in biological samples such as blood still need to be improved, although some preservatives, including diethyldithiocarbomate [48] and 2,3-dimercaptopropanesulph-onate [131], have been used to stabilize these metabolites in urine samples. As mentioned above, considerable amounts of arsenic species exist in clinical samples as a protein-bound complex. Although analysis of these protein-bound arsenic complexes has been conducted, the losses of these complexes from the sampling to the detection stage have not yet been resolved [131]. Therefore, the development of more applicable contemporary analytical protocols for these unstable arsenic species shall be explored. Furthermore, in order to achieve better therapeutic effects for individual APL patients and reduce side effects of arsenic compounds, not only detailed arsenic biomonitoring but also a predictive molecular biomarker for arsenic therapy is greatly desired. In this regard, we have recently investigated the correlation between the expression levels of AQP9 and sensitivity to ATO using NB4, HT93A, as well as primary APL cells from newly diagnosed and relapsed APL patients and provided

http://dx.doi.org/10.5772/60786

direct evidence that the expression of AQP9, rather than other biomarkers such as cell surface markers and chromosomal alteration, closely correlate with the sensitivity to ATO in both APL cell lines and primary blasts [132]. Our findings thus suggest that the AQP9 expression status of APL patients is a predictive marker for the successful outcome of ATO treatment. At the same time, we also showed that flow cytometry may be a new convenient and valuable tool for analyzing the AQP9 status of APL patients compared with current methods such as Western blotting [132]. Many naturally derived substances, including TCM, have been shown to be promising candidates endowed with potent antitumor activities in view of combination with arsenic compounds. In fact, many patients in Asian countries, especially those with end-stage cancer, prefer to choose traditional medicine therapy alone or in combination with chemotherapy, radiation therapy, as well as targeted therapy, aimed to palliate symptoms and improve the quality of life. Therefore, besides efforts in exploring the detailed molecular mechanism underlying their cytocidal effects against cancerous cells, systematic analyses aimed at understanding the pharmacology and toxicology profiles are eagerly awaited when used alone or in combination with other clinical drugs such arsenic compounds.

Acknowledgements

This work was supported in part by grants to Bo Yuan from the Japan–China Medical Association.

Author details

Bo Yuan[1,2*], Noriyoshi Iriyama[3], Xiao-Mei Hu[4], Toshihiko Hirano[5], Hiroo Toyoda[2] and Norio Takagi[1]

*Address all correspondence to: yuanbo@toyaku.ac.jp

1 Department of Applied Biochemistry, School of Pharmacy, Tokyo University of Pharmacy & Life Sciences, Horinouchi, Hachioji, Tokyo, Japan

2 Department of Clinical Molecular Genetics, School of Pharmacy, Tokyo University of Pharmacy & Life Sciences, Horinouchi, Hachioji, Tokyo, Japan

3 Department of Hematology and Rheumatology, Nihon University School of Medicine, Itabashi Hospital, Itabashi-ku, Tokyo, Japan

4 National Therapeutic Center of Hematology of Traditional Chinese Medicine, XiYuan Hospital, China Academy of Chinese Medical Sciences, Beijing, P. R. China

5 Clinical Pharmacology, School of Pharmacy, Tokyo University of Pharmacy & Life Sciences, Horinouchi, Hachioji, Tokyo, Japan

References

[1] de The H., Chomienne C., Lanotte M., Degos L., Dejean A. The t(15;17) translocation of acute promyelocytic leukaemia fuses the retinoic acid receptor alpha gene to a novel transcribed locus. Nature 1990; 347 558–561.

[2] Goddard A. D., Borrow J., Freemont P. S., Solomon E. Characterization of a zinc finger gene disrupted by the t(15;17) in acute promyelocytic leukemia. Science 1991; 254 1371–1374.

[3] Tong J. H., Dong S., Geng J. P., et al. Molecular rearrangements of the MYL gene in acute promyelocytic leukemia (APL, M3) define a breakpoint cluster region as well as some molecular variants. Oncogene 1992; 7 311–316.

[4] Yuan B., Yoshino Y., Kaise T., Toyoda H. Application of arsenic trioxide therapy for patients with leukemia. In: Sun, H.Z. (Ed.), Biological Chemistry of As, Sb and Bi. John Wiley & Sons, New York; 2011. p. 263–292. ISBN: 978-0-470-71390-7.

[5] Fang J., Chen S. J., Tong J. H., Wang Z. G., Chen G.Q., Chen Z. Treatment of acute promyelocytic leukemia with ATRA and As2O3: a model of molecular target-based cancer therapy. Cancer Biology & Therapy 2002; 1 614–620.

[6] Wang Z. Y., Chen Z. Acute promyelocytic leukemia: from highly fatal to highly curable. Blood 2008; 111 2505–2515.

[7] Zhang J. W., Wang J. Y., Chen S. J., Chen Z. Mechanisms of all-trans retinoic acid-induced differentiation of acute promyelocytic leukemia cells. Journal of Biosciences 2000; 25 275–284.

[8] Mueller B. U., Pabst T., Fos J., et al. ATRA resolves the differentiation block in t(15;17) acute myeloid leukemia by restoring PU.1 expression. Blood 2006; 107 3330–3338.

[9] Di Noto R., Lo Pardo C., Schiavone E.M., et al. All-trans retinoic acid (ATRA) and the regulation of adhesion molecules in acute myeloid leukemia. Leukemia & Lymphoma 1996; 21 201–209.

[10] Lin R. J., Nagy L., Inoue S., Shao W., Miller W. H. Jr., Evans R. M. Role of the histone deacetylase complex in acute promyelocytic leukaemia. Nature 1998; 391 811–814.

[11] Grignani F., De Matteis S., Nervi C., et al. Fusion proteins of the retinoic acid receptor-alpha recruit histone deacetylase in promyelocytic leukaemia. Nature 1998; 391 815–818.

[12] Melnick A., Licht J. D. Deconstructing a disease: RARalpha, its fusion partners, and their roles in the pathogenesis of acute promyelocytic leukemia. Blood 1999; 93 3167–3215.

[13] Cohen M. H., Hirschfeld S., Flamm Honig S., et al. Drug approval summaries: arsenic trioxide, tamoxifen citrate, anastrazole, paclitaxel, bexarotene. The Oncologist 2001; 6 4–11.

[14] Shen Z. X., Chen G. Q., Ni J. H., et al. Use of arsenic trioxide (As2O3) in the treatment of acute promyelocytic leukemia (APL) II: clinical efficacy and pharmacokinetics in relapsed patients. Blood 1997; 89 3354–3360.

[15] Soignet S. L., Maslak P., Wang Z. G., et al. Complete remission after treatment of acute promyelocytic leukemia with arsenic trioxide. New England Journal of Medicine 1998; 339 1341–1348.

[16] Wu J., Shao Y., Liu J., Chen G., Ho P. C. The medicinal use of realgar (As(4)S(4)) and its recent development as an anticancer agent. Journal of Ethnopharmacology 2011; 135 595–602.

[17] Hu X., Ma R., Xu Y., Guo X., Xu S., Liu F. Treatment of hematologic malignancies with Qinghuang Powder (in Chinese). International Journal of Traditional Chinese Medicine 2011; 33 568–570.

[18] Hu X. M., Liu F., Ma R. Application and assessment of Chinese arsenic drugs in treating malignant hematopathy in China. Chinese Journal of Integrative Medicine 2010; 16 368–377.

[19] Lu D. P., Qiu J. Y., Jiang B., et al. Tetra-arsenic tetra-sulfide for the treatment of acute promyelocytic leukemia: a pilot report. Blood 2002; 99 3136–3143.

[20] Wang F. R., Lou Y. Q., Lu D. P. [A clinical pharmacokinetic study of multi-dose oral tetra-arsenic tetra-sulfide combination therapy in acute promyelocytic leukemia]. Zhonghua Nei Ke Za Zhi 2005; 44 730–733.

[21] Styblo M., Del Razo L. M., Vega L., et al. Comparative toxicity of trivalent and pentavalent inorganic and methylated arsenicals in rat and human cells. Archives of Toxicology 2000; 74 289–299.

[22] Kumagai Y., Sumi D. Arsenic: signal transduction, transcription factor, and biotransformation involved in cellular response and toxicity. Annual Review of Pharmacology and Toxicology 2007; 47 243–262.

[23] Aposhian H. V. Enzymatic methylation of arsenic species and other new approaches to arsenic toxicity. Annual Review of Pharmacology and Toxicology 1997; 37 397–419.

[24] Kitchin K. T. Recent advances in arsenic carcinogenesis: modes of action, animal model systems, and methylated arsenic metabolites. Toxicology and Applied Pharmacology 2001; 172 249–261.

[25] Del Razo L. M., Styblo M., Cullen W. R., Thomas D. J. Determination of trivalent methylated arsenicals in biological matrices. Toxicology and Applied Pharmacology 2001; 174 282–293.

[26] Rossman T. G. Mechanism of arsenic carcinogenesis: an integrated approach. Mutation Research 2003; 533 37–65.

[27] Vahter M. Genetic polymorphism in the biotransformation of inorganic arsenic and its role in toxicity. Toxicology Letters 2000; 112–113 209–217.

[28] Fujisawa S., Ohno R., Shigeno K., et al. Pharmacokinetics of arsenic species in Japanese patients with relapsed or refractory acute promyelocytic leukemia treated with arsenic trioxide. Cancer Chemotherapy and Pharmacology 2007; 59 485–493.

[29] Kiguchi T., Yoshino Y., Yuan B., et al. Speciation of arsenic trioxide penetrates into cerebrospinal fluid in patients with acute promyelocytic leukemia. Leukemia Researc 2010; 34 403–405.

[30] Iriyama N., Yoshino Y., Yuan B., et al: Speciation of arsenic trioxide metabolites in peripheral blood and bone marrow from an acute promyelocytic leukemia patient. Journal of Hematology and Oncology 2012; 5 1.

[31] Yoshino Y., Yuan B., Miyashita S. I., et al. Speciation of arsenic trioxide metabolites in blood cells and plasma of a patient with acute promyelocytic leukemia. Analytical and Bioanalytical Chemistry 2009; 393 689–697.

[32] Fukai Y., Hirata M., Ueno M., et al. Clinical pharmacokinetic study of arsenic trioxide in an acute promyelocytic leukemia (APL) patient: speciation of arsenic metabolites in serum and urine. Biological and Pharmaceutical Bulletin 2006; 29 1022–1027.

[33] Lu M., Wang H., Li X. F., et al: Evidence of hemoglobin binding to arsenic as a basis for the accumulation of arsenic in rat blood. Chemical Research in Toxicology 2004; 17 1733–1742.

[34] Benramdane L., Accominotti M., Fanton L., Malicier D., Vallon J. J. Arsenic speciation in human organs following fatal arsenic trioxide poisoning—a case report. Clinical Chemistry 1999; 45 301–306.

[35] de Botton S., Sanz M. A., Chevret S., et al. Extramedullary relapse in acute promyelocytic leukemia treated with all-trans retinoic acid and chemotherapy. Leukemia 2006; 20 35–41.

[36] Specchia G., Lo Coco F., Vignetti M., et al. Extramedullary involvement at relapse in acute promyelocytic leukemia patients treated or not with all-trans retinoic acid: a report by the Gruppo Italiano Malattie Ematologiche dell'Adulto. Journal of Clinical Oncology 2001; 19 4023–4028.

[37] Au W. Y., Tam S., Fong B. M., Kwong Y.L. Elemental arsenic entered the cerebrospinal fluid during oral arsenic trioxide treatment of meningeal relapse of acute promyelocytic leukemia. Blood 2006; 107 3012–3013.

[38] Au W. Y., Tam S., Fong B.M., Kwong Y. L. Determinants of cerebrospinal fluid arsenic concentration in patients with acute promyelocytic leukemia on oral arsenic trioxide therapy. Blood 2008; 112 3587–3590.

[39] Helwig A., Klemm M., Schuttig R., et al. Arsenic-induced APL differentiation in cerebrospinal fluid. Leukemia Research 2007; 31 703–705.

[40] Knipp S., Gattermann N., Schapira M., Kaferstein H., Germing U. Arsenic in the cerebrospinal fluid of a patient receiving arsenic trioxide for relapsed acute promyelocytic leukemia with CNS involvement. Leukemia Research 2007; 31 1585–1587.

[41] Chen G. Q., Zhu J., Shi X. G., et al. In vitro studies on cellular and molecular mechanisms of arsenic trioxide (As2O3) in the treatment of acute promyelocytic leukemia: As2O3 induces NB4 cell apoptosis with downregulation of Bcl-2 expression and modulation of PML-RAR alpha/PML proteins. Blood 1996; 88 1052–1061.

[42] Jin Z., Ran M., Man Z. Arsenic trioxide entered cerebrospinal fluid with the help of mannitol overwhelm the meningeal relapse of acute promyelocytic leukemia. Haematologica 2007; 92 e82–84.

[43] Wang H., Cao F., Li J., et al. Arsenic trioxide and mannitol for the treatment of acute promyelocytic leukemia relapse in the central nervous system. Blood 2014; 124 1998–2000.

[44] Shen Y., Shen Z. X., Yan H., et al. Studies on the clinical efficacy and pharmacokinetics of low-dose arsenic trioxide in the treatment of relapsed acute promyelocytic leukemia: a comparison with conventional dosage. Leukemia 2001; 15 735–741.

[45] Miller W. H. Jr., Schipper H. M., Lee J. S., Singer J., Waxman S. Mechanisms of action of arsenic trioxide. Cancer Research 2002; 62 3893–3903.

[46] Kitchin K. T., Wallace K. The role of protein binding of trivalent arsenicals in arsenic carcinogenesis and toxicity. Journal of Inorganic Biochemistry 2008; 102 532–539.

[47] Naranmandura H., Suzuki N., Suzuki K. T. Trivalent arsenicals are bound to proteins during reductive methylation. Chemical Research in Toxicology 2006; 19 1010–1018.

[48] Wang Z., Zhou J., Lu X., Gong Z., Le X. C. Arsenic speciation in urine from acute promyelocytic leukemia patients undergoing arsenic trioxide treatment. Chemical Research in Toxicology 2004; 17 95–103.

[49] Shuzhen S., Rou M., Xiaomei H., et al. Karyotype and DNA-methylation responses in myelodysplastic syndromes following treatment with traditional chinese formula containing arsenic. Evidence-Based Complementary and Alternative Medicine 2012; 969476.

[50] Koch I., Sylvester S., Lai V. W., Owen A., Reimer K. J., Cullen W. R. Bioaccessibility and excretion of arsenic in Niu Huang Jie Du Pian pills. Toxicology and Applied Pharmacology 2007; 222 357–364.

[51] Kwan S. Y., Tsui S. K., Man T. O. Release of soluble arsenic from Realgar in simulated gastric juice. Analytical Letters 2001; 34 1431–1436.

[52] Wu X. H., Sun D. H., Zhuang Z. X., et al. Aanlysis and leaching characteristics of mercury and arsenic in Chinese medicinal material. Analytical Chimica Acta 2002; 453 311–323.

[53] Aposhian H. V., Gurzau E. S., Le X. C., et al. Occurrence of monomethylarsonous acid in urine of humans exposed to inorganic arsenic. Chemical Research in Toxicology 2000; 13 693–697.

[54] Wang J., Lin M., Zhang T., et al. Arsenic(II) sulfide quantum dots prepared by a wet process from its bulk. Journal of the American Chemical Society 2008; 130 11596–11597.

[55] Ye H. Q., Gan L., Yang X. L., Xu H. B. Membrane toxicity accounts for apoptosis induced by realgar nanoparticles in promyelocytic leukemia HL-60 cells. Biological Trace Element Research 2005; 103 117–132.

[56] Wang N., Wang L. W., Gou B. D., Zhang T. L. Preparation of realgar nanoparticle suspension and its inhibition effect on the proliferation of human myelocytic leukaemia HL-60 cells. Journal of Dispersion Science and Technology 2009; 30 237–240.

[57] Wang X. B., Gao H. Y., Hou B. L., Huang J., Xi R. G., Wu L. J. Nanoparticle realgar powders induce apoptosis in U937 cells through caspase MAPK and mitochondrial pathways. Archives of Pharmacal Research 2007; 30 653–658.

[58] Wu J. Z., Ho P. C. Evaluation of the in vitro activity and in vivo bioavailability of realgar nanoparticles prepared by cryo-grinding. European Journal of Pharmaceutical Sciences 2006; 29 35–44.

[59] Zhao Q. H., Zhang Y., Liu Y., et al. Anticancer effect of realgar nanoparticles on mouse melanoma skin cancer in vivo via transdermal drug delivery. Medical Oncology 2010; 27 203–212.

[60] Kaise T., Watanabe S., Itoh K. The acute toxicity of arsenobetaine. Chemosphere 1985; 14 1327–1332.

[61] Chen Z., Chen G. Q., Shen Z. X., Chen S. J., Wang Z. Y. Treatment of acute promyelocytic leukemia with arsenic compounds: in vitro and in vivo studies. Seminars in Hematology 2001; 38 26–36.

[62] Litzow M. R. Arsenic trioxide. Expert Opinion on Pharmacotherapy 2008; 9 1773–1785.

[63] Zhu J., Okumura H., Ohtake S., Nakamura S., Nakao S. Arsenic trioxide induces apoptosis in leukemia/lymphoma cell lines via the CD95/CD95L system. Oncology Reports 2003; 10 705–709.

[64] Szegezdi E., Cahill S., Meyer M., O'Dwyer M., Samali A. TRAIL sensitisation by arsenic trioxide is caspase-8 dependent and involves modulation of death receptor components and Akt. British Journal of Cancer 2006; 94 398–406.

[65] Kim E. H., Yoon M. J., Kim S. U., Kwon T. K., Sohn S., Choi K. S. Arsenic trioxide sensitizes human glioma cells, but not normal astrocytes, to TRAIL-induced apoptosis via CCAAT/enhancer-binding protein homologous protein-dependent DR5 upregulation. Cancer Research 2008; 68 266–275.

[66] Du Y., Wang K., Fang H., et al. Coordination of intrinsic, extrinsic, and endoplasmic reticulum-mediated apoptosis by imatinib mesylate combined with arsenic trioxide in chronic myeloid leukemia. Blood 2006; 107 1582–1590.

[67] Davison K., Mann K. K., Miller W. H. Jr. Arsenic trioxide: mechanisms of action. Seminars in Hematology 2002; 39 3–7.

[68] Ninomiya M., Kajiguchi T., Yamamoto K., Kinoshita T., Emi N., Naoe T. Increased oxidative DNA products in patients with acute promyelocytic leukemia during arsenic therapy. Haematologica 2006; 91 1571–1572.

[69] Wu J. Z., Ho P. C. Comparing the relative oxidative DNA damage caused by various arsenic species by quantifying urinary levels of 8-hydroxy-2'-deoxyguanosine with isotope-dilution liquid chromatography/mass spectrometry. Pharmaceutical Research 2009; 26 1525–1533.

[70] Pelicano H., Feng L., Zhou Y., et al. Inhibition of mitochondrial respiration: a novel strategy to enhance drug-induced apoptosis in human leukemia cells by a reactive oxygen species-mediated mechanism. Journal of Biological Chemistry 2003; 278 37832–37839.

[71] Wang J., Li L., Cang H., Shi G., Yi J. NADPH oxidase-derived reactive oxygen species are responsible for the high susceptibility to arsenic cytotoxicity in acute promyelocytic leukemia cells. Leukemia Research 2008; 32 429–436.

[72] Chou W. C., Jie C., Kenedy A. A., Jones R. J., Trush M. A., Dang C. V. Role of NADPH oxidase in arsenic-induced reactive oxygen species formation and cytotoxicity in myeloid leukemia cells. Proceedings of the National Academy of Sciences of the United States of America 2004; 101 4578–4583.

[73] Jing Y., Dai J., Chalmers-Redman R. M., Tatton W. G., Waxman S. Arsenic trioxide selectively induces acute promyelocytic leukemia cell apoptosis via a hydrogen peroxide-dependent pathway. Blood 1999; 94 2102–2111.

[74] Yi J., Gao F., Shi G., et al. The inherent cellular level of reactive oxygen species: one of the mechanisms determining apoptotic susceptibility of leukemic cells to arsenic trioxide. Apoptosis 2002; 7 209–215.

[75] Lin S., Del Razo L. M., Styblo M., Wang C., Cullen W. R., Thomas D. J. Arsenicals inhibit thioredoxin reductase in cultured rat hepatocytes. Chemical Research in Toxicology 2001; 14 305–311.

[76] Chouchane S., Snow E. T. In vitro effect of arsenical compounds on glutathione-related enzymes. Chemical Research in Toxicology 2001; 14 517–522.

[77] Hu X. M., Yuan B., Tanaka S., et al. Involvement of oxidative stress associated with glutathione depletion and p38 mitogen-activated protein kinase activation in arsenic disulfide-induced differentiation in HL-60 cells. Leukemia & Lymphoma 2014; 55 392–404.

[78] Hu X. M., Hirano T., Oka K. Arsenic trioxide induces apoptosis in cells of MOLT-4 and its daunorubicin-resistant cell line via depletion of intracellular glutathione, disruption of mitochondrial membrane potential and activation of caspase-3. Cancer Chemotherapy and Pharmacology 2003; 52 47–58.

[79] Yuan B., Ohyama K., Bessho T., Uchide N., Toyoda H. Imbalance between ROS production and elimination results in apoptosis induction in primary smooth chorion trophoblast cells prepared from human fetal membrane tissues. Life Sciences 2008; 82 623–630.

[80] Zhou Y., Hileman E. O., Plunkett W., Keating M. J., Huang P. Free radical stress in chronic lymphocytic leukemia cells and its role in cellular sensitivity to ROS-generating anticancer agents. Blood 2003; 101 4098–4104.

[81] Cai X., Shen Y. L., Zhu Q., et al. Arsenic trioxide-induced apoptosis and differentiation are associated respectively with mitochondrial transmembrane potential collapse and retinoic acid signaling pathways in acute promyelocytic leukemia. Leukemia 2000; 14 262–270.

[82] Gao F., Yi J., Shi G. Y., Li H., Shi X. G., Tang X. M. The sensitivity of digestive tract tumor cells to As2O3 is associated with the inherent cellular level of reactive oxygen species. World Journal of Gastroenterology 2002; 8 36–39.

[83] Park M. T., Kang Y. H., Park I. C., et al. Combination treatment with arsenic trioxide and phytosphingosine enhances apoptotic cell death in arsenic trioxide-resistant cancer cells. Molecular Cancer Therapeutics 2007; 6 82–92.

[84] Hu X. M., Yuan B., Song M. M., et al. Dose-dependent biphasic effects of arsenic disulfide on differentiation and apoptosis of HL-60 cells. Current Topics in Pharmacology 2013; 17 13–25.

[85] Chen G. Q., Shi X. G., Tang W., et al. Use of arsenic trioxide (As2O3) in the treatment of acute promyelocytic leukemia (APL) I: As2O3 exerts dose-dependent dual effects on APL cells. Blood 1997; 89 3345–3353.

[86] Kishi K., Toba K., Azegami T., et al. Hematopoietic cytokine-dependent differentiation to eosinophils and neutrophils in a newly established acute promyelocytic leukemia cell line with t(15;17). Experimental Hematology 1998; 26 135–142.

[87] Iriyama N., Yuan B., Hatta Y., et al. Granulocyte colony-stimulating factor potentiates differentiation induction by all-trans retinoic acid and arsenic trioxide and enhances arsenic uptake in the acute promyelocytic leukemia cell line HT93A. Oncology Reports 2012; 28 1875–1882.

[88] Hu X. M., Tanaka S., Onda K., et al. Arsenic disulfide induced apoptosis and concurrently promoted erythroid differentiation in cytokine-dependent myelodysplastic syndrome-progressed leukemia cell line F-36p with complex karyotype including monosomy 7. Chinese Journal of Integrative Medicine 2014; 20 387–393.

[89] Hu X. M., Yuan B., Tanaka S., et al: Arsenic disulfide-triggered apoptosis and erythroid differentiation in myelodysplastic syndrome and acute myeloid leukemia cell lines. Hematology 2014; 19 352–360.

[90] Bianchi N., Ongaro F., Chiarabelli C., et al. Induction of erythroid differentiation of human K562 cells by cisplatin analogs. Biochemical Pharmacology 2000; 60 31–40.

[91] Li X. F., Wu X. R., Xue M., et al. The role of DNA methylation in catechol-enhanced erythroid differentiation of K562 cells. Toxicology and Applied Pharmacology 2012; 265 43–50.

[92] Jiang Y., Dunbar A., Gondek L. P., et al. Aberrant DNA methylation is a dominant mechanism in MDS progression to AML. Blood 2009; 113 1315–1325.

[93] Tian Y., Liu Y., He P., et al. Arsenic sulfide promotes apoptosis in retinoid acid resistant human acute promyelocytic leukemic NB4-R1 cells through downregulation of SET protein. PLoS One 2014; 9 e83184.

[94] Sternsdorf T., Puccetti E., Jensen K., et al. PIC-1/SUMO-1-modified PML-retinoic acid receptor alpha mediates arsenic trioxide-induced apoptosis in acute promyelocytic leukemia. Molecular and Cellular Biology 1999; 19 5170–5178.

[95] Muller S., Matunis M. J., Dejean A. Conjugation with the ubiquitin-related modifier SUMO-1 regulates the partitioning of PML within the nucleus. Embo Journal 1998; 17 61–70.

[96] Tatham M. H., Geoffroy M. C., Shen L., et al. RNF4 is a poly-SUMO-specific E3 ubiquitin ligase required for arsenic-induced PML degradation. Nature Cell Biology 2008; 10 538–546.

[97] Wang J. Z., Liu Y. R., Qin Y. Z., et al. [Change of PML/PML-RARalpha protein during treatment with tetraarsenic tetrasulfide (As4S4) in patients with acute promyelocytic leukemia]. Zhongguo Shi Yan Xue Ye Xue Za Zhi 2003; 11 464–468.

[98] Hu J., Liu Y. F., Wu C. F., et al. Long-term efficacy and safety of all-trans retinoic acid/arsenic trioxide-based therapy in newly diagnosed acute promyelocytic leukemia. Proceedings of the National Academy of Sciences of the United States of America 2009; 106 3342–3347.

[99] Bhattacharjee H., Carbrey J., Rosen B. P., Mukhopadhyay R. Drug uptake and pharmacological modulation of drug sensitivity in leukemia by AQP9. Biochemical and Biophysical Research Communications 2004; 322 836–841.

[100] Liu Z., Shen J., Carbrey J. M., Mukhopadhyay R., Agre P., Rosen B. P. Arsenite transport by mammalian aquaglyceroporins AQP7 and AQP9. Proceedings of the National Academy of Sciences of the United States of America 2002; 99 6053–6058.

[101] Yoshino Y., Yuan B., Kaise T., et al. Contribution of aquaporin 9 and multidrug resistance-associated protein 2 to differential sensitivity to arsenite between primary cultured chorion and amnion cells prepared from human fetal membranes. Toxicology and Applied Pharmacology 2011; 257 198–208.

[102] Gottlicher M., Minucci S., Zhu P., et al. Valproic acid defines a novel class of HDAC inhibitors inducing differentiation of transformed cells. EMBO Journal 2001; 20 6969–6978.

[103] Quintas-Cardama A., Santos F. P., Garcia-Manero G. Histone deacetylase inhibitors for the treatment of myelodysplastic syndrome and acute myeloid leukemia. Leukemia 2011; 25 226–235.

[104] Bolden J. E., Peart M. J., Johnstone R. W. Anticancer activities of histone deacetylase inhibitors. Nat Reviews Drug Discovery 2006; 5 769–784.

[105] Iriyama N., Yuan B., Yoshino Y., et al. Enhancement of differentiation induction and upregulation of CCAAT/enhancer-binding proteins and PU.1 in NB4 cells treated with combination of ATRA and valproic acid. International Journal of Oncology 2014; 44 865–873.

[106] Cheng Y. C., Lin H., Huang M. J., Chow J. M., Lin S., Liu H. E. Downregulation of c-Myc is critical for valproic acid-induced growth arrest and myeloid differentiation of acute myeloid leukemia. Leukemia Research 2007; 31 1403–1411.

[107] Cimino G., Lo-Coco F., Fenu S., et al. Sequential valproic acid/all-trans retinoic acid treatment reprograms differentiation in refractory and high-risk acute myeloid leukemia. Cancer Research 2006; 66 8903–8911.

[108] Leiva M., Moretti S., Soilihi H., et al. Valproic acid induces differentiation and transient tumor regression, but spares leukemia-initiating activity in mouse models of APL. Leukemia 2012; 26 1630–1637.

[109] Ito K., Bernardi R., Morotti A., et al. PML targeting eradicates quiescent leukaemia-initiating cells. Nature 2008; 453 1072–1078.

[110] Imai M., Kikuchi H., Denda T., Ohyama K., Hirobe C., Toyoda H. Cytotoxic effects of flavonoids against a human colon cancer derived cell line, COLO 201: a potential natural anti-cancer substance. Cancer Letters 2009; 276 74–80.

[111] Imai M., Yuan B., Kikuchi H., et al. Growth inhibition of a human colon carcinoma cell, COLO 201, by a natural product, Vitex agnus-castus fruits extract, in vivo and in vitro. Advances in Biological Chemistry 2012; 02 20–28.

[112] Kikuchi H., Yuan B., Nishimura Y., et al. Cytotoxicity of Vitex agnus-castus fruit extract and its major component, casticin, correlates with differentiation status in leukemia cell lines. Internationa Journal of Oncology 2013; 43 1976–1984.

[113] Kikuchi H., Yuan B., Yuhara E., et al. Involvement of histone H3 phosphorylation via the activation of p38 MAPK pathway and intracellular redox status in cytotoxicity of HL-60 cells induced by Vitex agnus-castus fruit extract. Internationa Journal of Oncology 2014; 45 843–852.

[114] Kikuchi H., Yuan B., Yuhara E., Takagi N., Toyoda H. Involvement of histone H3 phosphorylation through p38 MAPK pathway activation in casticin-induced cytocidal effects against the human promyelocytic cell line HL-60. Internationa Journal of Oncology 2013; 43 2046–2056.

[115] Yuan B., Imai M., Kikuchi H., et al. Cytocidal effects of polyphenolic compounds, alone or in combination with, anticancer drugs against cancer cells: potential future application of the combinatory therapy. In: Apoptosis and Medicine. Ntuli TM (ed). InTech, Croatia; 2012. p155-174. DOI: 10.5772/50218.

[116] Ohyama K., Akaike T., Imai M., Toyoda H., Hirobe C., Bessho T. Human gastric signet ring carcinoma (KATO-III) cell apoptosis induced by Vitex agnus-castus fruit extract through intracellular oxidative stress. International Journal of Biochemistry and Cell Biology 2005; 37 1496–1510.

[117] Lane S. W., Scadden D. T., Gilliland D. G. The leukemic stem cell niche: current concepts and therapeutic opportunities. Blood 2009; 114 1150–1157.

[118] Hou D. X., Fujii M., Terahara N., Yoshimoto M. Molecular Mechanisms Behind the Chemopreventive Effects of Anthocyanidins. Journal of Biomedicine and Biotechnology 2004; 2004 321–325.

[119] Afaq F., Zaman N., Khan N., et al. Inhibition of epidermal growth factor receptor signaling pathway by delphinidin, an anthocyanidin in pigmented fruits and vegetables. International Journal of Cancer 2008; 123 1508–1515.

[120] Hafeez B. B., Siddiqui I. A., Asim M., et al. A dietary anthocyanidin delphinidin induces apoptosis of human prostate cancer PC3 cells in vitro and in vivo: involvement of nuclear factor-kappaB signaling. Cancer Research 2008; 68 8564–8572.

[121] Hou D. X., Ose T., Lin S., et al. Anthocyanidins induce apoptosis in human promyelocytic leukemia cells: structure-activity relationship and mechanisms involved. International Journal of Oncology 2003; 23 705–712.

[122] Hou D. X., Tong X., Terahara N., Luo D., Fujii M. Delphinidin 3-sambubioside, a Hibiscus anthocyanin, induces apoptosis in human leukemia cells through reactive oxygen species-mediated mitochondrial pathway. Archives of Biochemistry and Biophysics 2005; 440 101–109.

[123] Kitagawa S. Inhibitory effects of polyphenols on p-glycoprotein-mediated transport. Biological and Pharmaceutical Bulletin 2006; 29 1–6.

[124] Castro AF and Altenberg GA: Inhibition of drug transport by genistein in multidrug-resistant cells expressing P-glycoprotein. Biochemical Pharmacology 53: 89-93, 1997.

[125] Lee T. C., Ho I. C., Lu W. J., Huang J. D. Enhanced expression of multidrug resistance-associated protein 2 and reduced expression of aquaglyceroporin 3 in an arsenic-resistant human cell line. Journal of Biological Chemistry 2006; 281 18401–18407.

[126] Leslie E. M., Haimeur A., Waalkes M. P. Arsenic transport by the human multidrug resistance protein 1 (MRP1/ABCC1). Evidence that a tri-glutathione conjugate is required. Journal of Biological Chemistry 2004; 279 32700–32708.

[127] Yuan B., Ohyama K., Bessho T., Toyoda H. Contribution of inducible nitric oxide synthase and cyclooxygenase-2 to apoptosis induction in smooth chorion trophoblast cells of human fetal membrane tissues. Biochemical and Biophysical Research Communications 2006; 341 822–827.

[128] Yuan B., Ohyama K., Takeichi M., Toyoda H. Direct contribution of inducible nitric oxide synthase expression to apoptosis induction in primary smooth chorion trophoblast cells of human fetal membrane tissues. International Journal of Biochemistry and Cell Biology 2009; 41 1062–1069.

[129] Wang L., Zhou G. B., Liu P., et al. Dissection of mechanisms of Chinese medicinal formula Realgar-Indigo naturalis as an effective treatment for promyelocytic leukemia. Proceedings of the National Academy of Sciences of the United States of America 2008; 105 4826–4831.

[130] Kon A., Yuan B., Hanazawa T., et al. Contribution of membrane progesterone receptor alpha to the induction of progesterone-mediated apoptosis associated with mitochondrial membrane disruption and caspase cascade activation in Jurkat cell lines. Oncology Reports 2013; 30 1965–1970.

[131] Slejkovec Z., Falnoga I., Goessler W., et al. Analytical artefacts in the speciation of arsenic in clinical samples. Analytica Chimica Acta 2008; 607 83–91.

[132] Iriyama N., Yuan B., Yoshino Y., et al. Aquaporin 9, a promising predictor for the cytocidal effects of arsenic trioxide in acute promyelocytic leukemia cell lines and primary blasts. Oncology Reports 2013.

[133] Thomas D. J., Styblo M., Lin S. The cellular metabolism and systemic toxicity of arsenic. Toxicology and Applied Pharmacology 2001; 176 127–144.

Chapter 8

New Insights in Prognosis and Therapy of Chronic Lymphocytic Leukaemia

Isabel González Gascón y Marín, María Hernández-Sánchez, Ana-Eugenia Rodríguez.Vicente and José-Ángel Hernández-Rivas

Additional information is available at the end of the chapter

http://dx.doi.org/10.5772/60738

Abstract

Chronic lymphocytic leukaemia (CLL) is a heterogeneous disease with a very variable clinical outcome. New biological markers, such as cytogenetic abnormalities or mutation status, have become important prognostic factors. Whole-genome sequencing studies have revealed novel genomic mutations, *NOTCH1, SF3B1, BIRC3, TP53* and *MYD88* being the most important. All these mutations have also been associated with the disease outcome. The treatment of CLL has evolved favourably in recent years. However, adverse events or chemorefractoriness occurs in some cases. Luckily, an increasing number of compounds are under development with promising results. Some of these new targeted therapies include B-cell receptor inhibitors, new anti-CD20 antibodies, Bcl-2 inhibitors, immunomodulatory drugs or chimeric antigen receptors (CARs). In this chapter, we will conduct a review of the new prognostic markers of CLL, the relationship they have with each other to build prognostic scores, the role they have in guiding treatment decisions and the novel therapies that have emerged recently with immunologic, biochemical and genetic targets.

Keywords: Chronic lymphocytic leukaemia, genetic abnormalities, recurrent mutations, targeted therapy, signalling pathway

1. Introduction

Chronic lymphocytic leukaemia (CLL) is a neoplasm characterized by the proliferation and accumulation of monoclonal mature B lymphocytes in the peripheral blood, bone marrow, spleen and lymph nodes. It is the most frequent type of leukaemia in adults from Western countries, showing a predilection for the elderly, with a median age at diagnosis of 72 years old. It has been more prevalent in men than in women [1, 2].

The clinical course of CLL is highly heterogeneous. Some patients require treatment at the time of diagnosis, while others remain asymptomatic and may even never be treated. Therefore, median survival times range from a few months to many decades [3,4]. In order to define disease extent and prognosis, Rai and Binet staging systems were designed around 35–40 years ago and remain widely used in clinical practice [5,6]. They are based on physical examination and blood counts and are therefore inexpensive and easy to apply. However, some patients with early stages promptly progress and do not respond to therapy. For these reasons, over the last ten years, several biological markers such as immunoglobulin heavy-chain variable region (*IGHV*) mutation status, cytogenetic abnormalities or expression of specific proteins on CLL cells have become important prognostic factors for this disease [7–10]. They are available in routine clinical practice and may even guide treatment decisions. Recently, the improvements in the next-generation sequencing technologies have revealed novel genomic markers with important prognostic value highlighting *NOTCH1* (neurogenic locus notch homolog protein 1), *SF3B1* (splicing factor 3B subunit 1), *BIRC3* (baculoviral IAP repeat-containing protein 3), *TP53* (tumour protein p53) and *MYD88* (myeloid differentiation primary response 88). In the first part of this chapter, we will conduct a review of these markers, its implications on pathophysiology and prognosis of CLL, the relationship they have with other prognostic factors in order to establish new scores for clinical practice, and the role they have in guiding therapeutic choices.

CLL remains an incurable disease with the exception of allogeneic transplantation. Besides, some patients without treatment present survival rates similar to the normal population, and no benefit has been found when early treatment has been applied in this subset of patients. In addition, spontaneous cure has been reported in rare occasions [11]. For these reasons, only half of the patients diagnosed with CLL will require treatment during follow-up. Fortunately, survival rates of patients with CLL have improved significantly, thanks to the great advances in treatment over the past decades [12]. Glucocorticoids and alkylating drugs were the first treatments introduced, followed by purine analogues. Later, the arrival of targeted antibody therapy led by rituximab (anti-CD20) was the most revolutionary progress. Bendamustine, another alkylating agent used in Germany for more than 30 years, has also been approved for the treatment of CLL after showing its benefits for this disease in clinical trials [13,14]. All these drugs remain widely used in routine clinical practice, mainly in combination regimens. In fact, chemo-immunotherapy regimens are nowadays the standard approach to therapy of most patients with CLL, as they have demonstrated to produce a survival benefit with durable remissions [15–17]. Table 1 sums up approved drugs for the treatment of CLL by categories; and Table 2 summarizes the combination of suggested treatment regimens used for the treatment of CLL recommended by the NCCN (National Comprehensive Cancer Network) [17].

http://dx.doi.org/10.5772/60738

Alkylating agents
Chlorambucil
Cyclophosphamide
Bendamustine
Purine analogues
Fludarabine
Pentostatin
Cladribine
Monoclonal antibodies
Anti-CD20
Rituximab
Ofatumumab
Obinutuzumab
Anti-CD52
Alemtuzumab
B-cell receptor inhibitors
Ibrutinib
Idelalisib

Table 1. Approved drugs by categories for the treatment of CLL

Acronym	Drugs
FCR	Fludarabine, cyclophosphamide, rituximab
FR	Fludarabine, rituximab
PCR	Pentostatin, cyclophosphamide, rituximab
BR	Bendamustine, rituximab
Chlorambucil + anti-CD20	Rituximab/obinutuzumab/ofatumumab
HDMP + rituximab	High-dose methylprednisolone, rituximab
RR	Lenalidomide, rituximab
RCHOP	Rituximab, cyclophosphamide, doxorubicine, vincristine, prednisone
Idelalisib + rituximab	Idelalisib, rituximab
Alemtuzumab + rituximab	Alemtuzumab, rituximab

Table 2. Combination suggested treatment regimens used for the treatment of CLL recommended by the National Comprehensive Cancer Network (NCCN) Version 1-2015

Nevertheless, some of these regimens are not exempted from adverse events that limit their use in frail patients, especially the elderly. Moreover, some patients are chemo-resistant to these drugs, and a curative therapy is still absent for them. Knowledge of the pathogenesis of B-cell receptor (BCR) has led to the investigation of novel molecular targets like Bruton tyrosine kinase inhibitors or phosphatidylinositol 3-kinases (PI3Ks). New anti-CD20 antibodies such as ofatumumab or obinutuzumab have also been shown to have a promising activity in CLL. Other new target therapies under study include Bcl-2 inhibitors, immunomodulatory drugs (lenalidomide) or chimeric antigen receptors. The second part of this chapter will be dedicated to review novel therapies that have emerged recently with immunologic, biochemical and genetic targets.

2. Prognostic markers and risk stratification of CLL

The clinical course of CLL is extremely variable. Prognostic markers are important not only for patient management but also in understanding the disease biology. Many biological factors have been added to the classic staging systems of Rai and Binet with the intention to establish prognostic groups. However, as novel cytogenetic and molecular findings are discovered, our understanding on its prognostic value keeps in constant evolution. In this section, we will conduct a review of these "new" prognostic markers, focusing on genetic markers.

2.1. Genetic markers in CLL

2.1.1. Recurrent genomic abnormalities detected by interface fluorescence in situ hybridization (FISH)

FISH studies are able to detect clonal genomic aberrations in the majority (>80 %) of CLL patients. The most common recurrent chromosomal abnormalities include 13q deletion (13q-), 11q deletion (11q-), trisomy 12 (+12) and 17p deletion (17p-), defining five prognostic categories with different survival times [18].

2.1.1.1. 13q-

13q- is the most frequent chromosome aberration in CLL, observed in approximately 55 % of the cases, and entails the group of patients with a better prognosis. However, the deletions that occur at this chromosome are not homogeneous and neither is the prognosis for this subgroup of patients. The size of the deletion varies thumping. Two types of deletion have been proposed in accordance to their extent: 13q- type I or short deletions not comprising the *RB1* (retinoblastoma 1) locus and 13q- type II or large deletions including the *RB1* locus. The latter have been associated with a more aggressive clinical course [19,20]. 13q deletions are monoallelic in most cases, but biallelic losses have also been described in nearly 30 % of patients, and although it has been controversial, they do not seem to entail a worse clinical outcome [21–24]. The size of the clone harbouring 13q- has also implications on prognosis, with a significantly shorter time to first treatment (TTFT) and overall survival (OS), if a high proportion of cells carry 13q- [22,25,26]. With intent to explain the pathogenesis and clinical heterogeneity of 13q-, several genes located at 13q have been identified. Among them stand microRNAs (miRNAs) *miR15a and miR16-1, DLEU2, DLEU7* or *RB1*. *MiR15a* and miR16-1 exhibit a tumour suppressor function in CLL by targeting the *BCL-2* oncogene, being absent or downregulated in the majority of the cases [27,28].

2.1.1.2. 11q-

Prevalence of 11q deletions is estimated below 20 % [18]. The presence of 11q- entails bad prognosis, and often patients present with progressive disease, B symptoms, bulky lymphadenopathy, short TTFT and a reduced OS. In addition, 11q- is associated with unmutated *IGHV* status (U-CLL), which is consistent with the poor prognostic factors mentioned [29,30]. However, some evidence points out that the addition of immunotherapy to classic chemotherapy may overcome the effect of 11q- in previously untreated patients [15,31]. Analogously to 13q-, a high percentage of cells with 11q- has been associated with a worse outcome among 11q- patients [32,33]. 11q- usually implies the loss of the *ATM* (ataxia telangiectasia mutated) gene, albeit *ATM* mutations have been found in <30 % of 11q- cases. *ATM* gene is involved in the repair of damaged DNA; hence, its deficiency causes genomic instability and allows the accumulation of additional genetic mutations during disease course [34]. *BIRC3* gene is also located on 11q close to the *ATM* gene, and deletions and mutations of this gene lead to an unfortunate outcome as well, as they tend to appear in fludarabine-refractory patients [35].

2.1.1.3. +12

Trisomy 12 is the third most frequent cytogenetic aberration, occurring in up to 15 % of CLL cases. Patients with this aberration have been classically considered to have an intermediate prognosis; however, further work has considered this trisomy as a clinical heterogeneous entity [36]. +12 has been associated with an atypical morphology and immunophenotype [37] and has been connected with concurrent trisomy of chromosomes 18 and 19 [38]. Critical genes involved in this aberration remain unknown. *NOTCH-1* mutations were identified in 30–40 % of patients carrying +12, conferring a worse clinical outcome when present in this subset of patients [39–41]. Similarly to deletions, among patients with +12, a high percentage of cells carrying +12 is associated with a worse OS and TTFT [42].

2.1.1.4. 17p-

17p deletion is observed in around 7 % of untreated CLL cases, but its incidence may amount up to 45 % in cases of relapsed or refractory CLL [43]. 17p- is invariably associated with a very poor outcome because of the loss of *TP53* gene. In more than 75 % of the cases with 17p-, mutations in *TP53* are observed in the remaining allele [44]. In spite of that, monoallelic inactivation of *TP53* may be enough to confer a poor prognosis [45]. The tumour suppression p53 acts by inducing apoptosis or cell cycle arrest when DNA is damaged, and consequently genomic complexity is not a rare find in this setting [46]. As in other cytogenetic abnormalities, a high percentage of deleted cells has been associated with a worse outcome within 17p- patients [47]. Patients with 17p- usually do not respond to conventional therapies (fludarabine or alkylating agents), as they are based on p53-dependent mechanisms. Thus, these patients relapse more frequently and have a shorter OS [48]. Nowadays, 17p- is the only cytogenetic abnormality that defines a different treatment approach. Rational options for these patients include new B-cell receptor inhibitors or methylprednisolone +/- alemtuzumab or rituximab followed by allogeneic bone marrow transplantation in candidates for this procedure.

2.1.2. IGHV mutation status

The somatic hypermutation of the variable region of the immunoglobulin heavy-chain genes (*IGHV*) has become one of the most stable and reliable indicators of clinical outcome in CLL. Based on the cutoff value of 98 % identity with the closest germ line *IGHV*, two different subsets of CLL can be indentified: mutated CLL (M-CLL) and unmutated CLL (U-CLL) [8,9]. Somatic mutations of *IGHV* occur in approximately half of the cases and usually present with non-progressive disease, in contrast to patients with U-CLL who have a more aggressive disease with a shorter progression-free survival (PFS), TTFT and OS. U-CLL is also associated with unfavourable prognostic factors such as 11q-, 17p- or ZAP-70 positivity. Furthermore, irrespective of mutation status, some heavy-chain variable regions have been associated with specific clinical features, outcome and varying occurrences from country to country. For example, *IGHV1-69* gene has been observed to be one of the most frequently rearranged genes in Western patients and is almost always associated with the subset of U-CLL [49]. Other subgroups reported to be frequently used in Western patients are *IGHV3-23*, *IGHV4-34* and *IGHV3-07*. Moreover, an overrepresentation of the *IGHV3-21* gene has been reported in northern European countries compared to the Mediterranean region, and it has been associated with a worse prognosis despite the mutation status [50].

2.1.3. Mutations of key tumour suppressor genes

2.1.3.1. TP53 mutations

CLL harbours *TP53* mutations in around 5–10 % of the cases at diagnosis, but the incidence increases up to 40–50 % in refractory patients or Richter transformation. *TP53* mutations separate a group of patients with critical importance in CLL. This mutation is associated with an ominous outcome due to chemo-refractoriness and therefore is the only biomarker that currently drives treatment decisions in CLL. *TP53* mutations have a detrimental impact on therapy response, PFS and OS [45,48]. *TP53* is a tumour suppressor gene that induces apoptosis or cell cycle arrest after DNA damage. Chemo-refractoriness in patients with these mutations is explained by the mechanism of action of fludarabine or alkylant agents, based on a p53-dependent mechanism. Thus, analogously to 17p-, these patients should be treated, avoiding DNA-damaging chemotherapy agents. Very limited efficient options have been available in the last years in spite of allogeneic stem cell transplantation. Luckily, a number of novel biological drugs such as B-cell receptor inhibitors have been developed and incorporated in the treatment of these patients with encouraging results [51]. Although *TP53* mutations are usually accompanied by 17p-, some patients carry TP53 mutations in the absence of 17p-. However, the monoallelic *TP53* alteration has the same negative impact in prognosis than biallelic defects [44]. *TP53* mutations may appear in a nondominant clone of CLL cells. Ultradeep next-generation techniques were used with the purpose of identifying these subclones, and *TP53* mutations were observed in around 9 % of the cases. These patients showed the same poor survival than patients with *TP53* mutations in the predominant clone [52].

2.1.3.2. *ATM gene mutations*

ATM gene encodes for the ATM protein kinase, a member of the *PI3K* (phosphatidylinositol 3-kinase) family. *ATM* protein takes part in the DNA damage repair mechanism, mediating cellular response to DNA damage in the form of double-strand breaks [53]. The *ATM* gene is located on chromosome 11, and mutations in this gene occur in around 12 % of CLL cases [54]. As mentioned before, 11q- is not frequently associated with *ATM* mutations (30 % of cases), although 11q- almost always implies the loss of *ATM*. Similarly to TP53 and 17p-, mutations in the *ATM* gene entail bad prognosis despite its association with 11q-. Therefore, *ATM* mutations entail short OS, with a more aggressive disease and poor response to chemotherapy, and are related to U-CLL [54]. Another relevant finding concerning *ATM* gene is that biallelic inactivation carries a worse clinical outcome, with more treatment resistance compared to monoallelic alterations [55].

2.1.4. *Novel gene mutations*

New deep sequencing technologies have discovered in the last five years novel recurrent mutations in CLL, *NOTCH1, SF3B1, BIRC3* and *MYD88* being the most frequent [56–58]. These mutations can be observed in approximately 10–15 % of CLLs. Table 3 summarizes the most common mutations with their principal features.

Gene mutations	Chromosome	Association	Biologic function	Clinical outcome	Frequency
NOTCH1	9	+12	NOTCH1 signalling	Poor	10–15 %
SF3B1	2	11q-	mRNA splicing	Poor	5–10 %
BIRC3	11	11q-	NF-κB pathway	Poor	4 %
MYD88	3	13q-	NF-κB pathway	Good	3 %
ATM	11	11q-	DNA repair	Poor	12 %
TP53	17	17p-	DNA repair	Dreadful	5–10 %

Table 3. Most frequent recurrent mutations in CLL

2.1.4.1. NOTCH 1

NOTCH1 mutations occur in around 10–15 % of de novo CLL cases, being more frequent in advanced disease or Richter transformation [59]. These mutations result in the generation of a truncated protein which lacks the C-domain, becoming more stable in activating the *NOTCH-1* signalling pathway. This protein in its normal conformation regulates the transcription of *MYC, TP53* genes and molecules of the NF-κB pathway. Therefore, *NOTCH1* mutations allow, an up-regulation of the cell cycle, and consequently, an advantage in cell survival and apoptosis resistance [41,58]. *NOTCH1* mutations confer to CLL a worse clinical outcome with a shorter TTF, PFS, OS and less response to treatment even in the context of a rituximab-based regimen. In connection with this, bad prognostic markers have been associated with *NOTCH1* mutations. Among them, ZAP-70, CD38 and U-CLL stand out [60]. It is worth noting that approximately 30 % of cases with Richter transformation harbour NOTCH1 mutations. However, it is unclear whether this mutation is acquired during progression disease, as a consequence of clonal evolution or can be observed in early stages of CLL [41,59]. *NOTCH1* mutations have also been associated with +12, and when both alterations cluster, *NOTCH1* separates a subgroup of patients with poor outcome [40]. *NOTCH1* mutations have also been identified in 60 % of cases with T-acute lymphoblastic leukaemia and other non-haematological neoplasms, and its role among them can be ambiguous, acting not only as an oncogene but also as a tumour suppression gene. The relevance of these mutations is even greater as they can be used as a target for therapy. In fact, drugs for this purpose are under development [61].

2.1.4.2. SF3B1

SF3B1 gene is located at chromosome 2q33.1 and encodes for a splicing factor. Different mutations related to the splicing machinery have been associated with oncogenesis, pointing out that aberrant splicing constitutes an important pathway in malignant transformation. Nevertheless, the real mechanism underlying *SF3B1* dysfunction in CLL remains unknown. It is speculated that *SF3B1* mutations may trigger aberrant splicing of important proteins for the tumourigenesis process including cellular cycle control, angiogenesis or apoptosis. Somatic mutations of *SF3B1* can be found in around 10 % of CLL cases, but the incidence increases during disease evolution, probably determining the appearance of aggressive subclones [56]. *SF3B1* mutations in CLL entail bad prognosis with a more aggressive disease, advanced clinical stage at diagnosis and a worse OS, being more frequently observed in fludarabine refractory patients [62]. Bad prognosis markers such as ZAP-70 and U-CLL have also been associated with these mutations. In contrast, Richter transformation is not an often issue among *SF3B1* mutations [59]. In around 50 % of the cases, *SF3B1* mutations occur accompanied by 11q- or ATM mutations, and although unusual, mutations in *SF3B1* and *ATM* have been observed without 11q-. Other haematological diseases such as myelodysplastic syndromes and non-haematologic tumours may harbour *SF3B1* mutations, but they seem mutually exclusive from other lymphoid neoplasms. In contrast to CLL, *SF3B1* mutations confer a more favourable prognosis in myelodysplasia and identify a particular entity: refractory anaemia with ring sideroblasts [63,64].

2.1.4.3. BIRC3

BIRC3 mutations are unusual in CLL, with an incidence of 4 % approximately. The *BIRC3* gene, located near *ATM* gene at 11q33, together with *TRAF2* and *TRAF3* conforms a protein that negatively regulates the activation of the NF-κB signalling pathway. *BIRC3* mutations result in an activation of the NF-κB pathway, hence resistance to apoptosis and increased proliferation of cells. *BIRC3* mutations were found in cases of relapse or fludarabine resistance, especially in the absence of TP53 mutations. In this setting, the incidence of these mutations rises up to 25 %. Anyway, when they appear at diagnosis, a poor clinical outcome is also observed [35]. NF-κB inhibitors are under development in CLL cases harbouring *BIRC3* mutations with encouraging preclinical results [65].

2.1.4.4. MYD88

MYD88 protein takes part in the homeostasis of B human cells working as an adaptor protein of the toll-like/interleukine-1 receptor. *MYD88* mutations cause resistance to apoptosis after they activate the NF-κB pathway. *MYD88* mutations have been found in several lymphoid neoplasms, distinguishing lymphoplasmacytic lymphoma [66,67]. In CLL, they have been reported in a low proportion of cases (3–5 %) [57,58]. In contrast to previous recurrent mutations, mutations in *MYD88* have been associated with a good outcome in CLL patients. They have also been observed more frequently in young patients and detected in association with 13q- and M-CLL, maintaining the favourable prognosis in these populations [68].

2.1.5. Other genetic abnormalities with prognostic relevance

Other genetic abnormalities have been reported in CLL in a very low proportion of cases. These include deletion of 6q, trisomy 3, trisomy 8, trisomy 18, trisomy 19, deletion of 5q and gains of 2p, 3q, 17q and 8q. These alterations have also been related to disease outcome in a recent study that used array comparative genomic hybridization to identify genomic imbalance. Three groups of patients were made according to their prognostic outcome: good outcome (13q- without any of these alterations: gain, 1p, 7p, 12, 18p, 18q, 19, and loss, 4p, 5p, 6q, 7p), adverse outcome (gain, 2p, 3q, 8q, 17q, and loss, 7q, 8p, 11q, 17p, 18p) or intermediate outcome (remainder). This study also identified gain of 3q, 8q and 17p- as independent unfavourable prognostic biomarkers [69]. Translocations are also rare in CLL, but when present, they entail a negative prognostic impact [70]. Finally, complex karyotypes, defined by 3 or more alterations, whether deletions or gains, have also been associated with progressive or refractory disease and *ATM* and *TP53* defects [10,38].

2.2. Other prognostic biomarkers in CLL

Many non-genetic markers predict disease outcome in CLL. A brief enumeration of them and their implication in prognosis will be detailed below. Serum markers LDH and β_2-microglobulin have been widely used, indicating a more advance disease when their levels are high, and although they are not specific for CLL, they can be easily measured in clinical practice [71]. Lymphocyte double time, defined as the number of months that takes the lymphocyte count to double, is another classic prognostic marker that can be easily used in CLL. Hence, it has been proposed as one of the criteria to indicate therapy [72]. Several protein markers were investigated with the intention to find substitute markers for the arduous *IGHV* mutation status. Among them, CD38, ZAP70 (zeta-chain-associated protein) and CD49d stand out. CD38 and ZAP70 were first described as surrogate markers for U-CLL, but this has been controversial [7,9]. However, further studies demonstrated that both are independently associated with poor outcome regardless of mutation status [9,73,74]. CD49d has also been correlated with shorter survival times when expressed at high levels and has recently emerged as the strongest flow cytometry predictor for OS [75]. MicroRNAs are small non-coding RNA molecules which act as posttranscriptional regulators of gene expression. Its dysregulation is associated with tumour development, and in CLL, they might be used as prognostic markers, as some studies have demonstrated. For instance, reduced expression of *miR-29, mir-223, miR-34a* and *mir-181* or increased expression of *miR-21* and *mir-221/222* has been associated with poor prognosis [38]. However, to validate this data, corroboration in prospective studies is necessary.

2.3. Prognostic systems

Numerous prognostic markers have individually shown correlations with survival over the last decades. The current challenge is to build a prognostic model that is clinically relevant, easily applicable, oriented to take therapeutic decisions and feasible in the clinical practice setting. With these goals, some attempts have been done over time. A review of some of these models is summarized in Table 4 and detailed next [76].

Authors	Markers used	Prognostic groups
Rai et al.	-Haematological blood counts -Physical examination	Low: lymphocytosis Intermediate: lymphadenopathy, visceromegaly High: anaemia or thrombocytopenia
Binet et al.	-Haematological blood counts -Physical examination	A: < 3 areas lymphadenopathy B: no A, no B C: anaemia or thrombocytopenia
Döhner et al.	-FISH	13q-: median overall survival (OS) of 133 months Normal karyotype: 111 months +12: 114 months 11q-: 72 months 17p-: 32 months
Wierda et al.	-Age -Absolute lymphocyte count -β_2-microglobulin levels -Rai stage -Sex -Number of lymph node regions	Calculate the 5-year and 10-year survival probability with specific nomogram
Wierda et al.	-LDH -Number of lymph node regions -Size of lymph nodes on the neck -IGHV mutation status -FISH aberrations	Calculate the 2-year and 4-year treatment-free probability with specific nomogram

Authors	Markers used	Prognostic groups
Pflug et al.	-Sex -Age -ECOG status -17p- (six points) -11q- -*IGHV* mutation status -β_2-microglobulin levels -Thymidine kinase	Male, 1 point; TK >10 U/L, 2 points; β_2-microglobulin 1.7–3.5 mg/dL, 1 point; β_2-microglobulin >3.5 mg/dL, 2 points; unmutated-CLL (U-CLL), 1 point; ECOG >0, 1 point; 11q-, 1 point; age >60 years, 1 point Low risk: score 0 to 2 Intermediate risk: score 3 to 5 High risk: score 6 to 10 Very high: score 11 to 14
Rossi et al.	-FISH -New mutations	Very low risk: 13q- only Low risk: +12 or a normal FISH Intermediate risk: *NOTCH1* and/or *SF3B1* and/or 11q- High risk: *TP53* and/or *BIRC3* abnormalities
Haferlach et al.	-Age -Leucocyte count -*IGHV* mutation status -IgH translocations -Number of cytogenetic aberrations -*TP53* deletion -*ATM* mutations	Predicting OS: Age ≥ 65 years, 1 point; leucocyte count ≥20 × 10^9/l, 1 point; U-CLL,1 point; *TP53* deletion, 2 points; translocation involving the *IGH* locus on 14q32, 2 points; number of chromosome aberrations based on CBA 0, 0 points; 1 or 2, 1 point; and ≥3, 2 points Favourable risk: 0–3 points Intermediate risk: 4–5 points Unfavourable risk: "/>5 points Predicting TTFT: U-CLL, 1 point; *ATM* deletion, 1 point; translocation involving the IGH locus on 14q32, 2 points; number of chromosome aberrations based on CBA 0 or 1, 0 points; 2–4, 1 point; and ≥5, 2 points Favourable risk: 0–2 points Intermediate-1 risk: 3 points Intermediate-2 risk: 4 points Unfavourable risk: 5 points

Table 4. Summary of published prognostic indexes for CLL

Rai and Binet prognostic systems [5,6] were the initial scores intended to predict prognosis in patients with CLL. These score systems still stand in routine clinical practice nowadays as they are good predictors for prognosis, inexpensive and able to identify the need for therapy. The biggest disadvantage of them is that a notable amount of patients with early stages progress. *Wierda et al.* [71] developed a nomogram including age and absolute lymphocyte count, β_2-microglobulin levels, Rai stage, sex and number of involved lymph node regions. A specific punctuation was given to each independent covariate, and the summation of the points hurls a new score that can be extrapolated to calculate the 5- and

10-year probability of survival. This model may be useful for previously untreated patients, but its limitations include that it was performed in a young cohort of patients, not extrapolated to all CLL patients, and that new biological markers were not included. However, this nomogram has been validated later in an independent multicentre CLL population and improved by simplifying it into a four-variable model (age, sex, Binet staging, β-2-microglobulin) [77]. The development of FISH studies identified genomic aberrations in around 80 % of CLL patients and led to the stratification into a hierarchy of five prognostic subgroups with decreasing survival times: CLL cases with 17p- had the worst prognosis (median survival of 32 months), followed by cases harbouring 11q- (median survival of 72 months), +12 (median survival of 114 months), normal karyotype (median survival of 111 months) and 13q- (median survival of 133 months) [18]. This model supposed a great achievement to powerfully complement the Rai and Binet prognostic scores and allows to make therapeutic decisions such as to offer a different treatment to 17p- patients. The next step was to include classical and new biological and genetic markers in the same prognostic score. In line with this, *Wierda et al.* [78] proposed a new nomogram, this time including new prognostic markers, with the purpose to calculate the 2- and 4-year probability of TTFT. Along with LDH, the number of involved lymph node sites and large size of lymph nodes of the neck, new biological factors such as *IGHV* mutation status and FISH aberrations according to the hierarchal model were included. This model has not been validated in independent cohorts and has not been used to calculate OS. Nevertheless, it can be useful to identify patients at high risk for progression to treatment. The German CLL Study Group came up with another prognostic system based on 23 classical and novel biological and genetic markers [79]. Eight factors were finally independently associated with inferior survival: sex, age, ECOG status, 17p-, 11q-, *IGHV* mutation status, serum β_2-microglobulin levels and serum thymidine kinase. According to these factors, four risk categories could be separated with different survival times. This prognostic score was validated in an independent cohort. Comparing with classic staging systems, this prognostic score allows to identify early-stage patients who will sooner progress and to separate ultrahigh-risk patients. However, there are some barriers to adopt this score into clinical practice including that thymidine kinase is not available routinely; new data regarding novel mutations such as *NOTCH1, SF3B1* or *BIRC3* has not been incorporated; and p53 mutations in patients without 17p- were not represented. *Haferlach et al.* proposed two new scoring systems with a combination of genetic and classical markers. The parameters incorporated were age, leukocyte count, *IGHV* mutation status, IgH translocations, number of chromosomal aberrations detected with CBA (chromosome banding analysis) and *TP53* and *ATM* mutations. The applicability of these scores in the current setting is limited, as CBA is not commonly performed in clinical practice. *Rossi et al.* [80] were the first to propose a scoring system integrating both cytogenetic and mutational markers. This scoring system separates CLL patients into four prognostic risk groups: high risk, harbouring *TP53* and/or *BIRC3* abnormalities (10-year OS: 29 %); intermediate risk, harbouring *NOTCH1* and/or *SF3B1* mutations and/or 11q- (10-year OS: 37 %); low risk, harbouring +12 or a normal genetics (10-year OS: 57 %); and very low risk, harbouring 13q- only, whose 10-year OS

(69.3 %) did not significantly differ from a matched general population. This model exhibits superiority in discrimination patient outcome to the FISH-based model and can be used at any time point from diagnosis, maintaining its prognostic relevance. It emphasizes the importance of including new recurrent mutations, as these may reclassify patients into a higher-risk group. Other authors partially replicated this scoring system although finding some discrepancies that suggested that *NOTCH1* and *SF3B1* mutations should be considered as higher-risk alterations [81,82].

3. Targeted therapy for CLL

Immuno-chemotherapy is the initial approach to the majority of CLL patients who require therapy nowadays. However, some patients relapse, become refractory or suffer important secondary adverse events. For these reasons, the emergence of new targeted treatments has and will revolutionize the treatment model for CLL. Hopefully, targeted therapy will be not only more effective in improving survival of CLL patients but also less toxic, ameliorating quality of life of patients under treatment. This part of the chapter will be dedicated to review the novel targeted treatments that have been already approved or are being studied for the treatment of CLL.

3.1. Second-generation anti-CD20 monoclonal antibodies

CLL cells express antigen CD20 with a low intensity, but enough for the chimeric mouse anti-human CD20 monoclonal antibody rituximab to lyse these cells. Rituximab acts by different mechanisms including antibody-dependent cell-mediated cytotoxicity (ADCC), complement-mediated cytotoxicity and direct toxicity. When used in combination with chemotherapy, rituximab has demonstrated superiority over chemotherapy regimens and has therefore become a standard of care in the treatment of CLL patients either in front-line or salvage therapy [14,15].

3.1.1. Ofatumumab

Ofatumumab is a fully humanized anti-CD20 that binds to a different CD20 epitope than rituximab, generating a greater cytotoxic potential than rituximab by complement-mediated cytotoxicity with the same ADCC. It has been approved by the Food and Drug Administration (FDA) and the European Medicines Agency (EMA) for the treatment of fludarabine and alemtuzumab refractory CLL patients and recently by the FDA for previously untreated patients in combination with chlorambucil (Clb) in whom fludarabine-based therapy is considered inappropriate. The study that gave the indication of ofatumumab for previously treated patients consisted of a phase II trial including 138 patients with either fludarabine and alemtuzumab refractoriness or fludarabine refractoriness and bulky disease. Overall response (OR) rates were 58 % and 47 %, and median OS were 13.7 and 15.4 months, respectively. The most common adverse events were infusion reactions and infections, which were primarily grade 1 or 2 events [83]. The FDA approval of ofatumumab in combination with chlorambucil for previously untreated CLL patients was based on the results of a phase III trial only preliminary reported, comparing ofatumumab in combination with chlorambucil to single-agent chlorambucil in 447 patients in whom fludarabine-based therapy was considered to be inappropriate. The ofatumumab + chlorambucil arm demonstrated superiority with a higher OR (82 % vs. 69 %), CR (12 % vs. 1 %) and PFS (22.4 vs. 13.1 months) [84]. Anyway, a formal comparative trial of ofatumumab versus rituximab is missing, and therefore, the real value of ofatumumab remains to be determined.

3.1.2. Obinutuzumab (GA101)

Obinutuzumab is a new second-generation recombinant humanized anti-CD20, glycoengineered to increase its affinity in binding the type 2 CD20 epitope. Obinutuzumab produces an increased ADCC and direct cytotoxicity, with lower complement-mediated toxicity. The FDA approved this drug for its use in combination with chlorambucil for the treatment of patients with previously untreated CLL, in view of the primary results of the CLL-11 trial [85]. This study consisted of a phase III international clinical trial that compared chlorambucil (Clb) versus chlorambucil plus rituximab (R-Clb) versus chlorambucil plus obinutuzumab (O-Clb) in previously untreated CLL patients not candidates to receive fludarabine. Patients in the O-Clb arm achieved a higher OR rate and a prolonged PFS compared to patients in the R-Clb arm and a benefit in OS, PFS and OR rate than patients receiving Clb alone. Grade 3 and 4 neutropenia and infusion reactions were more common with O-Clb than with R-Clb, but the risk of infection was not increased. An updated analysis of this trial has been recently published, confirming the PFS benefit in the arm of O-Clb vs. R-Clb (29.2 versus 15.4 months, $P<0.001$) and reporting a longer TTFT in the arm of O-Clb vs. R-Clb (42.7 versus 32.7 months, $P<0.001$). The previously observed OS benefit of G-Clb over Clb monotherapy was confirmed [86].

3.2. B-Cell receptor signalling pathway

The B-cell receptor (BCR) signalling pathway is vital for CLL cell survival and proliferation and therefore constitutes an important new strategy for targeted therapy in CLL. Bruton tyrosine kinase (BTK) or phosphoinositide 3'-kinase (PI3K) constitutes some of the key kinases in this pathway. Inhibitors of these kinases have been under investigation in patients with CLL with promising clinical results and minimal toxicity. In fact, ibrutinib and idelalisib, two oral compounds given as continuous treatment, have been recently approved for treatment of CLL patients. They have demonstrated high efficacy even in the higher-risk patient subgroup. One important aspect of treatment with BCR inhibitors is the development of lymphocytosis, often transient, mediated by the migration of CLL cells from the bone marrow and lymph nodes to the peripheral blood, where cell survival is decreased.

3.2.1. Ibrutinib

Ibrutinib is an oral small molecule that acts as an irreversible covalent inhibitor of the BTK resulting in an inhibition of the BCR signalling pathway. It is the first BCR inhibitor approved by the FDA and EMA for the treatment of relapsed or refractory CLL and as a first-line treatment in cases of 17p- or *TP53* mutations in patients unsuitable for chemo-immunotherapy. Ibrutinib was approved in light of the results of a phase Ib/II multicentre clinical trial that included 85 refractory or relapsed CLL patients to receive ibrutinib at different doses [87]. The population represented at this trial had a high-risk disease with 33 % of 17p-, 36 % of 11q- and a median of four prior therapies. The results were encouraging with an OR rate independent of adverse risk factors of 71 % and an additional 15–20 % of patients with partial response with persistent lymphocytosis but reduced lymph nodes. The estimated 26-month PFS was 75 %, suggesting that ibrutinib responses are quite durable. Ibrutinib was well tolerated with predominant adverse events being grade 1 or 2 including transient diarrhoea, fatigue and upper respiratory tract infections. Subsequently, a multicentric randomized phase III compared ibrutinib with ofatumumab in a group of previously treated patients not candidates for purine analogues [88]. The trial was stopped early after interim analysis because of a significant improvement in OS and PFS in the ibrutinib arm. The promising results of these trials prompted out combination studies that are currently ongoing or have been completed. Combinations of ibrutinib plus rituximab or ibrutinib plus bendamustine and rituximab have also been explored in different trials that enrolled high-risk, refractory or relapsed CLL patients, obtaining OR rates between 93 % and 95%, with an acceptable toxicity profile and being effective even in the subgroups of patients with 17p- or *TP53* mutations [89,90]. In summary, ibrutinib is a well-tolerated drug that has been demonstrated to produce high response rates even in high-risk CLLs. The combination of ibrutinib with other drugs is under investigation and will hopefully change the actual paradigm of CLL treatment due to the encouraging preliminary results. Unfortunately, resistances and progressions to Richter syndrome have been described with a dismal prognosis in these cases.

3.2.2. Idelalisib (CAL-101)

Idelalisib is an oral selective inhibitor of PI3K that produces apoptosis in CLL cells. It has been approved by the FDA and EMA for use in combination with rituximab for patients who have received at least one prior therapy or as first-line treatment in the presence of 17p deletion or *TP53* mutation in patients unsuitable for chemo-immunotherapy. The efficacy of idelalisib in combination with rituximab was assessed in a multicentre randomized phase III trial that compared idelalisib plus rituximab with idelalisib plus placebo in patients with relapsed CLL. Most of the patients enrolled had adverse prognostic factors including 17p-, TP53 mutations or M-CLL. Idelalisib obtained a higher OR rate than placebo (81 % vs. 13 %, P> 0.001) and a superior OS (92 % vs. 80 % at 12 months, P=0.02). PFS at 24 weeks was 93 % in the idelalisib group compared with 46 % in the placebo group (P<0.001). Serious adverse events occurred in both groups in a proportion of 40 % (idelalisib) and 35 % (placebo). These included pneumonia, pyrexia and febrile neutropenia. The benefit of idelalisib was maintained among patients with adverse genetic features. Analogously to ibrutinib, lymphocytosis with node response was observed in some patients [91]. In view of this exciting results, further trials with idelalisib in combination with bendamustine, fludarabine or chlorambucil in patients with relapsed or refractory CLL are being performed, confirming the feasibility and benefits of these combinations [92].

3.3. Bcl-2 inhibitors

B-cell lymphoma-2 (Bcl-2) proteins, encoded by the Bcl-2 gene, are expressed at high levels in CLL cells. These proteins contribute to the regulation of the apoptotic process and therefore constitute an important therapeutic target for CLL.

3.3.1. ABT-263 (navitoclax)

Navitoclax is an orally bioavailable BCL-2 inhibitor that binds to several antiapoptotic BCL-2 family proteins including BCL-2, BCL-XL, BCL-x and BCL-B. A phase I trial conducted to evaluate the biologic activity, safety and pharmacokinetics of ABT-263 demonstrated encouraging results for this molecule as a single agent, even in patients with fludarabine-refractory disease, bulky adenopathy or 17p-. However, its therapeutic use was limited because of severe thrombocytopenia, observed as an important adverse effect in 28 % of the patients due to the inhibition of BCL-XL.

3.3.2. GDC-0199/ABT-199 (venetoclax)

GDC-0199/ABT-199 is a small molecule reengineered to decrease the thrombocytopenia side effect of navitoclax. ABT-199 produces a selective inhibition BCL-2 with a reduced effect on BCL-XL. It has shown promising results in a phase I trial that enrolled 56 refractory or relapsed CLL patients, 29 % with 17p- and 32 % with fludarabine resistance [93]. The major side effects included tumour lysis syndrome and neutropenia. Interestingly, ABT-199 yielded an OR rate of 85 %, with 13 % of complete responses and 72% of partial responses. These encouraging results were also observed in high-risk patients, with a response rate of 88 % and 75 % in patients with 17p- and fludarabine refractory, respectively. Clearly, these data indicate that Bcl-2 inhibitors will play an important role in the future for the treatment of CLL patients, and therefore, ABT-199 is currently being investigated in combination with immuno-chemotherapy.

3.4. Immunomodulatory drugs

Changes in the microenvironment of tumour cells promote the selective survival of malignant CLL cells preventing apoptosis. Immunomodulatory drugs act by altering cellular features and the cytokines of tumour microenvironment. In fact, lenalidomide has been shown to be effective in CLL.

3.4.1. Lenalidomide

Lenalidomide is an oral second-generation immunomodulatory drug with antiangiogenic, cytokine activity modulating, and immunomodule properties. It has been demonstrated to be active in MDS, multiple myeloma and lymphoproliferative disorders. The first phase II trials that tested lenalidomide in relapsed or refractory CLL obtained an OR rate between 32 % and 47 %. The major adverse effects reported were myelotoxicity, tumour flare and tumour lysis syndrome, all of them ameliorated with lower doses of lenalidomide [94,95]. Lenalidomide was also tested as a front-line therapy for CLL patients in another two trials with a different dosing, but both with a low initial dose (2.5–5 mg daily) and a further escalation to a target of 25 mg. These trials obtained an OR rate between 56 % and 65 %. A high proportion of tumour flare reactions were observed in one of them, although they were mild. Grade 3 or 4 neutropenia was also frequent but without serious consequences. A recent update of one of these studies showed that at a median follow-up of 4 years, time to treatment failure had not been reached and OS was 86 %. These studies showed that lenalidomide is effective as first-line therapy for CLL and is well tolerated when administered in a dose escalation plan [96–98]. Lenalidomide has also been tested in combination with other drugs. In a phase II trial, patients with relapsed or refractory CLL received a combination of rituximab and lenalidomide obtaining an OR rate of 66 % including 12 % of complete responses. Seventy-three percent of patients showed neutropenia (grade 3 or 4), and only 1 episode of grade 3 tumour lysis was reported. Another phase II study of lenalidomide and rituximab was performed, this time as a first-line therapy. The OR rate was 88 %, including 15 % of complete responses. Again, neutropenia was the most common adverse event [99,100]. Additional combinations are currently under study, as well as maintenance therapy after chemo-immunotherapy.

3.5. Chimeric antigen receptors

Chimeric antigen receptors (CARs) are engineered constructs that combine the antigen recognition domain of an antibody with intracellular signalling domains into a single chimeric protein. CD19 antigen is exclusively expressed in B-cells and therefore is a very suitable target for the treatment of CLL with CARs. Indeed, a pivot clinical trial proved the important antitumor activity of this CAR-modified autologous T-cells targeted to CD19 (CART19 cells) in three patients with refractory CLL [101]. Two out of the three patients achieved a complete response lasting longer than two years and the other patient a partial stable response. Toxicities included hypogammaglobulinemia, decreased number of plasma-cells and B-cell aplasia. The CART19 cells expanded > 1,000-fold in vivo and expressed functional CARs for at least six months, and a proportion of them persisted as memory CART19 cells. On average, each infused CAR-expressing T-cell was calculated to eradicate at least 1,000 CLL cells. In another study, ten patients with refractory CLL or relapsed B-cell acute lymphoblastic leukaemia (ALL) were treated with CART19 modified to express a second-generation CAR anti-CD19. Three of the four evaluable patients with bulky CLL who received prior treatment with cyclophosphamide experienced either a significant reduction or a mixed response in lymphadenopathy without development of B-cell aplasia. The short-term persistence of infused T-cells was enhanced by previous administration of cyclophosphamide and was inversely proportional to the tumour burden in peripheral blood [102]. In addition, a longer follow-up from ten patients treated with CART19 was reported. The study included nine adults with relapse or refractory CLL, three patients with p53 deletion and a child with relapsed and refractory ALL [103]. CLL patients received chemotherapy regimens 4–6 days before CART19 infusions. Four of the nine evaluable patients achieved a complete response, including three patients with CLL. Two additional patients from the CLL group had a partial response lasting from three to five months, and three patients did not respond. In the four patients who achieved complete response, maximal expanded cells in peripheral blood were detected at an average of 27-fold higher than the infused dose. No patients with complete response relapsed. Patients who responded developed a cytokine release syndrome manifested by fever, as well as variable degrees of anorexia, nausea, transient hypotension and hypoxia. In responding CLL patients, cytokine levels were increased, and five patients with cytokine release required treatment. In summary, CART19 can induce potent and sustained responses in patients with advance, refractory and high-risk CLL. However, further research is needed to ascertain the efficacy of this therapy and minimize associated cytokine-mediated toxicities.

Author details

Isabel González Gascón y Marín[1*], María Hernández-Sánchez[2], Ana-Eugenia Rodríguez.Vicente[2] and José-Ángel Hernández-Rivas[1,3]

*Address all correspondence to: igonzalezg@salud.madrid.org

1 Hospital Universitario Infanta Leonor, Madrid, Spain

2 Centro de Investigación del Cáncer. IBSAL. Universidad de Salamanca, Spain

3 Universidad Complutense, Madrid, Spain

References

[1] Rozman C, Montserrat E. Chronic lymphocytic leukemia. N Engl J Med. 1995 Oct 19;333(16):1052–7.

[2] Hallek M. Chronic lymphocytic leukemia: 2013 update on diagnosis, risk stratification and treatment. Am J Hematol. 2013 Sep;88(9):803–16.

[3] Dighiero G, Hamblin TJ. Chronic lymphocytic leukaemia. Lancet. 2008 Mar 22;371(9617):1017–29.

[4] Hernández JA, González M, Hernández JM. [Chronic lymphocytic leukemia]. Med Clínica. 2010 Jul 3;135(4):172–8.

[5] Rai KR, Sawitsky A, Cronkite EP, Chanana AD, Levy RN, Pasternack BS. Clinical staging of chronic lymphocytic leukemia. Blood. 1975 Aug;46(2):219–34.

[6] Binet JL, Auquier A, Dighiero G, Chastang C, Piguet H, Goasguen J, et al. A new prognostic classification of chronic lymphocytic leukemia derived from a multivariate survival analysis. Cancer. 1981 Jul 1;48(1):198–206.

[7] Crespo M, Bosch F, Villamor N, Bellosillo B, Colomer D, Rozman M, et al. ZAP-70 expression as a surrogate for immunoglobulin-variable-region mutations in chronic lymphocytic leukemia. N Engl J Med. 2003 May 1;348(18):1764–75.

[8] Hamblin TJ, Davis Z, Gardiner A, Oscier DG, Stevenson FK. Unmutated Ig V(H) genes are associated with a more aggressive form of chronic lymphocytic leukemia. Blood. 1999 Sep 15;94(6):1848–54.

[9] Damle RN, Wasil T, Fais F, Ghiotto F, Valetto A, Allen SL, et al. Ig V gene mutation status and CD38 expression as novel prognostic indicators in chronic lymphocytic leukemia. Blood. 1999 Sep 15;94(6):1840–7.

[10] Rodríguez-Vicente AE, Díaz MG, Hernández-Rivas JM. Chronic lymphocytic leukemia: a clinical and molecular heterogenous disease. Cancer Genet. 2013 Mar;206(3): 49–62.

[11] Del Giudice I, Chiaretti S, Tavolaro S, De Propris MS, Maggio R, Mancini F, et al. Spontaneous regression of chronic lymphocytic leukemia: clinical and biologic features of 9 cases. Blood. 2009 Jul 16;114(3):638–46.

[12] Brenner H, Gondos A, Pulte D. Trends in long-term survival of patients with chronic lymphocytic leukemia from the 1980s to the early 21st century. Blood. 2008 May 15;111(10):4916–21.

[13] Knauf WU, Lissichkov T, Aldaoud A, Liberati A, Loscertales J, Herbrecht R, et al. Phase III randomized study of bendamustine compared with chlorambucil in previously untreated patients with chronic lymphocytic leukemia. J Clin Oncol Off J Am Soc Clin Oncol. 2009 Sep 10;27(26):4378–84.

[14] Fischer K, Cramer P, Busch R, Böttcher S, Bahlo J, Schubert J, et al. Bendamustine in combination with rituximab for previously untreated patients with chronic lymphocytic leukemia: a multicenter phase II trial of the German Chronic Lymphocytic Leukemia Study Group. J Clin Oncol Off J Am Soc Clin Oncol. 2012 Sep 10;30(26):3209–16.

[15] Hallek M, Fischer K, Fingerle-Rowson G, Fink AM, Busch R, Mayer J, et al. Addition of rituximab to fludarabine and cyclophosphamide in patients with chronic lymphocytic leukaemia: a randomised, open-label, phase 3 trial. Lancet. 2010 Oct 2;376(9747): 1164–74.

[16] Hillmen P, Gribben JG, Follows GA, Milligan D, Sayala HA, Moreton P, et al. Rituximab plus chlorambucil as first-line treatment for chronic lymphocytic leukemia: Final analysis of an open-label phase II study. J Clin Oncol Off J Am Soc Clin Oncol. 2014 Apr 20;32(12):1236–41.

[17] NCCN Clinical Practice Guidelines in Oncology (NCCN Guidelines). Non-Hodgkin's Lymphomas. Version 1.2015 [Internet]. [cited 2015 Feb 1]. Available from: http://www.nccn.org/professionals/physician_gls/pdf/nhl.pdf

[18] Döhner H, Stilgenbauer S, Benner A, Leupolt E, Kröber A, Bullinger L, et al. Genomic aberrations and survival in chronic lymphocytic leukemia. N Engl J Med. 2000 Dec 28;343(26):1910–6.

[19] Mosca L, Fabris S, Lionetti M, Todoerti K, Agnelli L, Morabito F, et al. Integrative genomics analyses reveal molecularly distinct subgroups of B-cell chronic lymphocytic leukemia patients with 13q14 deletion. Clin Cancer Res Off J Am Assoc Cancer Res. 2010 Dec 1;16(23):5641–53.

[20] Parker H, Rose-Zerilli MJJ, Parker A, Chaplin T, Wade R, Gardiner A, et al. 13q deletion anatomy and disease progression in patients with chronic lymphocytic leukemia. Leukemia. 2011 Mar;25(3):489–97.

[21] Chena C, Avalos JS, Bezares RF, Arrossagaray G, Turdó K, Bistmans A, et al. Biallelic deletion 13q14.3 in patients with chronic lymphocytic leukemia: cytogenetic, FISH and clinical studies. Eur J Haematol. 2008 Aug;81(2):94–9.

[22] Van Dyke DL, Shanafelt TD, Call TG, Zent CS, Smoley SA, Rabe KG, et al. A comprehensive evaluation of the prognostic significance of 13q deletions in patients with B-chronic lymphocytic leukaemia. Br J Haematol. 2010 Feb;148(4):544–50.

[23] Puiggros A, Delgado J, Rodriguez-Vicente A, Collado R, Aventín A, Luño E, et al. Biallelic losses of 13q do not confer a poorer outcome in chronic lymphocytic leukaemia: analysis of 627 patients with isolated 13q deletion. Br J Haematol. 2013 Oct; 163(1):47–54.

[24] Garg R, Wierda W, Ferrajoli A, Abruzzo L, Pierce S, Lerner S, et al. The prognostic difference of monoallelic versus biallelic deletion of 13q in chronic lymphocytic leukemia. Cancer. 2012 Jul 15;118(14):3531–7.

[25] Dal Bo M, Rossi FM, Rossi D, Deambrogi C, Bertoni F, Del Giudice I, et al. 13q14 deletion size and number of deleted cells both influence prognosis in chronic lymphocytic leukemia. Genes Chromosomes Cancer. 2011 Aug;50(8):633–43.

[26] Hernández JA, Rodríguez AE, González M, Benito R, Fontanillo C, Sandoval V, et al. A high number of losses in 13q14 chromosome band is associated with a worse outcome and biological differences in patients with B-cell chronic lymphoid leukemia. Haematologica. 2009 Mar;94(3):364–71.

[27] Migliazza A, Bosch F, Komatsu H, Cayanis E, Martinotti S, Toniato E, et al. Nucleotide sequence, transcription map, and mutation analysis of the 13q14 chromosomal region deleted in B-cell chronic lymphocytic leukemia. Blood. 2001 Apr 1;97(7):2098–104.

[28] Calin GA, Dumitru CD, Shimizu M, Bichi R, Zupo S, Noch E, et al. Frequent deletions and down-regulation of micro- RNA genes miR15 and miR16 at 13q14 in chronic lymphocytic leukemia. Proc Natl Acad Sci U S A. 2002 Nov 26;99(24):15524–9.

[29] Döhner H, Stilgenbauer S, James MR, Benner A, Weilguni T, Bentz M, et al. 11q deletions identify a new subset of B-cell chronic lymphocytic leukemia characterized by extensive nodal involvement and inferior prognosis. Blood. 1997 Apr 1;89(7):2516–22.

[30] Neilson JR, Auer R, White D, Bienz N, Waters JJ, Whittaker JA, et al. Deletions at 11q identify a subset of patients with typical CLL who show consistent disease progression and reduced survival. Leukemia. 1997 Nov;11(11):1929–32.

[31] Tsimberidou A-M, Tam C, Abruzzo LV, O'Brien S, Wierda WG, Lerner S, et al. Chemoimmunotherapy may overcome the adverse prognostic significance of 11q deletion in previously untreated patients with chronic lymphocytic leukemia. Cancer. 2009 Jan 15;115(2):373–80.

[32] Marasca R, Maffei R, Martinelli S, Fiorcari S, Bulgarelli J, Debbia G, et al. Clinical heterogeneity of de novo 11q deletion chronic lymphocytic leukaemia: prognostic relevance of extent of 11q deleted nuclei inside leukemic clone. Hematol Oncol. 2013 Jun; 31(2):88–95.

[33] Jain P, Keating M, Thompson P, Trinh L, Wang X, Wierda W, et al. High FISH percentage of deletion 11q in patients with chronic lymphocytic leukemia is an independent predictor of adverse outcome. Am J Hematol. 2015 Feb 14.

[34] Rossi D, Gaidano G. ATM and chronic lymphocytic leukemia: mutations, and not only deletions, matter. Haematologica. 2012 Jan;97(1):5–8.

[35] Rossi D, Fangazio M, Rasi S, Vaisitti T, Monti S, Cresta S, et al. Disruption of BIRC3 associates with fludarabine chemorefractoriness in TP53 wild-type chronic lymphocytic leukemia. Blood. 2012 Mar 22;119(12):2854–62.

[36] Puiggros A, Blanco G, Espinet B. Genetic abnormalities in chronic lymphocytic leukemia: where we are and where we go. BioMed Res Int. 2014;2014:435983.

[37] Matutes E, Oscier D, Garcia-Marco J, Ellis J, Copplestone A, Gillingham R, et al. Trisomy 12 defines a group of CLL with atypical morphology: correlation between cytogenetic, clinical and laboratory features in 544 patients. Br J Haematol. 1996 Feb;92(2): 382–8.

[38] Rosenquist R, Cortese D, Bhoi S, Mansouri L, Gunnarsson R. Prognostic markers and their clinical applicability in chronic lymphocytic leukemia: where do we stand? Leuk Lymphoma. 2013 Nov;54(11):2351–64.

[39] Weissmann S, Roller A, Jeromin S, Hernández M, Abáigar M, Hernández-Rivas JM, et al. Prognostic impact and landscape of NOTCH1 mutations in chronic lymphocytic leukemia (CLL): a study on 852 patients. Leukemia. 2013 Dec;27(12):2393–6.

[40] Balatti V, Lerner S, Rizzotto L, Rassenti LZ, Bottoni A, Palamarchuk A, et al. Trisomy 12 CLLs progress through NOTCH1 mutations. Leukemia. 2013 Mar;27(3):740–3.

[41] Villamor N, Conde L, Martínez-Trillos A, Cazorla M, Navarro A, Beà S, et al. NOTCH1 mutations identify a genetic subgroup of chronic lymphocytic leukemia patients with high risk of transformation and poor outcome. Leukemia. 2013 Apr; 27(5):1100–6.

[42] González-Gascón Y Marín I, Hernández-Sánchez M, Rodríguez-Vicente A-E, Sanzo C, Aventín A, Puiggros A, et al. A high proportion of cells carrying trisomy 12 is associated with a worse outcome in patients with chronic lymphocytic leukemia. Hematol Oncol. 2015 Feb 17.

[43] Cramer P, Hallek M. Prognostic factors in chronic lymphocytic leukemia-what do we need to know? Nat Rev Clin Oncol. 2011 Jan;8(1):38–47.

[44] Zenz T, Kröber A, Scherer K, Häbe S, Bühler A, Benner A, et al. Monoallelic TP53 inactivation is associated with poor prognosis in chronic lymphocytic leukemia: results from a detailed genetic characterization with long-term follow-up. Blood. 2008 Oct 15;112(8):3322–9.

[45] Zenz T, Vollmer D, Trbusek M, Smardova J, Benner A, Soussi T, et al. TP53 mutation profile in chronic lymphocytic leukemia: evidence for a disease specific profile from a comprehensive analysis of 268 mutations. Leukemia. 2010 Dec;24(12):2072–9.

[46] Zenz T, Häbe S, Denzel T, Mohr J, Winkler D, Bühler A, et al. Detailed analysis of p53 pathway defects in fludarabine-refractory chronic lymphocytic leukemia (CLL): dissecting the contribution of 17p deletion, TP53 mutation, p53-p21 dysfunction, and miR34a in a prospective clinical trial. Blood. 2009 Sep 24;114(13):2589–97.

[47] Tam CS, Shanafelt TD, Wierda WG, Abruzzo LV, Van Dyke DL, O'Brien S, et al. De novo deletion 17p13.1 chronic lymphocytic leukemia shows significant clinical heterogeneity: the M. D. Anderson and Mayo Clinic experience. Blood. 2009 Jul 30;114(5): 957–64.

[48] Döhner H, Fischer K, Bentz M, Hansen K, Benner A, Cabot G, et al. p53 gene deletion predicts for poor survival and non-response to therapy with purine analogs in chronic B-cell leukemias. Blood. 1995 Mar 15;85(6):1580–9.

[49] Panovska-Stavridis I, Ivanovski M, Siljanovski N, Cevreska L, Efremov DG. Chronic lymphocytic leukemia patients with a V1-69 gene rearrangement do not have inferior survival with respect to patients that express other unmutated V(H) genes. Leuk Res. 2007 Feb;31(2):245–8.

[50] Thorsélius M, Kröber A, Murray F, Thunberg U, Tobin G, Bühler A, et al. Strikingly homologous immunoglobulin gene rearrangements and poor outcome in VH3-21-using chronic lymphocytic leukemia patients independent of geographic origin and mutational status. Blood. 2006 Apr 1;107(7):2889–94.

[51] Dreger P, Schetelig J, Andersen N, Corradini P, Van Gelder M, Gribben J, et al. Managing high-risk CLL during transition to a new treatment era: stem cell transplantation or novel agents? Blood. 2014 Dec 18;124(26):3841–9.

[52] Rossi D, Khiabanian H, Spina V, Ciardullo C, Bruscaggin A, Famà R, et al. Clinical impact of small TP53 mutated subclones in chronic lymphocytic leukemia. Blood. 2014 Apr 3;123(14):2139–47.

http://dx.doi.org/10.5772/60738

[53] Ouillette P, Li J, Shaknovich R, Li Y, Melnick A, Shedden K, et al. Incidence and clinical implications of ATM aberrations in chronic lymphocytic leukemia. Genes Chromosomes Cancer. 2012 Dec;51(12):1125–32.

[54] Austen B, Powell JE, Alvi A, Edwards I, Hooper L, Starczynski J, et al. Mutations in the ATM gene lead to impaired overall and treatment-free survival that is independent of IGVH mutation status in patients with B-CLL. Blood. 2005 Nov 1;106(9):3175–82.

[55] Rose-Zerilli MJJ, Forster J, Parker H, Parker A, Rodríguez AE, Chaplin T, et al. ATM mutation rather than BIRC3 deletion and/or mutation predicts reduced survival in 11q-deleted chronic lymphocytic leukemia: data from the UK LRF CLL4 trial. Haematologica. 2014 Apr;99(4):736–42.

[56] Quesada V, Conde L, Villamor N, Ordóñez GR, Jares P, Bassaganyas L, et al. Exome sequencing identifies recurrent mutations of the splicing factor SF3B1 gene in chronic lymphocytic leukemia. Nat Genet. 2012 Jan;44(1):47–52.

[57] Wang L, Lawrence MS, Wan Y, Stojanov P, Sougnez C, Stevenson K, et al. SF3B1 and other novel cancer genes in chronic lymphocytic leukemia. N Engl J Med. 2011 Dec 29;365(26):2497–506.

[58] Puente XS, Pinyol M, Quesada V, Conde L, Ordóñez GR, Villamor N, et al. Whole-genome sequencing identifies recurrent mutations in chronic lymphocytic leukaemia. Nature. 2011 Jul 7;475(7354):101–5.

[59] Rossi D, Rasi S, Spina V, Fangazio M, Monti S, Greco M, et al. Different impact of NOTCH1 and SF3B1 mutations on the risk of chronic lymphocytic leukemia transformation to Richter syndrome. Br J Haematol. 2012 Aug;158(3):426–9.

[60] Rossi D, Rasi S, Fabbri G, Spina V, Fangazio M, Forconi F, et al. Mutations of NOTCH1 are an independent predictor of survival in chronic lymphocytic leukemia. Blood. 2012 Jan 12;119(2):521–9.

[61] Paganin M, Ferrando A. Molecular pathogenesis and targeted therapies for NOTCH1-induced T-cell acute lymphoblastic leukemia. Blood Rev. 2011 Mar;25(2): 83–90.

[62] Rossi D, Bruscaggin A, Spina V, Rasi S, Khiabanian H, Messina M, et al. Mutations of the SF3B1 splicing factor in chronic lymphocytic leukemia: association with progression and fludarabine-refractoriness. Blood. 2011 Dec 22;118(26):6904–8.

[63] Visconte V, Makishima H, Maciejewski JP, Tiu RV. Emerging roles of the spliceosomal machinery in myelodysplastic syndromes and other hematological disorders. Leukemia. 2012 Dec;26(12):2447–54.

[64] Cazzola M, Rossi M, Malcovati L. Associazione Italiana per la Ricerca sul Cancro Gruppo Italiano Malattie Mieloproliferative. Biologic and clinical significance of so-

matic mutations of SF3B1 in myeloid and lymphoid neoplasms. Blood. 2013 Jan 10;121(2):260–9.

[65] Hertlein E, Wagner AJ, Jones J, Lin TS, Maddocks KJ, Towns WH, et al. 17-DMAG targets the nuclear factor-kappaB family of proteins to induce apoptosis in chronic lymphocytic leukemia: clinical implications of HSP90 inhibition. Blood. 2010 Jul 8;116(1):45–53.

[66] Ngo VN, Young RM, Schmitz R, Jhavar S, Xiao W, Lim K-H, et al. Oncogenically active MYD88 mutations in human lymphoma. Nature. 2011 Feb 3;470(7332):115–9.

[67] Treon SP, Xu L, Yang G, Zhou Y, Liu X, Cao Y, et al. MYD88 L265P somatic mutation in Waldenström's macroglobulinemia. N Engl J Med. 2012 Aug 30;367(9):826–33.

[68] Martínez-Trillos A, Pinyol M, Navarro A, Aymerich M, Jares P, Juan M, et al. Mutations in TLR/MYD88 pathway identify a subset of young chronic lymphocytic leukemia patients with favorable outcome. Blood. 2014 Jun 12;123(24):3790–6.

[69] Houldsworth J, Guttapalli A, Thodima V, Yan XJ, Mendiratta G, Zielonka T, et al. Genomic imbalance defines three prognostic groups for risk stratification of patients with chronic lymphocytic leukemia. Leuk Lymphoma. 2014 Apr;55(4):920–8.

[70] Cavazzini F, Hernandez JA, Gozzetti A, Russo Rossi A, De Angeli C, Tiseo R, et al. Chromosome 14q32 translocations involving the immunoglobulin heavy chain locus in chronic lymphocytic leukaemia identify a disease subset with poor prognosis. Br J Haematol. 2008 Aug;142(4):529–37.

[71] Wierda WG, O'Brien S, Wang X, Faderl S, Ferrajoli A, Do K-A, et al. Prognostic nomogram and index for overall survival in previously untreated patients with chronic lymphocytic leukemia. Blood. 2007 Jun 1;109(11):4679–85.

[72] Hallek M, Cheson BD, Catovsky D, Caligaris-Cappio F, Dighiero G, Döhner H, et al. Guidelines for the diagnosis and treatment of chronic lymphocytic leukemia: a report from the International Workshop on Chronic Lymphocytic Leukemia updating the National Cancer Institute-Working Group 1996 guidelines. Blood. 2008 Jun 15;111(12):5446–56.

[73] Ibrahim S, Keating M, Do KA, O'Brien S, Huh YO, Jilani I, et al. CD38 expression as an important prognostic factor in B-cell chronic lymphocytic leukemia. Blood. 2001 Jul 1;98(1):181–6.

[74] Dürig J, Nückel H, Cremer M, Führer A, Halfmeyer K, Fandrey J, et al. ZAP-70 expression is a prognostic factor in chronic lymphocytic leukemia. Leukemia. 2003 Dec; 17(12):2426–34.

[75] Bulian P, Shanafelt TD, Fegan C, Zucchetto A, Cro L, Nückel H, et al. CD49d is the strongest flow cytometry-based predictor of overall survival in chronic lymphocytic leukemia. J Clin Oncol Off J Am Soc Clin Oncol. 2014 Mar 20;32(9):897–904.

[76] Zenz T, Mohr J, Eldering E, Kater AP, Bühler A, Kienle D, et al. miR-34a as part of the resistance network in chronic lymphocytic leukemia. Blood. 2009 Apr 16;113(16): 3801–8.

[77] Bulian P, Tarnani M, Rossi D, Forconi F, Del Poeta G, Bertoni F, et al. Multicentre validation of a prognostic index for overall survival in chronic lymphocytic leukaemia. Hematol Oncol. 2011 Jun;29(2):91–9.

[78] Wierda WG, O'Brien S, Wang X, Faderl S, Ferrajoli A, Do K-A, et al. Multivariable model for time to first treatment in patients with chronic lymphocytic leukemia. J Clin Oncol Off J Am Soc Clin Oncol. 2011 Nov 1;29(31):4088–95.

[79] Pflug N, Bahlo J, Shanafelt TD, Eichhorst BF, Bergmann MA, Elter T, et al. Development of a comprehensive prognostic index for patients with chronic lymphocytic leukemia. Blood. 2014 Jul 3;124(1):49–62.

[80] Rossi D, Rasi S, Spina V, Bruscaggin A, Monti S, Ciardullo C, et al. Integrated mutational and cytogenetic analysis identifies new prognostic subgroups in chronic lymphocytic leukemia. Blood. 2013 Feb 21;121(8):1403–12.

[81] Jeromin S, Weissmann S, Haferlach C, Dicker F, Bayer K, Grossmann V, et al. SF3B1 mutations correlated to cytogenetics and mutations in NOTCH1, FBXW7, MYD88, XPO1 and TP53 in 1160 untreated CLL patients. Leukemia. 2014 Jan;28(1):108–17.

[82] Cortese D, Sutton L-A, Cahill N, Smedby KE, Geisler C, Gunnarsson R, et al. On the way towards a "CLL prognostic index": focus on TP53, BIRC3, SF3B1, NOTCH1 and MYD88 in a population-based cohort. Leukemia. 2014 Mar;28(3):710–3.

[83] Wierda WG, Kipps TJ, Mayer J, Stilgenbauer S, Williams CD, Hellmann A, et al. Ofatumumab as single-agent CD20 immunotherapy in fludarabine-refractory chronic lymphocytic leukemia. J Clin Oncol Off J Am Soc Clin Oncol. 2010 Apr 1;28(10):1749–55.

[84] Robak T, Janssens A, Govindbabu K, Grosicki S, Mayer J, Panagiotidis P, et al. Ofatumumab + Chlorambucil Versus Chlorambucil Alone in Patients with Untreated Chronic Lymphocytic Leukemia (CLL): Results of the Phase III Study Complement 1 (OMB110911). Hillmen P, editor. Blood. 2013 Dec 6;122(21):528.

[85] Goede V, Fischer K, Busch R, Engelke A, Eichhorst B, Wendtner CM, et al. Obinutuzumab plus chlorambucil in patients with CLL and coexisting conditions. N Engl J Med. 2014 Mar 20;370(12):1101–10.

[86] Goede V, Fischer K, Engelke A, Schlag R, Lepretre S, Montero LFC, et al. Obinutuzumab as frontline treatment of chronic lymphocytic leukemia: updated results of the CLL11 study. Leukemia. 2015 Jan 30.

[87] Byrd JC, Furman RR, Coutre SE, Flinn IW, Burger JA, Blum KA, et al. Targeting BTK with ibrutinib in relapsed chronic lymphocytic leukemia. N Engl J Med. 2013 Jul 4;369(1):32–42.

[88] Byrd JC, Brown JR, O'Brien S, Barrientos JC, Kay NE, Reddy NM, et al. Ibrutinib versus ofatumumab in previously treated chronic lymphoid leukemia. N Engl J Med. 2014 Jul 17;371(3):213–23.

[89] Barrientos JC, Barr PM, Flinn I, Burger JA, Salman Z, Clow F, et al. Ibrutinib in Combination with Bendamustine and Rituximab Is Active and Tolerable in Patients with Relapsed/Refractory CLL/SLL: Final Results of a Phase 1b Study. Brown JR, editor. Blood. 2013 Dec 6;122(21):525.

[90] Burger JA, Keating MJ, Wierda WG, Hartmann E, Hoellenriegel J, Rosin NY, et al. Safety and activity of ibrutinib plus rituximab for patients with high-risk chronic lymphocytic leukaemia: a single-arm, phase 2 study. Lancet Oncol. 2014 Sep;15(10): 1090–9.

[91] Furman RR, Sharman JP, Coutre SE, Cheson BD, Pagel JM, Hillmen P, et al. Idelalisib and rituximab in relapsed chronic lymphocytic leukemia. N Engl J Med. 2014 Mar 13;370(11):997–1007.

[92] Furman RR, Barrientos JC, Wagner-Johnston ND, Flinn I, Sharman JP, Boyd T, et al. Idelalisib, a Selective Inhibitor of PI3Kδ, in Combination with Bendamustine, Fludarabine or Chlorambucil in Patients with Relapsed or Refractory (R/R) Chronic Lymphocytic Leukemia (CLL). De Vos S, editor. Blood. 2013 Dec 6;122(21):2878.

[93] Eymour J. Updated results of a phase I first-in-human study of the BCL-2 inhibitor ABT-199 (GDC-0199) in patients with relapsed/refractory (R/R) chronic lymphocytic leukaemia (CLL). Hematol Oncol; 2013.

[94] Chanan-Khan A, Miller KC, Musial L, Lawrence D, Padmanabhan S, Takeshita K, et al. Clinical efficacy of lenalidomide in patients with relapsed or refractory chronic lymphocytic leukemia: results of a phase II study. J Clin Oncol Off J Am Soc Clin Oncol. 2006 Dec 1;24(34):5343–9.

[95] Ferrajoli A, Lee B-N, Schlette EJ, O'Brien SM, Gao H, Wen S, et al. Lenalidomide induces complete and partial remissions in patients with relapsed and refractory chronic lymphocytic leukemia. Blood. 2008 Jun 1;111(11):5291–7.

[96] Badoux XC, Keating MJ, Wen S, Lee B-N, Sivina M, Reuben J, et al. Lenalidomide as initial therapy of elderly patients with chronic lymphocytic leukemia. Blood. 2011 Sep 29;118(13):3489–98.

[97] Strati P, Keating MJ, Wierda WG, Badoux XC, Calin S, Reuben JM, et al. Lenalidomide induces long-lasting responses in elderly patients with chronic lymphocytic leukemia. Blood. 2013 Aug 1;122(5):734–7.

[98] Chen CI, Bergsagel PL, Paul H, Xu W, Lau A, Dave N, et al. Single-agent lenalidomide in the treatment of previously untreated chronic lymphocytic leukemia. J Clin Oncol Off J Am Soc Clin Oncol. 2011 Mar 20;29(9):1175–81.

[99] Badoux XC, Keating MJ, Wen S, Wierda WG, O'Brien SM, Faderl S, et al. Phase II study of lenalidomide and rituximab as salvage therapy for patients with relapsed or

http://dx.doi.org/10.5772/60738

refractory chronic lymphocytic leukemia. J Clin Oncol Off J Am Soc Clin Oncol. 2013 Feb 10;31(5):584–91.

[100] James DF, Werner L, Brown JR, Wierda WG, Barrientos JC, Castro JE, et al. Lenalidomide and rituximab for the initial treatment of patients with chronic lymphocytic leukemia: a multicenter clinical-translational study from the chronic lymphocytic leukemia research consortium. J Clin Oncol Off J Am Soc Clin Oncol. 2014 Jul 1;32(19):2067–73.

[101] Kalos M, Levine BL, Porter DL, Katz S, Grupp SA, Bagg A, et al. T cells with chimeric antigen receptors have potent antitumor effects and can establish memory in patients with advanced leukemia. Sci Transl Med. 2011 Aug 10;3(95):95-73.

[102] Brentjens RJ, Rivière I, Park JH, Davila ML, Wang X, Stefanski J, et al. Safety and persistence of adoptively transferred autologous CD19-targeted T cells in patients with relapsed or chemotherapy refractory B-cell leukemias. Blood. 2011 Nov 3;118(18): 4817–28.

[103] Porter DL, Grupp SA, Kalos M, Loren AW, Lledo L, Gilmore J, et al. Chimeric antigen receptor T cells directed against CD19 induce durable responses and transient cytokine release syndrome in relapsed, refractory CLL and ALL. ASH Annu Meet Abstr. 2012 Nov 16;120(21):717.

Chapter 9

Chronic Lymphocytic Leukemia — Microenvironment and B Cells

Rositsa Vladimirova, Dora Popova,
Elena Vikentieva and Margarita Guenova

Additional information is available at the end of the chapter

http://dx.doi.org/10.5772/60761

Abstract

Chronic lymphocytic leukemia (CLL) has been considered as an accumulative disease deriving from defects in apoptosis, but recent studies showed that CLL is a dynamic process in which monoclonal B cells proliferate within pseudofollicular proliferation centers. Microenvironmental interactions are essential for the survival and proliferation of CLL cells. The cell traffic between blood and secondary lymphoid tissues is controlled by tissue-specific chemokines and their specific receptors on B lymphocytes. Interstitial cell migration and adhesion events, predisposed by activational stimuli, determine CLL cell localization. Stimulation through the B cell receptor plays an important role in the expansion of the malignant clone in CLL. B cell receptors become activated either in an antigen-dependent or in an antigen-independent fashion in the secondary lymphatic tissues. However, low expression of the BCR correlates with reduced induction of protein tyrosine kinase activity and defective intracellular calcium mobilization and tyrosine phosphorylation. In contrast to normal B cells, leukemic cells are poor antigen presenting cells. This is due to the fact that leukemic cells have a reduced expression of costimulatory molecules and defects in the formation of immunological synapse with T cells. Increased surface expression of the costimulatory molecules on CLL cells correlates with their proliferation. At present, conventional treatments are not directed to interactions between CLL cells and their microenvironment, which is probably one of the reasons why, despite the significant progress in treatment, the disease still remains incurable. In this regard, identifying key biomarkers of intercellular interactions of neoplastic CLL population in comparison with clinical laboratory abnormalities in CLL enable clarification of essential processes in the development of the disease, and can be the basis for stratifying patient groups in order to optimize therapeutic approaches, which will make them relevant and promising.

Keywords: Chronic lymphocytic leukemia, Microenvironment, B cell receptor complex, Chemokine receptors, Cell adhesion molecules, Costimulatory receptors

1. Introduction

Chronic lymphocytic leukemia (CLL) is a disease with highly variable clinical manifestation and course ranging from an aggressive, life-threatening disease to an indolent form, which does not require treatment for many years. Current clinical staging systems are accessible and easy to apply; however, they do not allow a sufficiently accurate opportunity for individual assessment of the disease progression. Recently, significant progress has been made in our understanding of CLL pathogenesis. CLL has been considered as an accumulative disease deriving from an inherent defect in apoptosis, but recent studies showed that it is a dynamic process, wherein monoclonal B cells proliferate within pseudofollicular proliferation centers, hallmark of histopathology on this disease.

CLL cells interact with different types of cells, such as mesenchymal stromal cells (MSC), monocyte-derived nurse-like cells (NLC), follicular dendritic cells (FDC), and T cells. Microenvironmental interactions are critical for the survival and proliferation of the leukemic cells. A key role in the pathogenesis of the disease is given to the B cell receptors (BCRs), which in the secondary lymphatic tissues become activated either by antigen-dependent or in an antigen-independent fashion. The proliferative drive for the malignant cells is dependent from external microenvironmental signals, and the CLL cells undergo apoptosis unless their survival is reinforced by these external stimuli.

The cell traffic between the blood and secondary lymphoid tissues is controlled by tissue-specific chemokines and their specific receptors. B cells express CD184 (CXCR4) as a functional receptor, responsible for directing them mainly to the bone marrow (BM) environment. The specific ligand CXCL12 has been shown to have anti-apoptotic effects on CLL cells and protect them from spontaneous and chemotherapy-induced apoptosis in a contact-dependent manner via stromal cells or nurse-like cells. The chemokine receptor CD185 (CXCR5) plays an important role in lymphocyte homing guiding B cells into the B cell zone of secondary lymphoid organs and, together with CD197 (CCR7) (positioning in T cell zones of secondary lymphoid tissues), ensures the close contact between T and B cells and activation. CLL cells secrete chemokines as CCL3, CCL4, and CCL22, and therefore an autocrine way of stimulation on monoclonal B cells is also suggested.

Interstitial cell migration and adhesion events, influenced by activating stimuli, determine CLL cell localization. CD44 has been implicated in cell activation, migration, and tissue retention via binding to its extracellular matrix ligand hyaluronan. CD38, CD49d, MMP9, and CD44 are physically associated in a supramolecular cell surface complex; however, the complex is not

http://dx.doi.org/10.5772/60761

present in normal B cells. Taking into account the known properties of the individual molecules and their functional overlap, it seems that the complex CD38 / CD49d / MMP9 / CD44 plays a role in the migration into the tissues and in pro-survival signaling.

Stimulation through the BCR plays an important role in the selection and expansion of the malignant clone in CLL, and the prognostic impact of the mutational status of immunoglobulin heavy chain variable region (IGHV) genes could be considered as a consequence of the relevance of this process in CLL. Low expression of the BCR correlates with the reduced induction of protein tyrosine kinase activity and defective intracellular calcium mobilization and tyrosine phosphorylation. Although there are individual differences among patients, almost all CLL cases display very low levels of surface IgM and CD79b.

Costimulatory receptors on monoclonal B cells are expressed throughout B-cell development and are implicated in cell survival and differentiation. CD40/CD40L interaction stimulates B cells to proliferate, differentiate, upregulate costimulatory molecules, and increase antigen presentation. In contrast to normal B cells, leukemic cells are poor antigen presenting cells. This is due to the fact that leukemic cells have a reduced expression of costimulatory molecules such as CD80 and CD86 and they have a defect in the formation of immunological synapse with T cells. Surface expression of the costimulatory molecules CD80 and CD86 on CLL cells is increased with their proliferation. CD267 (transmembrane activator calcium modulator and cyclophilin ligand interactor - TACI) was identified as a receptor for B cell-activating factor (BAFF) and A proliferation-inducing ligand (APRIL), two members of the TNF ligand family. Both ligands induce proliferation, activation, and the survival of B cells, therefore the variable expression of CD267, detected in patients with CLL, is probably important for the disease characteristics.

The advances in fundamental understanding of the disease mechanisms in CLL will lead to improved therapies for patients. At present, conventional treatments are not directed to the interactions between CLL cells and their microenvironment, which is probably one of the reasons why, despite the significant progress in treatment, the disease still remains incurable. In this regard, studies on key biomarkers of intercellular interactions of the leukemic population enable clarification of key processes in the development of the disease, and can be the basis for defining a separate risk patient group to optimize therapeutic approaches, which will make them relevant and promising.

2. Microenvironment: Cells and interactions

Malignant B lymphocytes develop in the specific tissue microenvironment of the lymph node and eventually in the bone marrow (BM), where they interact with various cell populations - mesenchymal stromal cells (MSC), monocyte-derived nurse-like cells (NLC), follicular dendritic cells (FDC), and T cells. Unlike the non-dividing cells circulating in the peripheral blood (PB), tissue B cells proliferate (0.1–1% of the clone per day) [1]. This process occurs in pseudofollicular proliferation centers [2, 3]. The interaction of the leukemic cells with the microenvironment is similar to the model of normal B-cell engagement. Secondary lymphoid tissues are the place, where the B cell receptor (BCR) of monoclonal cells is activated [4] by microbial antigens, autoantigens [5], or independently of antigens [6, 7]. Activation triggers a signaling cascade facilitated by additional stimulatory signals, which results in the clone growth.

2.1. T lymphocytes

The interaction between monoclonal B lymphocytes and T lymphocytes is an important component of the malignant process. T cells are extremely important for malignant proliferation [8]. This was proven in a mouse xenograft model of CLL, in which activated CD41+ T cells proved to be a necessary condition for CLL cell proliferation. In patients suffering from this disease, T cells, mainly CD41+, often constitute a significant fraction of the lymphoid infiltrate in bone marrow and lymph nodes [9], located within and around proliferation centers [10, 11]. One of the factors mediating the migration to the particular location is the expression of the CD197 (CCR7) chemokine receptor on T cells, which facilitates recirculation through secondary lymphoid tissues, following the gradient of its specific ligands CCL19 and CCL21 secreted in the T-cell zone of the lymph node [12]. The CD40 receptor, a key modulator of the interaction between B- and T-lymphocytes, is stimulated by CD41+ T cells, which express its ligand CD154 (CD40L) [13] and are co-localized with leukemic cells in the proliferation centers [14]. In addition to the interactions through a direct intercellular contact, T lymphocytes secrete soluble active molecules, interleukins, cytokines, and chemokines, which stimulate proliferation and inhibit apoptosis of monoclonal B cells. Interleukin-4 (IL-4) inhibits spontaneous and drug-induced apoptosis through a mechanism causing hyperproduction of Bcl-2 [15]. The concurrent action of IL-2 [16] and Tumor Necrosis Factor-α (TNF-α) [17, 18] induces malignant proliferation. Interferon-γ (IFNγ) [19], IFNα [20], and IL-13 [21] have a similar effect. Leukemic cells also change the cellular component of the immune system by the production of immunosuppressive cytokines Tumor Growth Factor-β (TGF-β) [22] and IL-10 [23] and the expression of low levels of the adhesion and costimulatory molecules [24], thus leading to the increase and dysfunction of regulatory T lymphocytes [25, 26]. The gene expression profile (GEP) of T cells from patients with CLL shows multiple changes in the genes participating mostly in cellular differentiation, cytoskeleton, traffic, and cytotoxicity, which leads to an inhibited immune response [27].

2.2. Mesenchymal Stromal Cells (MSCs)

MSCs are another major cellular component of tissue microenvironment. These cells are a heterogeneous population, performing structural and functional interactions in normal hemopoiesis [28]. Stromal cells secrete cytokines, chemokines, proangiogenic factors, and extracellular matrix components. They express surface receptors, which mainly regulate migration and facilitate the survival of CLL lymphocytes. The interaction of the leukemic cells with MSC is in both directions. Not only monoclonal B cells migrate and are activated under the influence of MSC, but vice versa, they also activate them and induce stromal-cell proliferation and the secretion of mediators that increase the intensity of the malignant process [29, 30, 31, 32]. In the lymphoid tissues of patients with CLL, stromal cells are diffusely distributed within the entire tissue and in the perivascular spaces, where they are mixed with leukemic cells [33]. CLL lymphocytes cultured with bone-marrow stromal cells avoid both the spontaneous and drug-induced apoptosis [34, 35], through a mechanism dependent on direct intercellular contact [34]. CXCL12 secreted by the stromal cells directs the migration of the leukemic cells, which express the CXCR4 (CD184) receptor, through the stroma, and facilitate the penetration beneath it (a phenomenon called pseudoemperipolesis) [35]. Surface receptors and extracellular matrix elements induce anti-apoptotic stimuli in CLL lymphocytes, which are in contact with the stroma. Adhesion of tumor cells to stromal cells is mediated by the β1 and β2 integrins [36]. MSCs express Vascular Cell Adhesion Molecule 1 (VCAM-1) [37]. Attachment of α4β1 integrin (CD49d/CD29) to VCAM-1 or to the extracellular matrix component fibronectin protects CLL cells from a spontaneous or Fludarabine-induced apoptosis [36, 38] by means of PI3K/AKT signals and the increase of BCL-XL [39]. The interaction of the leukemic cell with the stroma also includes Matrix metalloproteinase-9 (MMP-9), Vascular Endothelial Growth Factor (VEGF), and endothelial cells. MMP-9 is the main matrix metalloproteinase produced by monoclonal B cells; it enhances extravasation and infiltration in lymphoid tissue by means of the proteolytic degradation of basal membranes and extracellular matrix components [40]. Regardless of its proteolytic activity, MMP-9 partially mediates anti-apoptotic signals in the leukemic clone when cultured with bone-marrow stromal cells [41]. The attachment of MMP-9 to α4β1 and CD44v in CLL lymphocytes leads to the activation of the Lck/Yes novel tyrosine kinase (LYN) and the Signal Transducer and Activator of Transcription 3 (STAT3) [39]. The expression of MMP-9 from leukemic cells is regulated by the α4β1 integrins and CXCL12 [40]. Monoclonal B lymphocytes in the bone marrow and lymph nodes express elevated levels of surface MMP-9, which shows the activation of tumor cells in tissues microenvironment [39].

2.3. Follicular dendritic cells

Follicular dendritic cells (FDC) are accessory cells in normal germinal centers, where they catch and retain antigen–antibody complexes on their cellular surfaces and present antigens to the B cells. After binding to immune complexes, normal B lymphocytes in the germinal center differentiate to memory B lymphocytes or plasma cells [42]. Normally, FDC are localized in secondary lymphoid tissues but not in the bone marrow [43], while in CLL these cells are localized in lymph node pseudofollicles [44, 45] and in nodular bone marrow infiltrates [46]. They secrete important anti-apoptotic and growth factors including BAFF, IL-15, and express adhesion molecules Vascular Cell Adhesion Molecule-1 (VCAM-1), Intercellular Adhesion Molecule-1 (ICAM-1), Plexin B1, and CD44 [42, 44]. The effects of FDC on malignant B lymphocytes have been studied on a follicular dendritic cell line (HK). There is evidence that HK cells facilitate the survival of B cells, protect them from a spontaneous or drug-induced apoptosis via the direct intercellular contact mechanism [47].

2.4. Tissue associated macrophages

Tissue associated macrophages have been studied in an in vitro model - NLC. In case of continuous culturing of peripheral blood mononuclear cells of CLL patients, large, rounded, rarely binuclear, CD68 expressing cells grow [48, 49]. NLC take this name since they contribute to the growth and survival of the CLL cells. Cells of a similar phenotype can be found in vivo

[49] in the secondary lymphoid organs of patients with CLL, but their number in the tissues is generally low [33]. NLC differentiate from monocytes as this differentiation depends on intercellular contacts with CLL lymphocytes. When monocytes from healthy individuals are co-cultured with leukemic cells, they differentiate to NLC; however normal B cells are unable to induce this differentiation [49]. NLC secrete chemokines (CXCL12 and CXCL13) and growth factors such as BAFF and APRIL, hold leukemic cells within tissues, and facilitate their survival and proliferation [50, 51, 52]. Malignant cells also express BAFF, APRIL, and their receptors, however, at a significantly lower rate [53, 54, 55], B-cell maturation antigen (BCMA) and CD267 (TACI). Two receptors connect APRIL–BCMA and TACI. Ligands BAFF and/or APRIL lower the spontaneous and drug-induced apoptosis of CLL cells [53, 54, 55]. In recent years, it has been proven experimentally that BAFF in cooperation with MYC protein, that plays a role in cell cycle progression, apoptosis and cellular transformation, causes the development of lymphocytic proliferation in mice that is similar to CLL [56]. MYC and its target genes are highly expressed in CLL cells in lymph nodes [4], which is stimulated by BAFF [56] and BCR activation in vitro [57].

2.5. Monoclonal B cells

The cell traffic between the blood and secondary lymphoid tissues is controlled by tissue-specific chemokines and their specific receptors on lymphocytes. The chemokine receptors expressed on neoplastic CLL cells drive migration to proliferation centers (Figure 1; Table 1).

3. Chemokine receptors on monoclonal B cells

3.1. CD184 (CXCR4) expression

The CD184 receptor binds CXCL12 (stromal cell-derived factor-1/SDF-1), a ligand characterized as a pre-B cell growth factor [58]. It is highly expressed on the peripheral blood leukemic cells surface, facilitates the chemotactic migration through vascular endothelium to bone marrow stromal cells following the CXCL12 gradient [35, 48, 55, 58, 59]. CD184 surface expression is regulated by the ligand CXCL12 through receptor endocytosis occurring as a result of activation [58]. This feature can be used to distinguish tissue leukemic cells expressing low levels of CD184 from blood CLL cells, which express high levels of CD184 [4, 58]. Proliferating CLL lymphocytes from bone marrow and lymphoid tissue show significantly lower levels of CXCR4 and CXCR5, compared to the non-proliferating ones [60, 61]. The BCR signals also decrease the expression of CD184 [62, 63]. As BCR signals may increase via Zap-70 [64], monoclonal B lymphocytes expressing Zap-70 have increased chemotaxis and survival as a response to CXCL12 compared to Zap-70 negative leukemic cells [65], the result of increased BCR signals. Leukemic cells expressing CD38 also show increased chemotaxis [66] compared to CXCL12, which can be inhibited by blocking with anti-CD38 monoclonal antibodies [67]. The signals conducted by CD184 induce mobilization of calcium, activation of PI3Ks [58], p44/42 MAPKs [48], and serine phosphorylation of STAT3 [35]. The signals conducted by CD184 can be inhibited by selective isomorphic inhibitors - the PI3K inhibitors [68] and the spleen tyrosine kinase (SYK) inhibitors [62], thus resulting in impaired migration of both the

http://dx.doi.org/10.5772/60761

normal B cells and the leukemic cells. According to some research teams, the levels of CXCR4 and its ligand CXCL12 correlate to well-established clinical parameters such as the Rai staging system, while other researchers do not observe correlation with the clinical stage of the disease or with the type of bone marrow infiltration, instead they report correlation with the lymphocyte count [69, 70]. It should be considered that CD184 is a constitutionally expressed receptor of B lymphocytes, which could explain the contradictory findings of the different research teams [71].

3.2. CD181 and CD182 expression

CD181 (CXCR1) and CD182 (CXCR2) have a common ligand - CXCL8. Monoclonal B cells secrete CXCL8 and express its receptors, which implies both the autocrine and paracrine stimulation of tumor cell through CXCL8. This stimulation leads to increased expression of anti-apoptotic protein Bcl-2 and survival of the clone [72].

3.3. CD183 expression

The chemokine receptor CD183 (CXCR3) interacts with three ligands (CXCL9, CXCL10, and CXCL11) [73]. CD183 is expressed on the surface of malignant cells as a functional receptor facilitating a directed drive and invasion [70, 73]. Leukemic cells express CXCL9, which constitutes proof of the autocrine way of a neoplastic growth stimulation, in addition to the paracrine way. Studies show correlation between the low expression of CD183 in the advanced stage of the disease (Rai III and Rai IV), non-mutated IGHV status, high CD38 expression, and the shortened general survival span of the patients. It is suggested that the lower levels of CD183 could be used as an independent adverse prognostic factor [74]. Nevertheless, the significance of CXCR3 remains disputable.

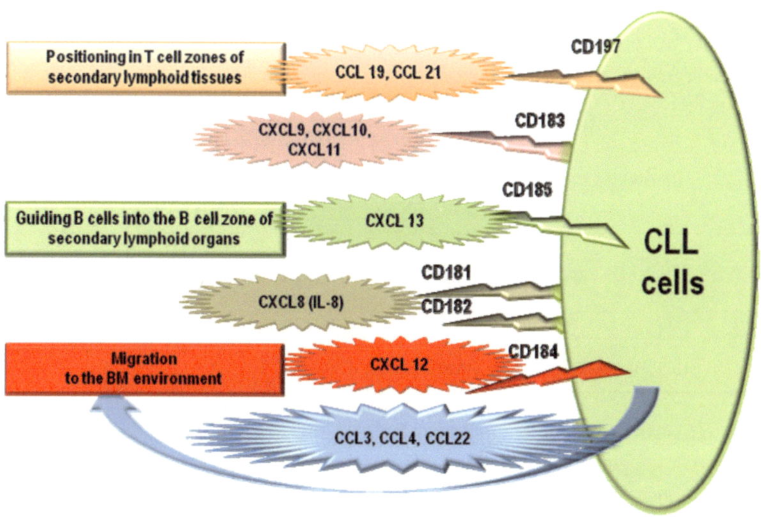

Figure 1. Chemokine receptors and chemokines involved in monoclonal B cell activation, migration, and proliferation

3.4. CD197 expression

CD197 (CCR7) is the main receptor responsible for the traffic of dendritic cells, the B- and T-lymphocytes through the high endothelial venules and their localization in the T cell zones of the secondary lymphoid organs. Its ligands - CCL19 and CCL21 are expressed in the T cell zone of secondary mucosa-associated tissues and high endothelial venules but not in the B cell zones, sinuses, and peripheral blood. CD197 is expressed mainly by naïve T lymphocytes but can be detected at certain levels also on B lymphocytes. The role of the receptor for the development of the secondary lymphoid organs has also been proven [12]. The expression of CD197 on leukemic B cells is significantly higher in patients with lymphadenopathy, compared to patients with organomegaly. The CD197-CCL21 binding activates intracellular signaling pathways, which lead to elevated expression of MMP-9 and infiltration of leukemic cells through basal membranes [12]. The increased expression of CD197 on Zap-70+ CLL cells enhances the response of CD197 to ligands [64], and the CD5 phosphorylation additionally stimulates its surface expression [75]. The binding of both CD197 and CD185 to the respective ligands elevates the expression of the partially expressed gene 10 (PEG10) in CD23+ CD5+ CLL cells. The increased synthesis of protein stabilizes caspase-3 and caspase-8 (which normally are pro-apoptotic proteins), protects them from degradation, thus leading to suppression of the TNF-α induced apoptosis [76, 77]. A correlation of CD197 with the Rai staging system has been found, which shows the need of further studies on the possible prognostic significance of this receptor [71].

RECEPTOR	LIGAND	CLL EXPRESSION	FUNCTION
CD181 (CXCR1) **CD182 (CXCR2)**	CXCL8 (IL-8)	Aberrant or activation expression	Inhibition of apoptosis by up-regulation of Bcl-2
CD183 (CXCR3)	CXCL9, CXCL10, CXCL11	Low to moderate continuous expression	Th1 response, inflammation, integrin activation, chemotaxis migration
CD184 (CXCR4)	CXCL12	High, low in receptor endocytosis as a result of interaction with CXCL12	Contact-dependent inhibition of apoptosis. Migration and homing
CD185 (CXCR5)	CXCL13	High	Migration, inhibition of apoptosis
CD197 (CCR7)	CCL19, CCL21	Moderate to high, correlates with lymphadenopathy	Inhibition of apoptosis

Table 1. Chemokine receptors and corresponding chemokines

3.5. Chemokines secreted by B cells

Activated monoclonal lymphocytes secrete the CCL3, CCL4 [59], and CCL22 [13] chemokines that participate in the adaptive immune response and are chemo-attractants for T lymphocytes and monocytes (Table 2). CCL3 and CCL4 are normally secreted by B cells after the activation through BCR and CD40–CD40L interaction [59, 62]. CCL3 secreted from tumor cells induces T cell traffic to the activated $CD38^{+}$/Ki-67^{+} leukemic lymphocytes for the purpose of enabling intercellular interactions, which enhance proliferation [62]. Similarly to CCL3 and CCL4, CCL22 participates in the process of attraction of T cells in tissues. It acts as a secondary signal to T lymphocytes; its secretion from malignant cells starts after attachment of CD40 to CD40L [13]. The monoclonal population in peripheral blood does not secrete CCL22; secretion is observed in lymph nodes and bone marrow, probably also as a result of the attachment to CD40. In classifying CLL patients on the basis of their response to CD40 ligation, it was found that the patients who did not show a response have less time until disease progression and a possibility for proliferation of B cells in conditions of lower stromal stimuli [78] (Figure 1).

CHEMOKINE	RECEPTOR	CLL EXPRESSION	SUPPOSED FUNCTIONS
CCL3	CCR1, CCR5	After activation by BCR, higher in Zap-70+ CLL-cells, SYK–dependent	In case of inflammation, activation of polymorphonuclear leukocytes and B cells
CCL4	CCR5		Supports T cells in T-B cell interactions
CCL22	CCR4	After CD40 ligation	Supports regulatory T cells

Table 2. Chemokine receptors and corresponding chemokines secreted from CLL cell [72]

4. Cell adhesion molecules on monoclonal B cells

Adhesion molecules facilitate the migration of leukemic cells to proliferation centers in bone marrow and secondary lymphoid tissues [79]; some of them show anti-apoptotic activity and a relation to drug resistance by binding to their receptors, which are expressed from bone-marrow stromal cells. The profile of CLL cells in regards to adhesion molecules has been the subject of studies in recent years since it determines the capacity of leukemic lymphocytes for response to chemokines and migration to regions, where antigens and additional activation stimuli influence B lymphocytes (Figure 2).

4.1. CD38 expression

The CD38 receptor performs and modulates a series of intracellular signals initiated by the cells of microenvironment. The percentage of CD38+ cells in the CLL clone is an indicator of the current level of cell activation; the cells with a higher expression of CD38 are better receivers of activation signals and hence the more aggressive portion of the malignant lymphocytes. Studies on patients with CLL using the incorporation in vivo of deuterium (^{2}H) in the form of heavy water ($^{2}H_2O$) in a cellular DNA have proved higher proliferation rate of $CD38^{+}$

lymphocytes in comparison to CD38⁻ cells [1]. CD38 + B lymphocytes react more effectively in binding to surface immunoglobulins (sIg), with Zap-70 also participating in this process. The ligand of CD38–CD31 is expressed on vascular endothelium cells and facilitates cell adhesion. The aggressiveness of CD38⁺ lymphocytes is mediated by their ability to migrate and interact with the cellular microenvironment. CD38 and Zap-70 are functionally related and define the cells with a higher migration potential [66]. In most of CLL patients, the proportion of CD38+ cells does not exceed a threshold of 30%, which defines the clone as positive. Disease progression is more common in the smaller proportion of patients with a CD38 expression defined as positive [80]. The higher proliferative potential of these lymphocytes suggests novel genomic disorders and clonal evolution [81, 82, 83, 84], which is supported by the increased incidence of the observed 11q and 17p deletions [85].

4.2. CD49d expression

The level of CD49d (VLA-4) positive B lymphocytes has been recognized as an independent prognostic factor in CLL. CD49d is α-integrin subunit (α4), which together with CD29 (β1 subunit) forms the $\alpha 4\beta 1$ integrin binding fibronectin and VCAM-1. Similarly to other integrins, $\alpha 4\beta 1$ mediates the adhesion of cells to the extracellular matrix, the first step of cell migration. CD49d and CD38 participate in the formation of a large macromolecular complex that includes CD49d, CD38, CD44v, and MMP-9 and has been observed in CLL cells without somatic mutations [86]. The physical and functional binding between CD49d/CD29 and CD38 has been proven in CLL [87].

In recent years, CD49d adhesion molecule facilitating both the intercellular contact and the adhesion to extracellular matrix has been established as a new prognostic marker. A multicenter study on 2,972 patients with CLL validated the prognostic significance of CD49d as an independent flow cytometric prognostic marker in terms of overall survival and time-to-treatment start, as defined over a threshold of 30% [88].

4.3. CD44 expression

The CD44 protein family comprises a large group of transmembrane glycoproteins obtained through alternative splicing and post-translational modification. The considerable degree of heterogeneity in molecular structure predetermines various essential functions. CD44 mediates interactions between cells and the extracellular matrix, delivers signals acting as a co-receptor for tyrosine kinases localized in cell membranes or by binding to intracellular signaling molecules and activating intracellular signaling pathways. The expression of different CD44 isoforms depends on the cell type, stage of activation, and differentiation. The participation of CD44 in the development and progression of hematological neoplasms is associated with the increase of apoptotic resistance, invasiveness, regulation of bone-marrow infiltration, and mobilization of leukemic cells in peripheral blood [89]. The surface levels of CD44v in CLL are associated with advanced clinical stage, resistance to therapy, and decreased survival [90]. Unlike other cooperating adhesion molecules such as CD11a, CD49d, CD54, CD58, and CD62L, the expression of CD44 and CD11c correlates with the splenal presentation of the disease [91]. Soluble CD44 is associated with shortened progression free survival [92],

http://dx.doi.org/10.5772/60761

while soluble CD44s and CD44v6 are associated with lymphadenopathy, advanced clinical stage, and resistance to chemotherapy [93]. The results of an in vitro study of the anti-apoptotic effects of CD44 in CLL cells showed protective action of cultured CLL cells with HK-cells against spontaneous apoptosis in increased levels of Mcl-1 (a member of the anti-apoptotic Bcl-2 family). In this study, the blocking of CD44 by monoclonal antibodies leads to a decrease of Mcl-1 and suppression of the protective effect of HK-cells, demonstrating that the anti-apoptotic mechanism is CD44-dependent [47]. The formation of macromolecular complexes from CD44v, CD49d, and MMP-9 on the cells of CLL, but not on normal B lymphocytes, as well as increased secretion of MMP-9 under the action of CD44 antibodies, reveals the molecular mechanism of regulation of invasion [94].

4.4. CD54 expression

CD54 is a glycoprotein that is expressed on the surface of vascular endothelium cells, macrophages, and lymphocytes. It binds type CD11a/CD18 and type CD11b/CD18 integrins. In case of cytokine stimulation by IL-1 and TNF-α, the concentrations of CD54 increase significantly [95]. Upon activation, cells connect to the endothelium via CD54–CD11a/CD18 and penetrate tissues [96]. A significant reduction of CD54 expression levels has been demonstrated in CLL patients compared to a control group of healthy subjects [97]. β1 and β2 integrins of the malignant B cell, acting simultaneously, mediate the connection of CD54 to bone-marrow stromal cells and protect them from apoptosis, while normal B lymphocytes cannot be protected by stromal cells due to the loss of this adhesion connection [36].

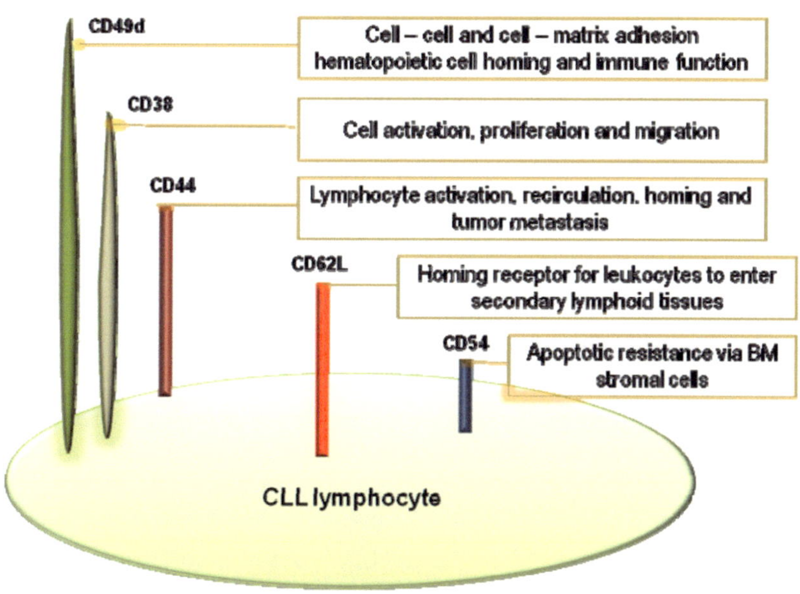

Figure 2. Adhesion molecules and their main functions directly relevant to CLL

4.5. CD62L expression

In the process of lymphocyte homing, B lymphocytes adhere and then enter sinusoidal endothelium before invasion in efferent lymph nodes, after which they leave the lymph nodes. CD62L (L-selectin), a member of the selectin family of adhesion molecules, plays an important role in the traffic and homing of lymphocytes to lymph nodes [98]. CD62L is considered the main adhesion molecule connecting B cell to sinusoidal endothelial cells through interaction with mannose receptor [99]; therefore it is believed that CD62L participates in mechanisms supporting the departure of lymphocytes from lymph nodes. In vitro studies of CLL cells demonstrated that stimulation through BCR causes a decrease of CD62L, in particular the expression on cells of patients with adverse prognostic factors and at risk of disease progression. The decreased level of surface CD62L is due to disaffiliation from the cell membrane and leads to an increase of its plasma levels [63]. A similar process is also seen in B cells activated by formyl peptides and phorbol 12-myristate 13-acetate [100, 101]. Functionally, leukemic lymphocytes, in which the expression of CD62L and CD184 decreases in a response to BCR signals, show reduction of migration to CXCL12 and adhesion to endothelial cells of the lymph node [63]. The adhesion molecule CD62L is the main factor for B cell departure from lymphatic tissue via connection with lymphatic endothelium [63]. After antigen activation, B lymphocytes lose surface expression of CD62L and do not adhere to the endothelium in lymph nodes [99, 102]. These cells remain in a close contact with the microenvironment and with the antigen stimulation, resulting in proliferation and lymph node enlargement. On the contrary, CLL cells, which do not respond to BCR stimuli, exit lymphoid organs quickly and recirculate like normal B lymphocytes, due to their ability to recognize a specific antigen [103]. In an in vitro study of CLL lymphocytes, increased expression of CD62L was associated with prolonged survival of the malignant cells. Since anti-apoptotic signals from the stromal cells were CD62L-dependent, the inhibition of CD62L by antibodies decreased the survival of the tumor cells. The study also showed over-expression of CD62L on malignant B lymphocytes localized in the proliferation centers of lymph nodes and bone marrow [104]. The immunophenotypic analysis of CLL cells in the process of culturing has demonstrated a change in the surface markers participating in intercellular contacts and conducting anti-apoptotic signals. Blockage of the activation and homing receptor CD62L induces cell death, equivalent to currently used chemotherapeutics [105].

5. B cell receptor complex

B cell receptor complex (BCRC) is a multimeric complex composed of a surface immunoglobulin homodimer and a non-covalently bound heterodimer Igα/Igβ (CD79a/CD79b). The signal pathway of BCRC supports cell proliferation and induces the production of antibodies in normal B lymphocytes. Binding to a specific antigen activates BCRC, which delivers a signal to kinases (spleen tyrosine kinase (SYK) and LYN), which phosphorylate and activate Igα/Igβ [106]. This phosphorylation step triggers a cascade of intracellular signals including activation of Bruton tyrosine kinase (BTK) and Phosphatidylinositaol 3-kinase (PI3K), which induce the mobilization and activation of further kinases (protein kinase C-β and mitogen-activated protein kinase - ERK) [107]. The activation of this cascade facilitates anti-apoptotic events and the proliferation of B cells through the enhancement of transcription factors such as the nuclear factor–κB (NF-κB) [108]. This signal pathway plays an important role in the pathogenesis of CLL, which has been supported by the following facts:

- Mutation status of BCR sequences is the best prognostic marker for disease progression [109].
- About 20% of untreated patients express very similar, sometimes identical, antigen receptors.
- Signals of BCRC play a significant role in trafficking, homing, and interactions in microenvironment [110].

There is a 10-fold decrease in the expression of membrane immunoglobulins [111] due to a critical defect in the formation of the BCR structure [112]. As a result, the stimulation of monoclonal B cells through BCR is impaired. Low expression of BCRC correlates with reduced induction of tyrosine kinase activity and affected intracellular mobilization of calcium and phosphorylation of tyrosine [113]. This low expression is a distinguishing feature of the disease, since similar expression is not found in other mature B cell lymphoproliferative diseases. What causes of this phenomenon is still unclear and is addressed in one study [114], while currently there is a consensus that no genetic defects are present in the components of BCRC [115]. Except in rare cases, surface IgM and CD79b are expressed on CLL cells in very low levels, compared to normal B lymphocytes, but the levels of mRNA and intracellular synthesis of the BCRC components are normal [112]. The correct binding is very important for proteins that consist of multiple subunits. This process takes place in the endoplasmic reticulum, where proteins are modified (split of signal peptides, N-glycosylation, formation of disulfide bridges). In case of failure of the maturation process sequence, various system control mechanisms are activated. They prevent the production of non-functional proteins. A study showed that a complete IgM is not transported to the membrane of the CLL cell [116, 117]. Monoclonal B lymphocytes have a phenotype, which is similar to naïve B cells from the mantle zone, they express CD5 and IgM/IgD and during a normal maturation process they should have expressed non-mutated immunoglobulin genes [118]. However, CLL cells in 50–70% of patients have somatic mutations of the IGHV genes [119], therefore they should have completed the stage of maturation in the lymph follicle. The nature of the leukemic clone is still not established [120, 121], and the absence or presence of somatic mutations is associated with the functioning of single IGHV genes [122].

6. Costimulatory receptors on monoclonal B cells

Cells proliferate in lymph nodes and bone marrow, where under the influence of microenvironment stimuli, they interact with stromal cells and T lymphocytes, resulting in apoptosis impairment and an increase of proliferation. The gene expression profile of CLL cells corresponds to that of activated B lymphocytes [4].

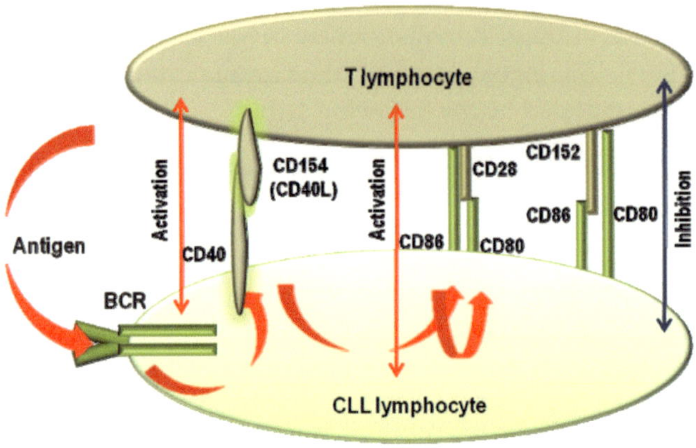

Figure 3. In case of binding of an antigen to the BCR, intracellular signals activate and increase the expression of CD40; the binding to the ligand leads to activation and increased expression of CD86. This in turn leads to activation and de novo expression of CD80. Both regulatory molecules have common ligands CD28 and CD152; these interactions modulate the proliferation of B and T cells

6.1. CD40 expression

CD40 is a molecule belonging to the tumor necrosis factor receptors (TNFR) family. It is expressed during B cell development and plays a major role in cell survival and differentiation [123, 124]. Its physiological ligand CD40L (CD154) is also a member of the TNFR family [125]. Interactions between CD40/CD40L stimulate the proliferation and differentiation of B cells, dendritic cells, and monocytes and enhance expression of costimulatory molecules and the antigenic presentation [126, 127]. After antigen recognition, the T cell receptor (TCR) induces increased CD154 expression on CD4+ T cells, enhances signals through CD40, and increases the expression of CD80/CD86 on antigen-presenting cells (Figure 3). This system enhances activation of T cells, their differentiation, and modulates humoral immune response [128]. The congenital deficit of CD154 in X-linked Hyper-IgM Syndrome leads to frequent bacterial infections due to impaired switching of immunoglobulin classes [129] similar to the immune disorders in CLL patients. Leukemic B lymphocytes express variably functional surface CD154, while CD4+ T cells in CLL patients do not express surface CD154 after CD3 ligation [130, 131]. Binding of CD40 induces expression of CD95, a receptor for apoptotic signals, but paradoxically it conducts a strong NF-κB mediated signal for the survival of leukemic cells in vitro [132]. CD40 activation of malignant cells reduces Fludarabine-induced apoptosis in vitro [133]. In patients with CLL, CD40 activation of B lymphocytes increases the expression of B7 molecules and these cells present alloantigens significantly better than non-stimulated CLL-cells (Figure 3) [24]. Surface expression of costimulatory molecules increases as the process is accompanied by an impaired T cell response to alloantigens and tumor antigens in many other B cell lymphoproliferative diseases [134, 135, 136]. In a study of antigen-presenting capacity of CD40-activated CLL lymphocytes and dendritic cells stimulated by apoptotic bodies of CLL cells, both kinds of antigen-presenting types generated specific T cells, proliferating in response to non-stimulated CLL lymphocytes. T cells isolated from patients with CLL recognize and produce allogenic stimulated and non-stimulated CLL lymphocytes, which shows that the cytotoxic T cells of the patients are functionally intact [137]. CLL lymphocytes activated through CD40 in the presence of IL-4 and INF-γ increase the expression of CD80 and Major histocompatibility complex-II (MHC-II) molecules. Antigen presentation of alloantigen from leukemic cells is comparable to that of normal CD40-activated B cells, as it increases in the presence of IL-4 and INF-γ [138].

6.2. CD80 and CD86 expression

CD80 and CD86 receptors belong to the B7 family, which is one of the most important secondary signaling mechanisms for maintaining the balance between adequate immune response, immunosuppression, and autoimmunity [139].

The expression of CD80 and CD86 is restricted to antigen-presenting cells, as both molecules play different roles in immune modulation due to different interactions with their ligands CD28 and CD152, respectively. The interaction of CD80 with CD152 has a higher affinity than the interaction of CD86 with CD152, while CD28 connects with CD86 more effectively than with CD80 [140]. Low expression of CD86 is registered on non-activated B cells, dendritic cells, and macrophages, in case of activation the levels of CD86 increase and CD80 is expressed de novo [141, 142]. These interactions form a costimulatory–co-inhibitory system that regulates immune responses (Figure 3). Mice with a CD80 and CD86 deficit are characterized with disorders in both the humoral and cell immune response [143]. Furthermore, in case of CD28 deficit, the receptor immune response to foreign antigens, infectious pathogens, and transplants is ineffective [144]. The interaction of CD80 and CD86 with its receptor CD28 generates costimulatory signals leading to a productive activation, expansion, differentiation, survival of the B- and T-cells and an effective antibody-mediated and cell immune response. This immune response is balanced by signals received through interactions with CD152. Mice with CD152 deficit develop an autoimmune phenotype and die rapidly due to multi-organ destruction [145]. The lack of signals from CD80 and CD86 precludes the development of autoimmune deficit in models of triple deficit of CD80, CD86, and CD152 [146]. The role of B7 in antitumor immunity is confirmed through a model system, where cytotoxic T lymphocytes remove mouse tumors, in which transfection of CD80 and CD86 was performed. Unlike solid tumors, both molecules are expressed in a number of hematologic diseases [147, 148]. For instance, cells from a follicular lymphoma increase their expression of CD80 and CD86 as well as other costimulatory and adhesion molecules after in vitro activation [149]. Malignant Reed Sternberg cells of classical Hodgkin's lymphoma also express high levels of CD80 and CD86 [150]. Expression in multiple myeloma is variable and correlates with prognosis [151]. In CLL, the expression levels are low in non-stimulated malignant lymphocytes and increase after stimulation [148, 152].

6.3. CD267 (TACI) expression

The CD267 receptor binds to two ligands - BAFF and APRIL, thus inducing activation, proliferation, and survival of B cells [52, 153, 154, 155]. CD267 is expressed on subsets of B lymphocytes and activated T cells [156] and the expression varies in different B cell subpopulations, the strongest being on marginal-zone B cells and memory CD27+ B lymphocytes [157, 158, 159], and increases after stimulation [160, 161]. In human B cells, BAFF and APRIL induce IgG and IgA immunoglobulin classes switch in the presence of IL-10 or TGF-β [162]. After the discovery of the mutations in TNFRSF13b, the regulatory role of expression of CD267 in final B cell differentiation and binding to Common variable immunodeficiency (CVID) in humans was established [163, 164]. The binding of BAFF to CD267 stimulates NF-κB activation in B lymphoma cells in vitro, while soluble forms of CD267 inhibit this induction as well as the production of IgM by B lymphocytes [165]. CD267 (TACI) was initially defined as a receptor interacting with Calcium modulating ligand (CAML) meaning that it conducts signals through both NF-κB and NFAT/AP-1. The binding of BAFF and APRIL to CD267 can also conduct negative regulatory signals for B cell maturation and activation. In a study on the expression of CD267 in CLL, a significant decrease of the levels compared to healthy control indicators was found [166], which raises the question of the significance of CD267 in the pathogenesis of CLL. The observed lymphocytic proliferation and development of autoimmune diseases in mice with CD267 deficit suggests that this receptor could conduct pro-apoptotic signals in activated B cells [167, 168]. In humans, the higher is the expression of CD267 on monoclonal B lymphocytes the higher is the percentage of apoptotic leukemic cells [166], therefore it was presumed that the decreased receptor expression reduces the negative regulatory signal to B cells. The authors also found inverse correlation between CD267 and Bcl-2 expression of the leukemic cells and a positive correlation between TACI and the expression of prostate apoptosis response-4 (PAR-4), which is a unique pro-apoptotic protein, selectively inducing apoptosis in tumor cells [169]. Based on the observation of increased numbers of circulating and splenal B lymphocytes in TACI–/– deficit mice [167, 170], it can be speculated that CD267 is an inhibitor of B cell proliferation [167]. Similarly, a study of 62 untreated patients with CLL showed inverse correlation between the amount of CD5+ B cells, leukocyte count, and the expression of CD267. The study also showed significantly lower expression of the receptor in Rai stages III and IV patients, as well as in Zap-70+ and CD38+ positive patients, compared to Zap-70 and CD38– negative [166]. Further studies on the expression of CD267 and the clinical course of the disease are needed to establish the precise role of this receptor in the progression of CLL.

7. Conclusion

The phenotypic profile of malignant lymphocytes is of pathological and biological significance. It reflects the relationship between B cells, the tumor microenvironment, and the importance of intercellular interactions. Variations in the expression profile of CLL patients reflect different mutations and impaired regulatory mechanisms. The existence of a complex network of antiapoptotic and prosurvival molecules, including cell adhesion, proinflammatory, angiogenic, and proto-oncogenic molecules, is responsible for supporting the infiltrating malignant cells and for the maintenance of the neoplastic tissue in CLL. Many prosurvival signaling pathways potentially sustaining CLL cell maintenance interact with one another. Thus, it appears that developing new classes of drugs affecting simultaneously various signaling pathways, and therefore abrogating signaling redundancy-associated chemoresistance to classical drugs, is feasible.

http://dx.doi.org/10.5772/60761

Author details

Rositsa Vladimirova[1*], Dora Popova[1], Elena Vikentieva[1] and Margarita Guenova[2]

*Address all correspondence to: rossy_vladimirova@yahoo.com

1 Department of Clinical Laboratory and Immunology, Military Medical Academy, Sofia, Bulgaria

2 Laboratory of Haematopathology and Immunology, National Specialised Hospital for Active Treatment of Hematological Diseases, Sofia, Bulgaria

References

[1] Messmer BT, Messmer D, Allen SL, et al. In vivo measurements document the dynamic cellular kinetics of chronic lymphocytic leukemia B cells. J Clin Invest. 2005; 115(3): 755–64.

[2] Stein H, Bonk A, Tolksdorf G, et al. Immunohistologic analysis of the organization of normal lymphoid tissue and non-Hodgkin's lymphomas. J Histochem Cytochem. 1980; 28(8): 746–60

[3] Burger JA, Ghia P, Rosenwald A, et al. The microenvironment in mature B-cell malignancies: a target for new treatment strategies. Blood. 2009; 114(16): 3367–75.

[4] Herishanu Y, Perez-Galan P, Liu D, et al. The lymph node microenvironment promotes B-cell receptor signaling, NF-kappaB activation, and tumor proliferation in chronic lymphocytic leukemia. Blood. 2011; 117(2): 563–74.

[5] Chiorazzi N, Rai KR, Ferrarini M. Chronic lymphocytic leukemia. N Engl J Med. 2005; 352(8): 804–15.

[6] Duhren-von Minden M, Ubelhart R, Schneider D, et al. Chronic lymphocytic leukaemia is driven by antigen-independent cell-autonomous signalling. Nature. 2012; 489(7415): 309–12.

[7] Chiorazzi N, Efremov DG. Chronic lymphocytic leukemia: a tale of one or two signals? Cell Res. 2013; 23:182–5.

[8] Bagnara D, Kaufman MS, Calissano C, et al. A novel adoptive transfer model of chronic lymphocytic leukemia suggests a key role for T lymphocytes in the disease. Blood. 2011; 117(20): 5463–72.

[9] Pizzolo G, Chilosi M, Ambrosetti A, et al. Immunohistologic study of bone marrow involvement in B-chronic lymphocytic leukemia. Blood. 1983; 62(6): 1289–96.

[10] Patten PE, Buggins AG, Richards J, et al. CD38 expression in chronic lymphocytic leukemia is regulated by the tumor microenvironment. Blood. 2008; 111(10): 5173–81.

[11] Giné E, Martinez A, Villamor N et al. Expanded and highly active proliferation centers identify a histological subtype of chronic lymphocytic leukemia ("accelerated" chronic lymphocytic leukemia) with aggressive clinical behavior. Haematologica 2010; 95(9): 1526-33.

[12] Till KJ, Lin K, Zuzel M, et al. The chemokine receptor CCR7 and alpha4 integrin are important for migration of chronic lymphocytic leukemia cells into lymph nodes. Blood. 2002; 99: 2977–84.

[13] Ghia P, Strola G, Granziero L, et al. Chronic lymphocytic leukemia B cells are endowed with the capacity to attract CD41, CD40L1 T cells by producing CCL22. Eur J Immunol. 2002; 32(5):1403–13.

[14] Granziero L, Ghia P, Circosta P, et al. Survivin is expressed on CD40 stimulation and interfaces proliferation and apoptosis in B-cell chronic lymphocytic leukemia. Blood. 2001; 97(9): 2777–83.

[15] Dancescu M, Rubio-Trujillo M, Biron G, et al. Interleukin 4 protects chronic lymphocytic leukemic B cells from death by apoptosis and upregulates Bcl-2 expression. J Exp Med. 1992; 176(5): 1319–26.

[16] Trentin L, Cerutti A, Zambello R, et al. Interleukin-15 promotes the growth of leukemic cells of patients with B-cell chronic lymphoproliferative disorders. Blood. 1996; 87(8): 3327–35.

[17] Foa R, Massaia M, Cardona S, et al. Production of tumor necrosis factor-alpha by B-cell chronic lymphocytic leukemia cells: a possible regulatory role of TNF in the progression of the disease. Blood. 1990; 76(2): 393–400.

[18] Reittie JE, Yong KL, Panayiotidis P, et al. Interleukin-6 inhibits apoptosis and tumour necrosis factor induced proliferation of B-chronic lymphocytic leukaemia. Leuk Lymphoma. 1996; 22(1–2): 83–90.

[19] Buschle M, Campana D, Carding SR, et al. Interferon gamma inhibits apoptotic cell death in B cell chronic lymphocytic leukemia. J Exp Med. 1993; 177(1): 213–18.

[20] Panayiotidis P, Ganeshaguru K, Jabbar SA, et al. Alpha-interferon (alpha-IFN) protects B-chronic lymphocytic leukaemia cells from apoptotic cell death in vitro. Br J Haematol. 1994; 86(1): 169–73.

[21] Chaouchi N, Wallon C, Goujard C, et al. Interleukin-13 inhibits interleukin-2- induced proliferation and protects chronic lymphocytic leukemia B cells from in vitro apoptosis. Blood. 1996; 87(3): 1022–29.

[22] Lotz M, Ranheim E, Kipps TJ. Transforming growth factor beta as endogenous growth inhibitor of chronic lymphocytic leukemia B cells. J Exp Med. 1994; 179(3): 999–1004.

[23] Fayad L, Keating MJ, Reuben JM, et al. Interleukin-6 and interleukin-10 levels in chronic lymphocytic leukemia: correlation with phenotypic characteristics and outcome. Blood. 2001; 97(1): 256–63.

[24] Ranheim EA, Kipps TJ. Activated T cells induce expression of B7/BB1 on normal or leukemic B cells through a CD40-dependent signal. J Exp Med.1993; 177(4): 925-35.

[25] Beyer M, Kochanek M, Darabi K, et al. Reduced frequencies and suppressive function of CD41CD25hi regulatory T cells in patients with chronic lymphocytic leukemia after therapy with fludarabine. Blood. 2005; 106(6): 2018–25.

[26] Biancotto A, Dagur PK, Fuchs JC, et al. Phenotypic complexity of T regulatory subsets in patients with B-chronic lymphocytic leukemia. Mod Pathol. 2012; 25(2): 246–59.

[27] Gorgun G, Holderried TA, Zahrieh D, et al. Chronic lymphocytic leukemia cells induce changes in gene expression of CD4 and CD8 T cells. J Clin Invest. 2005; 115(7): 1797–805.

[28] Kurtova AV, Balakrishnan K, Chen R, et al. Diverse marrow stromal cells protect CLL cells from spontaneous and drug-induced apoptosis: development of a reliable and reproducible system to assess stromal cell adhesion-mediated drug resistance. Blood. 2009; 114(20): 4441–50.

[29] Ding W, Knox TR, Tschumper RC, et al. Platelet-derived growth factor (PDGF)-PDGF receptor interaction activates bone marrow-derived mesenchymal stromal cells derived from chronic lymphocytic leukemia: implications for an angiogenic switch. Blood. 2010; 116(16): 2984–93.

[30] Ding W, Nowakowski GS, Knox TR, et al. Bi-directional activation between mesenchymal stem cells and CLL B-cells: implication for CLL disease progression. Br J Haematol. 2009; 147(4): 471–83.

[31] Ghosh A, Secreto C, Knox T, et al. Circulating microvesicles in B-cell chronic lymphocytic leukemia can stimulate marrow stromal cells: implications for disease progression. Blood. 2010; 115(9): 1755–64.

[32] Schulz A, Toedt G, Zenz T, et al. Inflammatory cytokines and signaling pathways are associated with survival of primary chronic lymphocytic leukemia cells in vitro: a dominant role of CCL2. Haematologica. 2011; 96(3): 408–16.

[33] Ruan J, Hyjek E, Kermani P, et al. Magnitude of stromal hemangiogenesis correlates with histologic subtype of non-Hodgkin's lymphoma. Clin Cancer Res. 2006; 12(19): 5622–31.

[34] Panayiotidis P, Jones D, Ganeshaguru K, et al. Human bone marrow stromal cells prevent apoptosis and support the survival of chronic lymphocytic leukaemia cells in vitro. Br J Haematol. 1996; 92(1): 97–103.

[35] Burger M, Hartmann T, Krome M, et al. Small peptide inhibitors of the CXCR4 chemokine receptor (CD184) antagonize the activation, migration and antiapoptotic responses of CXCL12 in chronic lymphocytic leukemia B cells. Blood. 2005; 106(5): 1824–30.

[36] Lagneaux L, Delforge A, De Bruyn C, et al. Adhesion to bone marrow stroma inhibits apoptosis of chronic lymphocytic leukemia cells. Leuk Lymphoma. 1999; 35(5–6): 445–53.

[37] Pittenger MF, Mackay AM, Beck SC, et al. Multilineage potential of adult human mesenchymal stem cells. Science. 1999; 284(5411): 143–7.

[38] De la Fuente MT, Casanova B, Moyano JV, et al. Engagement of alpha4beta1 integrin by fibronectin induces in vitro resistance of B chronic lymphocytic leukemia cells to fludarabine. J Leukoc Biol. 2002; 71(3): 495–502.

[39] Redondo-Munoz J, Ugarte-Berzal E, Terol MJ, et al. Matrix metalloproteinase-9 promotes chronic lymphocytic leukemia b cell survival through its hemopexin domain. Cancer Cell. 2010; 17(2): 160–72.

[40] Redondo-Munoz J, Escobar-Diaz E, Samaniego R, et al. MMP-9 in B-cell chronic lymphocytic leukemia is up-regulated by alpha4beta1 integrin or CXCR4 engagement via distinct signaling pathways, localizes to podosomes, and is involved in cell invasion and migration. Blood. 2006; 108(9): 3143–51.

[41] Ringshausen I, Dechow T, Schneller F, et al. Constitutive activation of the MAPkinase p38 is critical for MMP-9 production and survival of B-CLL cells on bone marrow stromal cells. Leukemia. 2004; 18(12): 1964–70.

[42] Park CS, Choi YS. How do follicular dendritic cells interact intimately with B cells in the germinal centre? Immunology. 2005; 114(1): 2–10.

[43] Chilosi M, Pizzolo G, Fiore-Donati L, et al. Routine immunofluorescent and histochemical analysis of bone marrow involvement of lymphoma/leukaemia: the use of cryostat sections. Br J Cancer. 1983; 48(6): 763–75.

[44] Stevenson FK, Caligaris-Cappio F. Chronic lymphocytic leukemia: revelations from the B-cell receptor. Blood. 2004; 103(12): 4389–95.

[45] Schmid C, Isaacson PG. Proliferation centres in B-cell malignant lymphoma, lymphocytic (B-CLL): an immunophenotypic study. Histopathology. 1994; 24(5): 445–51.

[46] Chilosi M, Pizzolo G, Caligaris-Cappio F, et al. Immunohistochemical demonstration of follicular dendritic cells in bone marrow involvement of B-cell chronic lymphocytic leukemia. Cancer. 1985; 56(2): 328–32.

[47] Pedersen IM, Kitada S, Leoni LM, et al. Protection of CLL B cells by a follicular dendritic cell line is dependent on induction of Mcl-1. Blood. 2002; 100(5): 1795-801.

[48] Burger JA, Tsukada N, Burger M, et al. Blood-derived nurse-like cells protect chronic lymphocytic leukemia B cells from spontaneous apoptosis through stromal cell-derived factor-1. Blood. 2000; 96(8): 2655–63.

[49] Tsukada N, Burger JA, Zvaifler NJ, et al. Distinctive features of "nurselike" cells that differentiate in the context of chronic lymphocytic leukemia. Blood. 2002; 99(3): 1030–7.

[50] Schiemann B, Gommerman JL, Vora K, et al. An essential role for BAFF in the normal development of B cells through a BCMA-independent pathway. Science. 2001; 293(5537): 2111–4.

[51] Schneider P, Takatsuka H, Wilson A, et al. Maturation of marginal zone and follicular B cells requires B cell activating factor of the tumor necrosis factor family and is independent of B cell maturation antigen. J Exp Med. 2001; 194(11): 1691–7.

[52] Mackay F, Schneider P, Rennert P, et al. BAFF and APRIL: a tutorial on B cell survival. Annu Rev Immunol. 2003; 21: 231-64.

[53] Kern C, Cornuel JF, Billard C, et al. Involvement of BAFF and APRIL in the resistance to apoptosis of B-CLL through an autocrine pathway. Blood. 2004; 103(2): 679–88.

[54] Novak A, Bram R, Kay N, et al. Aberrant expression of B-lymphocyte stimulator by B chronic lymphocytic leukemia cells: a mechanism for survival. Blood. 2002; 100(8): 2973–9.

[55] Nishio M, Endo T, Tsukada N, et al. Nurselike cells express BAFF and APRIL, which can promote survival of chronic lymphocytic leukemia cells via a paracrine pathway distinct from that of SDF-1alpha. Blood. 2005; 106(3): 1012–20.

[56] Zhang W, Kater AP, Widhopf GF, et al. B-cell activating factor and v-Myc myelocytomatosis viral oncogene homolog (c-Myc) influence progression of chronic lymphocytic leukemia. Proc Natl Acad Sci U S A. 2010; 107(44): 18956–60.

[57] Krysov S, Dias S, Paterson A, et al. Surface IgM stimulation induces MEK1/2-dependent MYC expression in chronic lymphocytic leukemia cells. Blood. 2012; 119(1): 170–9.

[58] Burger JA, Burger M, and Kipps TJ. Chronic lymphocytic leukemia B cells express functional CXCR4 chemokine receptors that mediate spontaneous migration beneath bone marrow stromal cells. Blood. 1999; 94(11): 3658–67.

[59] Burger JA, Quiroga MP, Hartmann E, et al. High-level expression of the T-cell chemokines CCL3 and CCL4 by chronic lymphocytic leukemia B cells in nurse-like cell cocultures and after BCR stimulation. Blood. 2009; 113(13): 3050–58.

[60] Bürkle A, Niedermeier M, Schmitt-Graff A, et al. Overexpression of the CXCR5 chemokine receptor and its ligand, CXCL13 in B-cell chronic lymphocytic leukemia. Blood. 2007; 110(9): 3316–25.

[61] Bennett F, Rawstron A, Plummer M, et al. B-cell chronic lymphocytic leukaemia cells show specific changes in membrane protein expression during different stages of cell cycle. Br J Haematol. 2007; 139(4): 600–4.

[62] Quiroga MP, Balakrishnan K, Kurtova AV, et al. B-cell antigen receptor signaling enhances chronic lymphocytic leukemia cell migration and survival: specific targeting with a novel spleen tyrosine kinase inhibitor, R406. Blood. 2009; 114(5): 1029–37.

[63] Vlad A, Deglesne PA, Letestu R, et al. Down-regulation of CXCR4 and CD62L in chronic lymphocytic leukemia cells is triggered by B-cell receptor ligation and associated with progressive disease. Cancer Res. 2009; 69(16): 6387-95.

[64] Chen L, Widhopf G, Huynh L, et al. Expression of ZAP-70 is associated with increased B-cell receptor signaling in chronic lymphocytic leukemia. Blood. 2002; 100(13): 4609-14.

[65] Richardson SJ, Matthews C, Catherwood MA, et al. ZAP-70 expression is associated with enhanced ability to respond to migratory and survival signals in B-cell chronic lymphocytic leukemia (B-CLL). Blood. 2006; 107(9): 3584–92.

[66] Deaglio S, Vaisitti T, Aydin S, et al. CD38 and ZAP-70 are functionally linked and mark CLL cells with high migratory potential. Blood. 2007; 110(12): 4012–21.

[67] Vaisitti T, Aydin S, Rossi D, et al. CD38 increases CXCL12-mediated signals and homing of chronic lymphocytic leukemia cells. Leukemia. 2010; 24: 958-69.

[68] Niedermeier M, Hennessy BT, Knight ZA, et al. Isoform-selective phosphoinositide 3′-kinase inhibitors inhibit CXCR4 signaling and overcome stromal cell-mediated drug resistance in chronic lymphocytic leukemia: a novel therapeutic approach. Blood. 2009; 113(22): 5549–57.

[69] Barretina J, Junca J, Llano A, et al. CXCR4 and SDF-1 expression in B-cell chronic lymphocytic leukemia and stage of the disease. Ann Hematol. 2003; 82: 500–5.

[70] Dao-Ung LP, Sluyter R, Fuller SJ, et al. CXCR4 but not CXCR3 expression correlates with lymphocyte counts in B-cell chronic lymphocytic leukemia. Ann Hematol. 2004; 83: 326–7.

[71] Ghobrial I, Bone N, Stenson M, et al. Expression of the chemokine receptors CXCR4 and CCR7 and disease progression in B-cell chronic lymphocytic leukemia/ small lymphocytic lymphoma. Mayo Clin Proc. 2004; 79: 318–25.

[72] Schröttner P, Leick M, Burger M. The role of chemokines in B cell chronic lymphocytic leukaemia: pathophysiological aspects and clinical impact. Ann Hematol. 2010; 89: 437–46.

[73] Jones D, Benjamin RJ, Shahsafaei A, et al. The chemokine receptor CXCR3 is expressed in a subset of B-cell lymphomas and is a marker of B-cell chronic lymphocytic leukemia. Blood. 2000; 95: 627–32.

[74] Ocana E, Delgado-Perez L, Campos-Caro A, et al. The prognostic role of CXCR3 expression by chronic lymphocytic leukemia B cells. Haematologica. 2007; 92: 349–56.

[75] Gary-Gouy H, Sainz-Perez A, Marteau JB, et al. Natural phosphorylation of CD5 in chronic lymphocytic leukemia B cells and analysis of CD5-regulated genes in a B cell line suggest a role for CD5 in malignant phenotype. J Immunol. 2007; 179: 4335–44.

[76] Chunsong H, Yuling H, Li W, et al. CXC chemokine ligand 13 and CC chemokine ligand 19 cooperatively render resistance to apoptosis in B cell lineage acute and chronic lymphocytic leukemia CD23+ CD5+ B cells. J Immunol. 2006; 177: 6713–22.

[77] Ticchioni M, Essafi M, Jeandel PY, et al. Homeostatic chemokines increase survival of B-chronic lymphocytic leukemia cells through inactivation of transcription factor FOXO3a. Oncogene. 2007; 26: 7081–91

[78] Scielzo C, Apollonio B, Scarfò L, et al. The functional in vitro response to CD40 ligation reflects a different clinical outcome in patients with chronic lymphocytic leukemia. Leukemia. 2011; 25: 1760-7.

[79] Reif K, Ekland EH, Ohl L, et al. Balanced responsiveness to chemoattractants from adjacent zones determines B-cell position. Nature. 2002; 416: 94–9.

[80] Malavasi F, Deaglio S, Damle R, et al. CD38 and chronic lymphocytic leukemia: a decade later. Blood. 2011; 118(13): 3470-78.

[81] Rai KR, Döhner H,. Keating :J, et al. Chronic Lymphocytic Leukemia: Case-Based Session. Hematol 2001; 1:141-56

[82] Gunnarsson R, Mansouri L, Isaksson A, et al. Array-based genomic screening at diagnosis and during follow-up in chronic lymphocytic leukemia. Haematologica. 2011; 96(8): 1161-9.

[83] Braggio E, Kay NE, Vanwier S, et al. Longitudinal genome wide analysis of patients with chronic lymphocytic leukemia reveals complex evolution of clonal architecture at disease progression and at the time of relapse. Leukemia. 2012; 26(7): 1698-701

[84] Zhang L, Znoyko I, Costa LJ, et al. Clonal diversity analysis using SNP microarray: a new prognostic tool for chronic lymphocytic leukemia. Cancer Genet. 2011; 204(12): 654-65.

[85] Kröber A, Seiler T, Benner A, et al. V(H) mutation status, CD38 expression level, genomic aberrations and survival in chronic lymphocytic leukemia. Blood. 2002; 100(4): 1410-6.

[86] Buggins AG, Levi A, Gohil S, et al. Evidence for a macromolecular complex in poor prognosis CLL that contains CD38, CD49d, CD44 and MMP-9. Br J Haematol. 2011; 154(2): 216-22.

[87] Zucchetto A, Vaisitti T, Benedetti D, et al. The CD49d/CD29 complex is physically and functionally associated with CD38 in B-cell chronic lymphocytic leukemia cells. Leukemia. 2012; 26(6): 1301-12.

[88] Bulian P, Shanafelt T, Fegan C, et.al. CD49d is the strongest flow cytometry-based predictor of overall survival in chronic lymphocytic leukemia. J Clin Oncol. 2014; 32(9): 897-904.

[89] Hertweck MK, Erdfelder F, Kreuzer KA. CD44 in hematological neoplasias. Ann Hematol. 2011; 90(5): 493-508.

[90] Zarcone D, De Rossi G, Tenca C, et al. (1998) Functional and clinical relevance of CD44 variant isoform expression on B-cell chronic lymphocytic leukemia cells. Haematologica. 1998; 83(12): 1088-98.

[91] Bairey O, Zimra Y, Rabizadeh E, et al. Expression of adhesion molecules on leukemic B cells from chronic lymphocytic leukemia patients with predominantly splenic manifestations. Isr Med Assoc. 2004; J 6(3): 147-51.

[92] Molica S, Vitelli G, Levato D, et al. Elevated serum levels of soluble CD44 can identify a subgroup of patients with early B-cell chronic lymphocytic leukemia who are at high risk of disease progression. Cancer. 2001; 92(4): 713-9.

[93] Eisterer W, Bechter O, Söderberg O, et al. Elevated levels of soluble CD44 are associated with advanced disease and in vitro proliferation of neoplastic lymphocytes in B-cell chronic lymphocytic leukaemia. Leuk Res. 2004; 28(10): 1043-51.

[94] Redondo-Muñoz J, Ugarte-Berzal E, García-Marco JA, et al. Alpha4beta1 integrin and 190- kDa CD44v constitute a cell surface docking complex for gelatinase B/MMP-9 in chronic leukemic but not in normal B cells. Blood. 2008; 112(1): 169-78.

[95] Rothlein RD. A human intercellular adhesion molecule (ICAM-1) distinct from LFA-1. J Immunol. 1986; 137(4): 1270–4.

[96] Yang L, Froio RM, Sciuto TE, et al. ICAM-1 regulates neutrophil adhesion and transcellular migration of TNF-α-activated vascular endothelium under flow. Blood. 2005; 106(2): 584–92.

[97] Khorshed A, Abdelhamid T, Wahab NA, et al. The impact of selected apoptotic markers and adhesion molecules on response to chemotherapy and prognosis of chronic lymphocytic leukemia. Nature Sci. 2010; 8(8): 229-35.

[98] Rosen SD. Ligands for L-selectin: homing, inflammation, and beyond. Annu Rev Immunol. 2004; 22: 129–56.

[99] Irjala H, Johansson EL, Grenman R, et al. Mannose receptor is a novel ligand for L-selectin and mediates lymphocyte binding to lymphatic endothelium. J Exp Med. 2001; 194: 1033–42.

[100] Alexander SR, Kishimoto TK, Walcheck B. Effects of selective protein kinase C inhibitors on the proteolytic down-regulation of L-selectin from chemoattractant-activated neutrophils. J Leukoc Biol. 2000; 67: 415–22.

[101] Smalley DM, Ley K. L-selectin: mechanisms and physiological significance of ectodomain cleavage. J Cell Mol Med. 2005; 9: 255–66.

[102] Reichert RA, Gallatin WM, Weissman IL, et al. Germinal center B cells lack homing receptors necessary for normal lymphocyte recirculation. J Exp Med. 1983; 157: 813–27.

[103] Qi H, Egen JG, Huang AY, et al. Extrafollicular activation of lymph node B cells by antigen-bearing dendritic cells. Science. 2006; 312: 1672–6.

[104] Burgess M, Gill D, Singhania R, et al. CD62L as a therapeutic target in chronic lymphocytic leukemia. Clin Cancer Res. 2013; 19: 5675-85.

[105] Burgess M, Mollee P, Singhania R, et Al. CD62L expression is associated with chronic lymphocytic leukemia (CLL) Cell survival in vitro and represents a novel therapeutic target in CLL. Blood. 2013; 122(21): 4136-42.

[106] Suljagic M, Laurenti L, Tarnani M, et al. Reduced expression of the tumor suppressor PHLPP1 enhances the antiapoptotic B-cell receptor signal in chronic lymphocytic leukemia B-cells. Leukemia. 2010; 24: 2063–71.

[107] Davids MS, Brown JR. Targeting the B cell receptor pathway in chronic lymphocytic leukemia. Leuk Lymphoma. 2012; 53: 2362–70.

[108] Herishanu Y, Polliack A. B-cell receptor signaling in chronic lymphocytic leukemia leans on Lyn. Leuk Lymphoma. 2013; 54: 1125–6.

[109] Hamblin TJ, Davis Z, Gardiner A, et al. Unmutated Ig VH genes are associated with a more aggressive form of chronic lymphocytic leukemia. Blood. 1999; 94(6): 1848-54.

[110] Cesano A, Perbellini O, Evensen E, et al. Association between B-cell receptor responsiveness and disease progression in B-cell chronic lymphocytic leukemia: results from single cell network profiling studies. Haematologica. 2013; 98: 626–34.

[111] Ternynck T, Dighiero G, Follezou J, et al. Comparison of normal and CLL lymphocyte surface Ig determinants using peroxidase-labeled antibodies. I. Detection and quantitation of light chain determinants. Blood, 1974; 43: 789–95.

[112] Vuillier F, Dumas G, Magnac C, et al. Lower levels of surface B-cell-receptor expression in chronic lymphocytic leukemia are associated with glycosylation and folding defects of the mu and CD79a chains. Blood. 2005; 105: 2933–40.

[113] Oppezzo P, Dighiero G. Role of the B-cell receptor and the microenvironment in chronic lymphocytic leukemia. Blood Cancer Journal. 2013; 3: e149. doi:10.1038/bcj. 2013.45.

[114] Thompson AA, Talley JA, Do HN, et al. Aberrations of the B-cell receptor B29 (CD79b) gene in chronic lymphocytic leukemia. Blood. 1997; 90: 1387–94.

[115] Rassenti LZ, Kipps TJ. Expression of Ig-beta (CD79b) by chronic lymphocytic leukemia B cells that lack immunoglobulin heavy-chain allelic exclusion. Blood. 2000; 95: 2725–7.

[116] Payelle-Brogard B, Magnac C, Alcover A, et. al. Defective assembly of the B-cell receptor chains accounts for its low expression in B-chronic lymphocytic leukaemia. Br J Haematol. 2002; 118: 976–85.

[117] Payelle-Brogard B, Magnac C, Oppezzo P, et al. Retention and defective assembly of the B-cell receptor in the endoplasmic reticulum of chronic lymphocytic leukaemia B cells cannot be reverted upon CD40 ligand stimulation. Leukemia. 2003; 17: 1196–99.

[118] Dighiero G, Hamblin TJ. Chronic lymphocytic leukaemia. Lancet. 2008; 371: 1017–29.

[119] Schroeder HW, Dighiero G. The pathogenesis of chronic lymphocytic leukemia: analysis of the antibody repertoire. Immunol Today. 1994; 15: 288–94.

[120] Oppezzo P, Magnac C, Bianchi S, et al. Do CLL B cells correspond to naive or memory B-lymphocytes? Evidence for an active Ig switch unrelated to phenotype expression and Ig mutational pattern in B-CLL cells. Leukemia. 2002; 16: 2438–46.

[121] Chiorazzi N, Ferrarini M. Cellular origin(s) of chronic lymphocytic leukemia: cautionary notes and additional considerations and possibilities. Blood. 2011; 117: 1781–91.

[122] Darzentas N, Hadzidimitriou A, Murray F, et al. A different ontogenesis for chronic lymphocytic leukemia cases carrying stereotyped antigen receptors: molecular and computational evidence. Leukemia. 2010; 24: 125–32.

[123] Foy T, Shepherd D, Durie F, et al. In vivo CD40-gp39 interactions are essential for thymus-dependent humoral immunity. II. Prolonged suppression of the humoral immune response by an antibody to the ligand for CD40, gp39. J Exp Med. 1993; 178: 1567–75.

[124] Van Kooten C, Banchereau J. Functions of CD40 on B cells, dendritic cells and other cells. Curr Opin Immunol. 1997; 9: 330–7.

[125] Castle BE, Kishimoto K, Stearns C, et al. Regulation of expression of the ligand for CD40 on T helper lymphocytes. J Immunol. 1993; 151: 1777– 88.

[126] Yellin MJ, Sinning J, Covey LR et al. T lymphocyte T cell–B cell activation molecule/ CD40-L molecules induce normal B cells or chronic lymphocytic leukemia B cells to

http://dx.doi.org/10.5772/60761

express CD80 (B7/BB1) and enhance their costimulatory activity. J Immunol. 1994; 153: 666–74.

[127] Von Bergwelt-Baildon M, Vonderheide R, Maecker B, et al. Human primary and memory cytotoxic T lymphocyte responses are efficiently induced by means of CD40-activated B cells as antigen-presenting cells: potential for clinical application. Blood. 2002; 99: 3319–25.

[128] Van Essen D, Kikutani H, Gray D. CD40 ligand-transduced co-stimulation of T cells in the development of helper function. Nature. 1995; 378: 620–23.

[129] Aruffo A, Farrington M, Hollenbaugh D, et al. The CD40 ligand, gp39, is defective in activated T cells from patients with X-linked hyper-IgM syndrome. Cell. 1993; 72: 291–300.

[130] Cantwell M, Hua T, Pappas J, et al. Acquired CD40-ligand deficiency in chronic lymphocytic leukemia. Nat Med. 1997; 3: 984–9.

[131] Schattner EJ, Mascarenhas J, Reyfman I, et al. Chronic lymphocytic leukemia B cells can express CD40 ligand and demonstrate T-cell type costimulatory capacity. Blood. 1998; 91: 2689–97.

[132] Schattner EJ. CD40 ligand in cell pathogenesis and therapy. Leuk Lymphoma. 2000; 37: 461–72.

[133] Romano MF, Lamberti A, Tassone P, et al. Triggering of CD40 antigen inhibits fludarabine-induced apoptosis in B chronic lymphocytic leukemia cells. Blood. 1998; 92: 990–5.

[134] Schultze JL, Seamon MJ, Michalak S, et al. Autologous tumor infiltrating T cells cytotoxic for follicular lymphoma cells can be expanded in vitro. Blood. 1997; 89: 3806–16.

[135] Cardoso A, Schultze J, Boussiotis V, et al. Pre-B acute lymphoblastic leukemia cells may induce T-cell anergy to alloantigen. Blood. 1996; 88: 41–8.

[136] Schmitter D, Bolliger U, Hallek M, et al. Involvement of the CD27- CD70 co-stimulatory pathway in allogeneic T-cell response to follicular lymphoma cells. Br J Haematol. 1999; 106: 64–70.

[137] Krackhardt AM, Harig S, Witzens M, et al. T-cell responses against chronic lymphocytic leukemia cells: implications for immunotherapy. Blood. 2002; 100: 167–73.

[138] Schultze JL, Michalak S, Lowne J, et al. Human non-germinal center B cell interleukin (IL)-12 production is primarily regulated by T cell signals CD40 ligand, interferon gamma, and IL-10: role of B cells in the maintenance of T cell responses. J Exp Med. 1999; 189: 1–12.

[139] Greaves P and Gribben J. The role of B7 family molecules in hematologic malignancy. Blood. 2013; 121(5): 734–44.

[140] Collins A, Brodie D, Gilbert R, et al. The interaction properties of costimulatory molecules revisited. Immunity. 2002; 17: 201–10.

[141] Carreno BM, Collins M. The B7 family of ligands and its receptors: new pathways for costimulation and inhibition of immune responses. Annu Rev Immunol. 2002; 20: 29–53.

[142] Aicher A, Hayden-Ledbetter M, Brady WA, et al. Characterization of human inducible costimulator ligand expression and function. J Immunol. 2000; 164: 4689–96.

[143] Borriello F, Sethna MP, Boyd SD, et al. B7-1 and B7-2 have overlapping, critical roles in immunoglobulin class switching and germinal center formation. Immunity. 1997; 6:303–13.

[144] Lenschow DJ, Walunas TL, Bluestone JA. CD28/B7 system of T cell costimulation: A comprehensive review of B7, CD28 and CTLA4 functions. Annu Rev Immunol. 1996; 14: 233–58.

[145] Tivol EA, Borriello F, Schweitzer AN, et al. Loss of CTLA-4 leads to massive lymphoproliferation and fatal multiorgan tissue destruction, revealing a critical negative regulatory role of CTLA-4. Immunity. 1995; 3: 541-7.

[146] Mandelbrot DA, McAdam AJ, Sharpe AH. B7-1 or B7-2 is required to produce the lymphoproliferative phenotype in mice lacking cytotoxic T lymphocyte-associated antigen 4 (CTLA-4). J Exp Med. 1999; 189: 435–40.

[147] Dorfman DM, Schultze JL, Shahsafaei A, et al. In vivo expression of B7-1 and B7-2 by follicular lymphoma cells can prevent induction of T-cell anergy but is insufficient to induce significant T-cell proliferation. Blood.1997; 90(11): 4297-306.

[148] Vyth Dreese FA, Boot H, Dellemijn TA, et al. Localization in situ of costimulatory molecules and cytokines in B-cell non-Hodgkin's lymphoma. Immunology. 1998; 94(4): 580–6.

[149] Schultze JL, Cardoso AA, Freeman GJ, et al. Follicular lymphomas can be induced to present alloantigen efficiently: a conceptual model to improve their tumor immunogenicity. Proc Natl Acad Sci U S A. 1995; 92(18): 8200–4.

[150] Delabie J, Ceuppens JL, Vandenberghe P, et al. The B7/BB1 antigen is expressed by Reed-Sternberg cells of Hodgkin's disease and contributes to the stimulating capacity of Hodgkin's disease-derived cell lines. Blood. 1993; 82(9): 2845–52.

[151] Pope B, Brown RD, Gibson J, et al. B7-2-positive myeloma: incidence, clinical characteristics, prognostic significance and implications for tumor immunotherapy. Blood. 2000; 96(4): 1274–9.

[152] Dakappagari N, Ho SN, Gascoyne RD, et al. CD80 (B7.1) is expressed on both malignant B cells and nonmalignant stromal cells in non-Hodgkin lymphoma. Cytometry B: Clin Cytom. 2012; 82(2): 112–9.

[153] Bossen C, Schneider P. BAFF, APRIL and their receptors: structure, function and signaling. Semin Immunol. 2006; 18: 263–75.

[154] Tangye SG, Bryant VL, Cuss AK, et al. BAFF, APRIL and human B cell disorders. Semin Immunol. 2006; 18: 305–17.

[155] Dang L, White DW, Gross S, et al. Cancer-associated IDH1 mutations produce 2-hydroxyglutarate. Nature. 2009; 462: 739–44.

[156] Von Bulow G, Bram R. NF-AT activation induced by CAML interacting member of the tumor necrosis factor receptor superfamily. Science. 1997; 278: 138–41.

[157] Ng L, Sutherland A, Newton R, Qian F, et al. B cell-activating factor belonging to the TNF family (BAFF)-R is the principal BAFF receptor facilitating BAFF costimulation of circulating T and B cells. J Immunol. 2004; 173: 807–17.

[158] Avery DT, Kalled SL, Ellyard, JI, et al. BAFF selectively enhances the survival of plasmablasts generated from human memory B cells. J Clin Invest. 2003; 112: 286–97.

[159] Novak, A, Darce J, Arendt B, et al. Expression of BCMA, TACI and BAFF-R in multiple myeloma: a mechanism for growth and survival. Blood. 2004; 103: 689–94.

[160] Batten M, Fletcher C, Ng L, et al. TNF deficiency fails to protect BAFF transgenic mice against autoimmunity and reveals a predisposition to B cell lymphomas. J Immunol. 2004; 172: 812–22.

[161] Sakurai D, Kanno Y, Hase H, et al. TACI attenuates antibody production costimulated by BAFF-R and CD40. Eur J Immunol. 2007; 37. DOI 10.1002/eji.200636623.

[162] Litinskiy MB, Nardelli B, Hilbert, DM, et al. DCs induce CD40-independent Immunoglobulin class switching through BLyS and APRIL. Nat Immunol. 2002; 3: 822–9.

[163] Castigli E, Wilson S, Garibyan L, et al. TACI is mutant in common variable immunodeficiency and IgA deficiency. Nat Genet. 2005; 37: 829–34.

[164] Chapel S, Webster H, Pan-Hammarstrom D, et al. Mutations in TNFRSF13B encoding TACI are associated with common variable immunodeficiency in humans. Nat Genet. 2005; 37: 820–8.

[165] Xia XZ, Treanor J, Senaldi G, et al. TACI is a TRAF-interacting receptor for TALL-1, a tumor necrosis factor family member involved in B cell regulation. J Exp Med. 2000; 192: 137–43.

[166] Bojarska-Junak A, Hus I, Sieklucka M, et al. The role of TACI expression in chronic lymphocytic leukemia. Centr Eur J Immunol. 2011; 36(1): 46–50.

[167] Yan M, Wang H, Chan B, et al. Activation and accumulation of B cells in TACI-deficient mice. Nat Immunol. 2001; 2: 638–43.

[168] Seshasayee D, Valdez P, Yan M, et al. Loss of TACI causes fatal lymphoproliferation and autoimmunity, establishing TACI as an inhibitory BLyS receptor. Immunity. 2003; 18: 279–88.

[169] Ranganathan P, Rangnekar V. Regulation of cancer cell survival by Par-4. Ann NY Acad Sci. 2005; 1059: 76–85.

[170] Von Bülow G, Van Deursen J, Bram R. Regulation of the T-independent humoral response by TACI. Immunity. 2001; 14: 573–82.

Chapter 10

Zinc Oxide Nanoparticles and Photodynamic Therapy for the Treatment of B-chronic Lymphocytic Leukemia

Sandra Loydover Peña Luengas, Gustavo H. Marin, Luis Rivera, Adrian Tarditti, Gustavo Roque and Eduardo Mansilla

Additional information is available at the end of the chapter

http://dx.doi.org/10.5772/61796

Abstract

The generation of singlet oxygen (SO) in the presence of specific photosensitizers (PS) or semiconductor nanoparticles (NPs) and its application in photodynamic therapy (PDT) has great interest for the development of new cancer therapies. Our work focused on the identification of factors leading to the enhancement of B-Chronic Lymphocytic Leukemia (B-CLL) intracellular SO production and cell killing using Manganese (Mn) doped and undoped Zinc Oxide (ZnO) NPs as potential photosensitizers with and without PDT. Mn can enhance ZnO NPs generation of SO by targeted cells. Multi drug resistant B-Chronic Lymphocytic Leukemia (B-CLL) cells spontaneously produce high amounts of Reactive Oxygen Species (ROS) having an altered redox state in relation to that of normal B lymphocytes. These little variations of its SO intracellular concentrations could allow ZnO NPs to execute specific deadly programs against these leukemic cells with no significant damage to normal lymphocytes. A 0.5% Mn Doped ZnO NP was finally selected for further probes as it had the best killing activity in fludarabine resistant B-CLL cells, especially when combined with PDT. This could be an innovative specific therapy against resistant B-CLL probably contributing in the near future for the definitive benefit of these bad prognostic patients.

Keywords: ZnO, Naoparticles, PDT, Leukemia

1. Introduction

B-chronic lymphocytic leukemia (B-CLL) and other chronic indolent hematologic malignancies like B lymphomas are diseases that usually originate from hematopoietic B cells with abnormal alterations in the processes of development, maturation, and/or apoptosis. They usually manifest as progressive accumulations of morphologically mature B lymphocytes although immunologically dysfunctional [1, 2]. B-CLL is the most common adult leukemia in the western world, and currently it has no available curative strategy [1]. Beside many new discoveries for its treatment, advanced stages of B-CLL usually derived in drug resistance and aggressive progression with the death of the majority of patients [3, 4]. Chemotherapy is still a valid alternative for its temporary improvement or just for tumor mass reduction but not for a definitive healing treatment modality as it has been said [3]. The gold standard of any antineoplastic drug should be to submit the malignant cells to an apoptotic or cytotoxic program, without involving healthy ones, thereby minimizing adverse effects and maximizing the expected results, especially in those situations where drug resistance has developed [5, 6, 7]. Therefore, it is essential to have new treatment modalities in order to increase the anti-B-CLL effects, providing greater biological activity and much more specificity for this kind of disease. New drugs as well as monoclonal antibodies and other biologics have shown real improvements as antineoplastic therapies [8, 9]. However, in general, the side effects are also frequent, and the development of resistance or relapse is usually inevitable for these kind of diseases [3, 5, 10, 11]. In order to minimize adverse effects, new drug delivery strategies should be designed for therapeutic or diagnostic purposes in oncology. Thus, when such an agent is desired to be specifically delivered inside a tumor mass, innovations are needed. In our present state of knowledge, the systemic administration of antineoplastic drugs usually faces problems related to nondesired effects in healthy tissues and incomplete distribution inside the targeted tumor [12]. Then "specific targeted therapies" (STT) could be the new hope for solid and hematological tumors [13]. Advancements in materials science and the ever-increasing miniaturization of technology have led to the development of nanotechnology, a discipline concerned with the development and utilization of nanomaterials, structures with dimensions in the 1- to 100-nm range [14, 15, 16]. Nanoparticles (NPs) are increasingly being recognized for their utility in the field of medicine, including use as drug carriers and imaging tools [17, 18, 19]. Investigations of reactive species (free atoms, clusters, and reactive particles) throughout the 1970s and 1980s, coupled with new techniques and instruments (innovations in mass spectrometry, vacuum technology, microscopes, and more), brought nanotechnology to different fields, including chemistry, physics, material science, engineering, and biology [20]. Today, nanoscale materials represent real and widespread possibilities for interesting fundamental science as well as useful technologies [21, 22]. Nanotechnology and nanoscience are multidisciplinary fields between chemistry, which deals with atoms, molecules, and condensed matter physics, which deals with solids of an essentially infinite array of bound atoms or molecules of dimension no greater than 100 nm [23]. We have now the unique opportunity to change some properties of materials through the management of size and shape. This is a central point of nanoscience that will permit us the control of some electronic as well as magnetic conditions of matter by which it can become much more active and useful for cancer treatments [24, 25, 26, 27, 28, 29]. Although the 8 physical and chemical properties of substances have been well characterized, an intriguing facet of nanotechnology is that materials reduced to the nanoscale in size begin to display different physical and chemical properties. This can include changes in optical properties, such as color and light diffraction, solubility, hardness and strength, magnetism, heat, and electrical conductivity, and surface reactivity [21, 30]. As NP size is reduced, the surface area-to-volume ratio increases, and a large number of the atoms

http://dx.doi.org/10.5772/61796

composing the particle are found on the particle surface [31]. This can render substances previously thought inert suddenly highly reactive. These changes in properties mean that researchers cannot rely upon expectations of chemical behavior based on the previously understood characteristics of these substances [20, 32]. In NPs made of semiconducting materials, the band gap can be modified with NP size [33, 34, 35]. The band gap is the amount of energy required for an electron in the material to be liberated from the allowed valence band and become a charge carrier. If enough energy is supplied, an electron jumps from the valence band to the conductance band, leaving behind a vacancy called an electron hole in the valance band. In NPs, a large portion of the atoms are found at the surface, and consequently so too are the highly reactive valence electrons and holes. This has strong implications for the potential of NP to have toxic reactivity in biological systems [36, 37, 38, 39]. The formation of vesicles or capsules that are small enough to be delivered into the human body by means of inhalation, injection, or permeation through the skin has received significant attention [40]. The outer shell of the vesicles may be chemically functionalized with receptors and other species to selectively target certain organs [41]. In this way, it is possible to think between some other strategies, in the use of delivery/antineoplastic systems that could be delivered easily straight into the tumor's cells. By using nanoparticle systems, it is possible now to provide more precisely many drugs and peptides specifically inside the tumors [7, 42, 43]. These nanoparticles can be made of biodegradable as well as nonbiodegradable materials. Some of their effects could be derived from its abilities to transport and deliver drugs, reducing toxicity as well as increasing bioavailability or even by a direct effect of their molecular and electrical properties as it is the case for some metallic nanoparticles [8, 44]. When they are designed to transport drugs, it is clear that they can specifically deliver them in huge amounts and very specifically inside neoplastic cells without much harm to healthy ones [9, 45]. This has been described for cisplatin in which a higher apoptosis process was observed than with a free drug [10]. These nanopharmaceuticals as multifunctional drugs and imaging agents with a very wide repertoire of action will surely be the next generation of antineoplastic therapeutic and diagnostic agents [11, 46]. There is some previous but limited published experience with NPs in lymphomas, including in vivo studies in lymphoproliferative diseases [42–44]. We have already published [47] the possibility of using these pharmaceutical new systems to overcome drug resistance of B-chronic lymphocytic leukemia (B-CLL) cells. Nanotechnology, the science that studies, develops, and employs nanometer-scale complex systems, has claimed to be the key to improve treatment outcomes in oncology [33, 48, 49]. Then NPs, objects of a size of tens to hundreds of nanometers as it has been said, constructed with different materials such as natural or synthetic polymers or even metals, could be custom designed for almost every disease, including B-CLL and other lymphomas [47, 50]. These elements when made of zinc oxide (ZnO) are plausible to be coated and modified by other metals like manganese (Mn) and could generate apoptotic and/or cytotoxic changes in malignant cells, especially in the shape of autophagy. This specialized way of tumor cell death seems to be the specific result of metal NPs action and could be an interesting and innovative mechanism to be full discovered and achieved in cancer treatment [51, 52]. ZnO NPs doped with metals such as Mn may have their optical and electronic properties modified as Mn is known to increase metal NP's surface defects, thus generating photooxidation reactions that could be enhanced by PDT [53, 54, 55].

In this way, we thought that these NPs made of Mn-doped ZnO could be used in the treatment of B-CLL and other indolent lymphomas, alone or in combination with PDT. These NPs, by itself or even more if excited by light emission, may generate ROS especially one of its kind, singlet oxygen (SO), which could lead to an induced apoptotic process or some other kind of death pathway like autophagy in B-CLL cells, including those with resistant phenotypes to conventional therapies [56, 57]. This strategy could be a very specific one, considering that the oxidative stress found in leukemic cells is supposed to be a lot much higher than that of normal B lymphocytes [6, 7]. Based on a growing body of evidence, ROS production is proposed as a key cytotoxic mechanism mediated by ZnO NPs leading to cell death [58, 59]. The photoactivation of these ZnO NPs is predicted to induce greater levels of ROS, including intracellular SO release which, if effectively targeted to cancer cells, could produce their selective final destruction [48, 60]. The use of ZnO nanoparticles (NPs) for biomedical applications, particularly PDT, relies on the fact that semiconductor nanomaterials could generate reactive oxygen species (ROS) and are promising candidates to become the new generation of photosensitizers (PS) [61]. ZnO is an excellent PS candidate due to its nontoxicity and ability to biodegrade [62, 63]. Moreover, it displays high thermal and chemical stabilities [64]. Furthermore, ZnO is a high-quality semiconductor material with a band gap of 3.37 eV, is transparent in the UV region, and has a large excitation binding energy at room temperature (60 meV) [65]. ZnO has the hexagonal wurtzite structure with lattice parameters $a = 3.29$Å and $c = 5.24$ Å) [65]. Cancer disease has been one of the principal causes of death worldwide for many years [66, 67]. Photodynamic therapy (PDT) has been successful in the treatment of skin tumors and superficial skin health conditions [68, 69, 70]. We propose to expand the applicability of PDT for therapeutic purposes on other cancer types, which involve internal organs, including the hematological system, and in this respect, NPs possess various physical characteristics, which make them ideal for cancer targeting and treatment using them as PS with PDT [48, 71]. Some of these physical characteristics are size in the nanometer scale for cell membrane internalization, intense emission for illumination, and stability. In addition, they can be prepared with absorption at definite wavelengths to tune them to penetrate into deep seated tumors. Nanotechnology, in fact, has recently been utilized for specific targeting to tumor cells [60, 71] as opposed to current technology based on drug diffusion upon systemic drug uptake, which only reaches a maximum of 30% to the intended site and with the added secondary harmful effects on health. In PDT, a nanoparticle sensitizer is excited at its maximum absorption wavelength, thereby being promoted to its singlet excited state, which then is converted into its triplet state by intersystem crossing [72, 73]. Then the triplet state of the NP transfers energy to the ground state triplet oxygen, which is converted to singlet oxygen (SO) [74, 75]. The search for efficient sensitizers for in situ SO generation is currently of utmost importance for use in PDT [73, 74]. Diverse organic molecules have been synthesized, incorporating different structural features that have been identified with enhanced SO production. NPs have recently been identified as potential sensitizer candidates for SO generation due to their high extinction coefficients, and a few reports have been published [48, 71]. We proposed to use nontoxic functionalized water-soluble ZO and zinc sulfide (ZS) NPs as enhanced SO photosensitizers and to identify factors for their enhanced SO production for improved cancer treatment especially for B-CLL.

2. PDT and metal NPs for cancer treatment

Photodynamic therapy (PDT) is a form of phototherapy using nontoxic light-sensitive compounds that are exposed selectively to light, whereupon they become toxic to targeted malignant and other diseased cells [21, 22]. It is used clinically to treat a wide range of medical conditions, including wet age-related macular degeneration and malignant cancers [23] and is recognized as a treatment strategy, which is both minimally invasive and minimally toxic. Most modern PDT applications involve three key components: [21] a photosensitizer, a light source, and tissue oxygen. The combination of these three components leads to the chemical destruction of any tissues, which either have selectively taken up the photosensitizer or have been locally exposed to light [22]. The wavelength of the light source needs to be appropriate for exciting the photosensitizer to produce ROS [22]. These ROS generated through PDT are free radicals (Type I PDT) generated through electron abstraction or transfer from a substrate molecule and highly reactive state of oxygen known as SO (Type II PDT) [22, 70]. A photosensitizer is a chemical compound that can be promoted to an excited state upon absorption light and undergo intersystem crossing with oxygen to produce SO. The photosensitizer should not be harmful to the target tissue until the treatment beam is applied and preferential uptake in target tissue. Some of these physical characteristics are size in the nanometer scale for cell membrane internalization as well as intense emission for illumination and stability [21, 22]. In PDT, a nanoparticle sensitizer is excited at its maximum absorption wavelength, thereby being promoted to its singlet excited state, which then is converted into its triplet state [23]. Then the triplet state of the nanoparticle transfers energy to the ground state triplet oxygen, which is converted to singlet oxygen (SO) [22]. Metal oxides (MO) play a very important role in many areas of chemistry, physics, and materials science. MO NPs can exhibit unique physical and chemical properties due to their limited size and a high density of corner or edge surface sites [23]. MO NPs include materials such as TiO_2, CeO_2, Al_2O_3, Fe_2O_3, and ZnO and are already found in many products. TiO_2 and ZnO nanomaterials are used in topically applied products such as sunscreens and cosmetics, as are pure gold NPs [76]. Their remarkable physical properties form the basis for motivation of metal NPs synthesis and large effort has especially been focused on the design, characterization, and medical applications of ZnO nanomaterials [77]. Inorganic semiconductor nanocrystals have unique properties resulting from quantum confinement [78]. For semiconductor nanocrystals, the energy gap increases with decreasing size [79]. The excitation tracks the absorbance, resulting in a tunable fluorophore that can be excited efficiently at any wavelength shorter than the emission peak but will emit with the same characteristic narrow, symmetric spectrum regardless of the excitation wavelength [80]. ZnO, also known as zincite, is an inorganic compound, nearly insoluble in water that occurs rarely in nature. It is mostly produced synthetically for its commercial used [65,81]. ZnO is actually a wideband gap semiconductor of the II–VI semiconductor group [76]. At a nanoscale, size exhibits quantum confinement as its electrons are contained in discrete energy bands. In this way and when sufficient energy is supplied, electrons can move from the valence to the conductance band, being able to act as powerful reductants in aqueous solutions as well as mobile charge carriers donating electrons to oxygen to generate superoxide radicals [81, 82]. When this electron movement into the conductance band occurs, there are electron vacancies that can produce powerful oxidation reactions in water. This production of hydrogen peroxide and photocatalysis of ROS by NP-sized ZnO in water can be 100–1000 times faster than bulk ZnO [83, 84].

2.1. Methodology and experimental procedures

2.1.1. Synthesis of NPs

Eight different types of Zn NPs were synthesized by different methods as described here: NP1 ZnO, NP2 ZnO:Mn^{+2} 0.5%, NP3 ZnO:Mn^{+2} 1.0%, NP4 ZnO:Mn^{+2} 1.5%, NP5 ZnO:Mn^{+2} 2.0%, NP6 ZnS, NP7 ZnS:Mn^{+2} 1.0%, and NP8 ZnO/ZnS. NPs were finally diluted and prepared for all experiments by vigorous sonication and addition of human serum albumin.

a. Synthesis of ZnO and Mn-doped ZnO NPs: These NPs were synthesized via wet-chemical techniques [53, 85]. The different Mn doping percentages applied on the surface of NPs were 0.5%, 1.0%, 1.5%, and 2.0%. Undoped ZnO NPs were synthesized with a similar procedure except for the addition of manganese acetate [53].

b. Synthesis of colloidal ZnS semiconductor nanocrystals capped with PVP and prepared using 1% concentration of Mn^{+2} ion as a dopant: The NPs were synthesized via wet-chemical techniques [86]. Undoped ZnS NPs were synthesized with a similar procedure except for the addition of manganese acetate [87].

c. Synthesis of ZnO/ZnS core shell NPs: The preparation of ZnO/ZnS core shell NPs was performed by the thermal decomposition of Zn-MPA complexes [88, 89]. ZnS shell was grown on ZnO nanoparticle by the decomposition of the complex Zn-MPA(3-mercapto-propionic acid) at 100°C. The S atoms originating from the thermal decomposition are deposited slowly.

2.1.2. Characterization of NPs

We characterized all NPs by transmission electron microscopy (TEM) (JEM-2100F, JEOL Inc.) and scanning electron microcopy (SEM) (JEOL-JSM 6500 instrument and a Philips/FEI, XL30s, FEG SEM/Phoenix EDAX) observation after the deagglomeration of NPs with human serum albumin (HSA) 1.5 mg/mL and intense sonication, as well as by elemental composition analysis by energy-dispersive X-ray spectroscopy (EDS). Also, X-ray diffraction (XRD) measurements were carried out with a diffractometer (D500/Siemens) using Cu-Kα radiation with $\lambda = 0.154315$ nm to determine the crystalline nature of the selected NPs. A UV-Vis spectrophotometer (DU 800, Beckman Coulter) was used to study the optical absorption of NPs. Luminescence properties and SO generation by NPs were determined by photoluminescence (PL) spectroscopy, using a spectrofluorometer (FluoroMax-2/Horiba Scientific) at room temperature with a 150-mW continuous ozone-free Xe lamp. Fourier-transformed infrared (FTIR) spectra was recorded using an attenuated total reflection Fourier transform infrared (FTIR-Varian 3100 FTIR/Bio-Rad) to evaluate and characterized the presence of functional groups on the surface of these NPs. The excitation wavelength for photoluminescence measurements was set at 350 nm for ZnO and manganese-doped ZnO NPs, and the excitation wavelengths for ZnS NPs were 320 and 340 nm for manganese-doped ZnS NPs. The excitation wavelength for ZnO/ZnS core shell nanoparticles was 310 nm. For book space reasons, we will only describe here the characterization in full detail only of that type of NP with the best B-CLL cytotoxic effects when applying PDT and tested in vitro for viability and mortality of leukemic cells as later will be described.

2.1.3. *Penetration of cells by NPs*

Amounts of 0.1, 0.2, and 0.3 mg/mL of each of the eight NPs produced were incubated with 4 million cells in 2 mL of culture medium for a maximum period of 3 h, under conditions already described. NP penetration of cells was determined by TEM and by fluorescence microscopy (Motic Inverted Microscope AE30-31 with Episcopic-Fluorescence Attachment EF-INV-II) using a DAPI filter. The degree of penetration was determined by 3 independent pathologists observers trained in cell observation with TEM by evaluation of 5 pictures taken at every each time point (0, 30, 60, 120, and 180 min) of incubation of the cells with the different NPs and its selected concentrations mentioned before. For this purpose, cells with NPs were submitted to two washing cycles and finally to a resuspension step in PBS before TEM observation was performed. Results were the mean of the penetration scores given by all the observers to the 5 pictures for each specific NP and its different concentrations at every time point. Finally, the level of penetration was ranked in relation of the total cell surface covered with NPs as none (0–5%), discrete (6–45%), moderate (46–75%), or intense (76–100%), as seen in each TEM picture by each observer. The time at which the highest level of cell penetration by NPs occurred was later used as the best time point for all laser irradiation experiments. When maximum NP penetration of cells was determined by TEM, the confirmation of these data was done by observation of cells under fluorescence microscopy using a DAPI filter in which the cells were supposed to fluorescence when penetrated by NPs.

2.1.4. *Enhanced singlet oxygen production by PDT*

Since we wanted to have a simple, precise, and reproducible energy source, our approach was to first evaluate different light sources with diverse characteristics in the following order, i.e., broad wavelengths of excitation, unique wavelengths, tailored to requirements of the specific photosensitizer. We wanted to evaluate the robustness of the light sources, so we chose two well-known sensitizers to assess the accuracy and reproducibility of the measurements by calculating the rate of photooxidation and the quantum yield of SO production. Thus, we undertook the task of optimizing the SO production by varying the reaction parameters, such as, concentration of PS, concentration of quencher, solvent, nature and potency of irradiation source, and irradiation time. We used the most commonly quenchers described in the specialized scientific literature: 1,3-diphenylisobenzofuran (DPBF), 2,5-dimethylfuran (DMF), and 2,5-diphenylfuran (DPF) [90, 91]. After optimizing the conditions for PSs to produce SO, we moved to experiments with NPs in order to quantify the production of SO for all the NPs mentioned before, using three methods: spectrophotometry, fluorometry analysis of DPBF oxidation, and analysis of fluorescent probe: singlet oxygen sensor green (SOSG). We choose the standard with the highest production of SO (RB) and a laser on a wavelength of 532 nm because excited nanoparticles and RB are found at this wavelength to trigger photochemical reactions, which produced reactive SO. We measured the intracellular production of SO after the internalization of NPs with and without PDT by a fluorometric analysis of DPBF and analysis of fluorescent probe: singlet oxygen sensor green (SOSG) using a novel method first described by us, which measured the efficiency of the intracellular production of SO by the use of the different NPs with and without PDT. All experiments were made in triplicate.

2.1.5. Apoptosis and cytotoxicity assays of NPs on B-CLL cells

Each of the NPs was tested for apoptotic and cytotoxic effects on B-CLL cells by flow cytometry and propidium iodide/acridine orange vital staining with fluorescent microscopy observation as well as MTT assays, with and without PDT.

2.1.6. Measurement of free ion Zn

Free levels of ion Zn in ultrapure distilled water after incubation with NPs for 24 and 48 h were evaluated by a classical method.

2.1.7. Morphological cell changes after treatment

B-CLL cells and normal lymphocytes were evaluated by light and TEM observation after treatment for cell morphological changes.

3. Results and discussion

3.1. UV-Vis NPs absorption

The optical absorption spectra were recorded in the wavelength region of 200–800 nm. Doping with Mn could increase surface defects of NPs affecting the optical and electronic properties of nanoparticles as well as improving the action of PDT when visible light is used as source. UV-Vis absorption of undoped ZnO and 0.5% Mn-doped ZnO showed a difference in the optical absorption of both the undoped and the Mn-doped ZnO NPs, which could indicate that Mn generates more active sites for reaction at energy level lower than the conduction band of undoped ZnO, and thus absorbs more visible light via these defects sites. Absorption wavelength varies according to the different percentages of doping (Table 1) the optical band gap of undoped and Mn-doped ZnO NPs. Doping ZnO NPs with 0.5% of Mn would contribute with tail states in the vicinity of the valence band owing to the defect sites and reduces its effective band gap.

NPs	**Estimated optical band gap (eV)**
ZnO	3.5
ZnO:Mn^{+2} 0.5% doping	3.4
ZnO:Mn^{+2} 1.0% doping	3.6
ZnO:Mn^{+2} 1.5% doping	3.54
ZnO:Mn^{+2} 2.0% doping	3.50

Table 1. Optical band gap of undoped ZnO and Mn-doped ZnO NPs at different percentages

3.2. Photoluminescence measurements

The emission spectra of all these NPs had one weak band in the UV region around 397 nm that could be attributed to their band gap as well as another broad one at 542 nm in the visible region, which could be related to oxygen defects. The visible emission is the dominant feature of the luminescence of ZnO and Mn-doped ZnO NPs and results from recombination involving trap states [92]. This increase of fluorescence intensity probably indicates that the incorporation of Mn ions into ZnO NPs may suppress some nonradioactive recombinations of free excitation that is near the band gap emission [92].

3.3. Infrared analysis

An FTIR spectrum of ZnO NPs showed an absorption band centered at 451 cm^{-1} corresponding to the stretching vibration of Zn-O, confirming the formation of a ZnO bound [53, 93], and a vibration band at 1021 corresponding to a C-O bond. The O-H broad stretching band at 3438 cm^{-1} is shown in the spectrum [92, 94]. The intense absorption bands at 1405 cm^{-1} and 1586 cm^{-1} were due to C-C and CH_3COO^- stretching vibrations of carboxylic acid, respectively [95]. The strong presence of those bands at 1405 and 1586 could be attributed to the formation of a zinc acetate solution complex in ethanol, occurring during the synthesis process [96]. The Fourier transform infrared (FTIR) spectrum of the 0.5% Mn-doped ZnO NPs has an intense band at 446 cm^{-1}. This peak confirms substitution of Zn^{+2} ions by Mn^{+2} ions in the crystal structure. The photoluminescence studies illustrated that the doping with Mn modifies the emission properties of ZnO NPs.

3.4. XRD analysis

The average crystalline size of NPs was 7.78 ± 0.9 nm and was determined using the Debye–Scherrer formula [97, 98]. The average crystallite sizes are presented in Table 2. From the results of the XRD analysis of Mn-doped ZnO NPs, we observed that the crystal size increases with doping up to 0.5%, indicating the incorporation of Mn in the ZnO lattice. This phenomenon is shown in Table 4, where the lattice parameters of Mn-doped NPs at different atomic percentages in the 0–2 at.% range were slightly higher than those of undoped ZnO NPs. Any other impurities were detected. In Table 3, the average crystallite sizes of Mn-doped ZnO NPs synthesized at all the different dopant atomic percentages in the 0–2 at.% range are presented.

Percentage of Mn doping of ZnO NPs	Average crystallite size ± standard deviation (nm)
ZnO undoped	7.78 ± 0.9
0.5% Mn^{+2}-doped ZnO NPs	14.41 ± 0.8
1.0% Mn^{+2}-doped ZnO NPs	13.25 ± 0.8
1.5% Mn^{+2}-doped ZnO NPs	11.45 ± 0.7
2.0% Mn^{+2}-doped ZnO NPs	10.95 ± 0.6

Table 2. Average crystallite size of ZnO NPs doped at different Mn atomic percentages in the 0–2 at.% range

Lattice Constants (A°)	ZnO	ZnO:Mn 0.5%	ZnOMn 1.0%	ZnO:Mn 1.5%	Zno:Mn 2.0%
a=b	3.231	3.232	3.245	3.260	3.271
c	5.092	5.174	5.193	5.212	5.236

Table 3. The lattice constants calculated from XRD data of ZnO and different Mn atomic cm^{-1} with percentages in the 0–2 at.% range

3.5. TEM, SEM, and EDS analysis of NPs

By scanning electron microscopy (SEM) and transmission electron microscopy (TEM) after being well deagglomerated using human serum albumin (HSA) and intense sonication [99], most of the nanoparticles had spherical shapes and a well-ordered morphology. Highly monodispersed NPs with an average size of 22.4 ± 1.6 nm were clearly observed (Figures 1 and 2). The resulting ZnO and 0.5% Mn-doped ZnO NP morphology was quite similar when observed by both analysis (TEM and SEM), constituting a homogeneous population of NPs of that mentioned size (Figures 1 and 2). TEM and SEM images showed that the NPs appeared a little larger in size than the same estimated result from Scherrer analysis [100]. In Table 4, the experimental Mn concentration was compared to that obtained by the EDS analysis; being quite similar, this confirms the atomic percentage of Mn present in the ZnO nanoparticles.

% Mn (Theorical)	%Mn (EDS)
0	0
0.5	0.4

Table 4. Theoretical Mn content of 0.5% Mn-doped ZnO NPs and that determined by EDS in the same NPs.

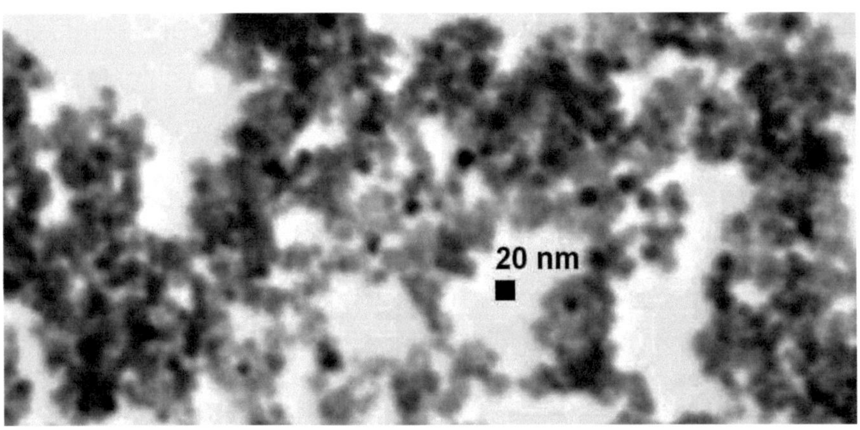

Figure 1. TEM picture of 0.5% Mn-doped ZnO NPs, where they are seen with strong black color, with spherical morphology and uniform size. The gray background is produced by the human albumin used to disperse the particles.

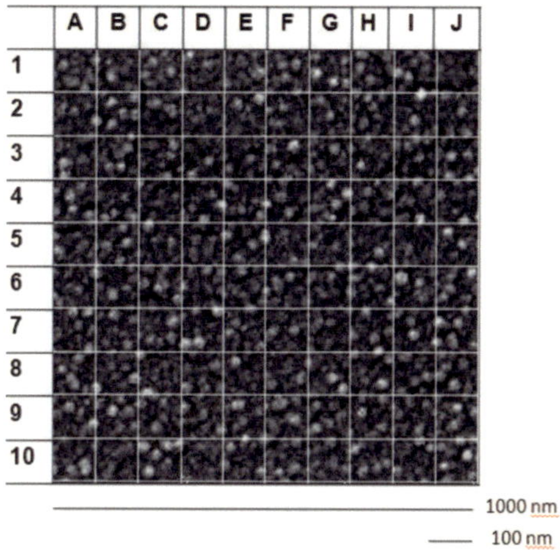

Figure 2. SEM observation of 0.5% Mn-doped ZnO NPs with a counting grid of 1000 × 1000 nm with small square sections of 100 × 100 nm to characterize NPs distribution and size.

3.6. Analytical methods for determination of SO production

Similar results were obtained by the three analytical methods for NPs of 1.0 Mn-doped ZnO. Comparing the spectrophotometric method and fluorometry analysis of DPBF oxidation, similar results were obtained for NPs of 1.0% and 1.5% Mn-doped ZnO and 1.0% Mn-doped ZnS NPs. Core shell ZnO/ZnS did not produce SO at all (Table 5). The measurement of singlet oxygen was similar for ZnO nanoparticles and 1.0% and 2.0% Mn-doped ZnO NPs by both fluorescence methods. Comparing the spectrophotometric method and analysis of fluorescent probe, singlet oxygen sensor green (SOSG), similar results were obtained for NPs of 1.0% Mn-doped ZnO and ZnS.

NPs	**Φ_Δ SO by Spectrophotometry analysis**	**Φ_Δ SO by fluorometry analysis of DPBF oxidation**	**Φ_Δ SO by analysis of fluorescent probe: SOSG**
ZnO	N.R	0.71 $p<0.05$ *	0.66 $p<0.05$ *
ZnO:Mn 0.5% doping	0.60 $p<0.05$ *	0.48	0.74
ZnO:Mn 1.0% doping	0.32	0.28	0.32
ZnO:Mn 1.5% doping	0.17	0.17	0.30
ZnO:Mn 2.0% doping	N.R	0.1	0.17
ZnS	0.36	0.22	0.39
ZnS:Mn 1.0% doping	0.20	0.23	0.52

Table 5. SO quantum yield of NPs by spectrophotometric and fluorometric analysis of DPBF oxidation and by analysis of fluorescent probe: singlet oxygen sensor green (SOSG) in water

We measured the generation of SO in all experiments using NPs and laser irradiation at a wavelength of 532 nm following three different analytical methods: spectrophotometry and fluorometry analysis of DPBF oxidation as well as by the use of a fluorescent probe: singlet oxygen sensor green (SOSG). A standard photosensitizer, RB, of a known SO quantum yield was used to calculate the SO QY of the NPs. Singlet oxygen quantum yield of rose bengal was always significantly higher compared with the QY of any of the NPs used. Anyway, as NPs could have several advantages, that will be explained later on when compared to PSs such as RB. Our results will surely be of great importance for the future clinical application of ZnO NPs. It was clearly demonstrated that the decomposition of DPBF by SO induced by 1.0% Mn-doped ZnO and ZnS NPs at 1.0 mg/mL under laser irradiation conditions was always a time-dependent phenomenon. Comparing both the spectrophotometric method and the fluorometry analysis of DPBF oxidation, similar results were obtained for NPs of 1.0% and 1.5% Mn-doped ZnO and 1.0% Mn-doped ZnS NPs. Our core shell ZnO/ZnS NPs did not produce SO at all. The measurement of SO generation was similar for ZnO nanoparticles and 1.0% and 2.0% Mn-doped ZnO NPs by both fluorescence methods. Comparing the spectrophotometric method and singlet oxygen sensor green (SOSG) routes, similar results were obtained for NPs of 1.0% Mn-doped ZnO and ZnS NPs. In all the other experiments performed in similar conditions, we always found a significant higher generation of SO when 0.5% Mn-doped ZNO NPs were used, and these results seem to indicate that this kind of NP could be the most appropriate to use in living models when SO generation could be needed as a therapeutic strategy. Then the most interesting sample tested in order to use in further experiments with living cells, animal models, or even patients as a potential intracellular SO generator should be 0.5% Mn-doped ZnO NPs, which generated the highest amounts of SO compared to the other Mn-doped samples at 1%, 1.5%, and 2%. These features make 0.5% Mn-doped ZnO nanoparticles potential potent photosensitizers for a combine treatment with PDT. Results for all NPs by the three analytical methods are presented in Table 6. The highest values of SO QY was 0.60 by the spectrophotometric method and 0.74 by SOSG using 0.5% Mn-doped ZnO NPs ($p < 0.05$) and 0.71 by the fluorescence method of DPBF oxidation using ZnO NPs ($p < 0.05$). When a dopant is introduced into a nanoparticle like the ones presented here, a range of percent doping may be most effective in a specific desire clinical action like anticancer selective activity. Additionally, it may be the case that the most effective percent range depends on the nanoparticle composition and the dopant composition. In our case, 0.5% Mn^{+2}-doped NPs had the highest effectiveness in the production of SO. This may be explained in terms of their optical properties with the presence of this doping. Higher fluorescence in the visible region as compared to those Mn^{+2}-doped NPs at 1.0%, 1.5%, and 2.0%. 0.5% Mn^{+2}-doped ZnO NPs generated more SO due of the special transitions in the d orbitals of Mn^{+2}, favoring the photocatalytic processes. At this percentage, the optical and electronic properties of the NPs were favorable for PDT. In this way, there is more energy transfer between the excited NPs with triplet oxygen to produce SO. It is known that these NPs have a good capacity to donor energy and can act as novel PSs in the use of PDT for cancer treatment [28, 50, 101]. The QY of SO by spectrophotometry was 0.60 and 0.48 by fluorometry analysis of DPBF oxidation and 0.74 by analysis of fluorescent probe, respectively. With increasing doping of ZnO NPs from 1.0% to 2.0%, the production of SO decreased in all methods. ZnS NPs without Mn doping when compared to 1.0% Mn-doped ZnS NPs showed an increased SO production by the spectrophotometric method. The results were similar for ZnS and 1.0% Mn-doped ZnS by the fluorometric method using DPBF oxidation. In the SO detection method using the Sensor Green, Mn-doped ZnS NPs show a considerable increase in the production of singlet oxygen compared to undoped NPs. In general, all NPs have a good production of SO and can be used as efficient PS in PDT except ZnO/ZnS core shell. We made a comparative extensive study with 3 different analytical methods: spectrophotometry, fluorometry analysis of DPBF oxidation, and analysis of fluorescent probe: singlet oxygen sensor green (SOSG), using a novel method first described by us, which measured the efficiency of the intracellular production of SO by the use of the different NPs with and without PDT. There is no current scientific literature of this kind doing comparative studies of the intracellular production of SO, making our group the pioneers worldwide. For the results obtained with our 0.5% Mn-doped ZnO NPs, we certainly believe that this specific doping level generates new unique electrical and luminescence properties in our ZnO NPs for this particular concentration of Mn most probably related to a specialized way of tumor cell death called autophagy, which seems to be the specific result of the intracellular action of metal ZnO NPs at this Mn doping level. The Mn^{+2} dopant atomic percentage of 0.5% for ZnO NPs should be interacting with the molecular and electrical configurations of these Zn NPs in such a way that SO generation is clearly enhanced especially when PDT is used. This could be an interesting and innovative mechanism to be fully discovered and achieved in cancer treatment, especially when low concentrations of Mn doping are used in ZnO NPs associated to PDT [33, 48]. It could be important to look in future studies into the behavior of ZnO NPs when doped with concentrations lower than 0.5% especially at the mitochondrial cell level where many of the respiratory and energy generation processes of the cell are taken place. As shown in our experiments, higher concentrations over 0.5% seem not to improve SO generation or leukemic cell death. In this way, it was thought that these NPs made of Mn-doped ZnO could be used in the treatment of B-CLL and other indolent lymphomas, alone or in combination with PDT. These NPs, when excited by light emission, may generate ROS, especially SO, which could lead to an induced apoptotic process or some other kind of death pathway like autophagy in B-CLL cells, including those with resistant phenotypes to conventional therapies [57]. This strategy could be a very specific one, considering that the oxidative stress found in leukemic cells is supposed to be a lot much higher than that of normal B lymphocytes [102, 103]. Based on a growing body of evidence, ROS production is proposed as a key cytotoxic mechanism mediated by ZnO NPs leading to cell death [104, 105]. The photoactivation of these ZnO NPs was predicted to induce greater levels of ROS, including intracellular SO that we measured by an innovative method developed in this research. This enhanced intracellular generation of SO, if effectively targeted to cancer cells by our Mn-doped ZnO NPs, could produce their selective final destruction [106, 107].

3.7. Intracellular measurement of so production after treatment with NPs with and without PDT

Each of the NPs was tested for apoptotic and cytotoxic effects in B-CLL cells as assayed by flow cytometry and propidium iodide/acridine orange staining as well as MTT assays. It is clear by the results of our experiments that the lowest concentration of Mn doping (0.5%) could play the most important role in enhancing the cytotoxic effects of our NPs of the present research. These NPs seem to be very selective in their cytotoxic effects toward diseased B-CLL. Our most effective NPs have been synthesized or modified by a method that affects its biological behavior by the addition of a dopant in a concentration that basically could change their redox potential [85, 108]. These parameters could allow for influence same NPs and/or a preferential association of the NPs with a diseased cell. Fluorescence spectra photooxidation of DPBF in the presence of NPs inside B-CLL cells and DPT treatment showed that DPBF reacts with SO, causing a progressive decrease in the intensity of the quencher again. This decomposition of DPBF by SO produced by the use of 1.0% Mn-doped ZnO NPs 3 and ZnS NPs 6 in B-CLL cells was a time-dependent phenomenon (Figures 3 and 4) with an increased production of intracellular SO in B-CLL cells when PDT was delivered. The intracellular singlet oxygen QY of RB was significantly higher compared with QY of NPs (Figures 3 and 4; $p < 0.05$). The quantum yield of SO for B-CLL cells was 0.16 for NPs3 and 0.21 for NPs6 using DPBF as the chemical quencher (Table 6).

SO QY	B-CLL Lymphocytic cells
NP 3	0.16
NP 6	0.21

Table 6. Singlet oxygen (SO) quantum yield (QY) of NPs in B-CLL lymphocytic cells

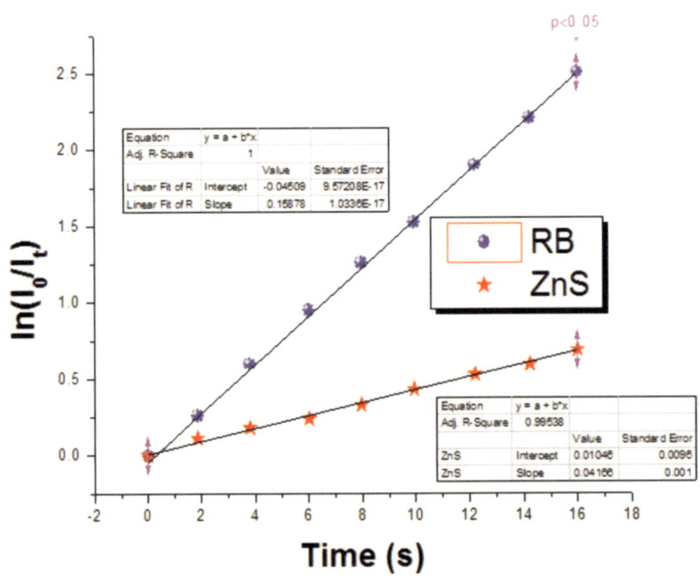

Figure 3. Time-dependent decomposition of DPBF at 6.0 × 10^{-5} M by SO produced by ZnS NPs at 15 μg/mL and RB at 1.0 × 10^{-5} M and incubated with B-CLL cells (4 million/2 mL PBS) and irradiated with a green laser 532 nm at a distance of 40 cm up to 16 s every 2 s compared to that produced by RB under same experimental conditions.

http://dx.doi.org/10.5772/61796

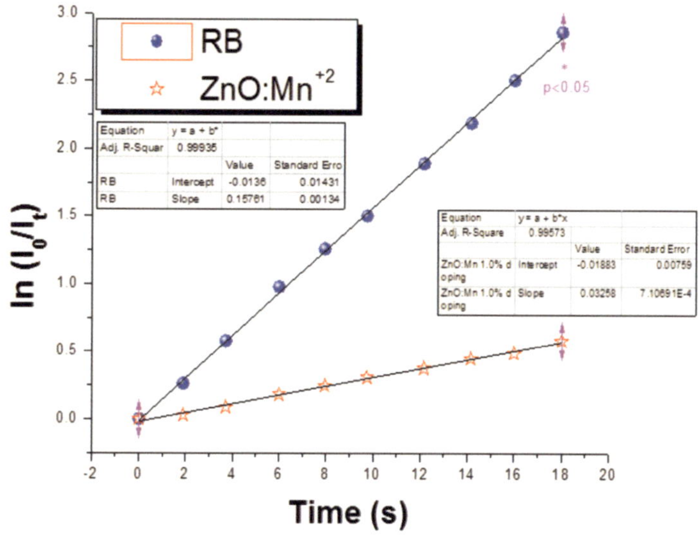

Figure 4. Time-dependent decomposition of DPBF at 6.0 × 10^{-5} M by SO produced by 1.0% Mn-doped ZnO NPs at 15 µg/mL and RB at 1.0 × 10^{-5} M and incubated with B-CLL cells (4 million/2 mL PBS) and irradiated with a green laser 532 nm at a distance of 40 cm up to 18 s every 2 s compared to that produced by RB under same experimental conditions.

3.8. Penetration of cells by NPs

We first evaluated the effect of three different doses (0.1, 0.2, and 0.3 mg/mL) of each of the 8 NPs produced by testing them in their penetration capacity into B-CLL cells as well as into normal B lymphocytes during a total culture period of 3 h (Fig 5). The results of these experiments indicated that 0.2 mg/mL of each of the analyzed NPs resulted in an intense cell penetration activity that was not further increased by its rising to a higher concentration of 0.3 mg/mL. Because of this, the concentration of 0.2 mg/mL of NPs was used in all further experiments. At zero time, no particles were seen inside any of the cells (Fig 6a), but at 2 h time point, all observers agreed that there was a maximum "intense" similar penetration of all NPs in both types of cells (Figure 6b). Normal lymphocytes as well as B-CLL cells were well and maximally penetrated by NPs at 0.2 mg/mL concentration when cultured at 37°C during 2 h and observed under TEM (Figure 6b). At 3 h culture time, no further significant increase in the amount of total NP penetration into cells was observed in either leukemic or normal ones. B-CLL cells as well as normal B lymphocytes when incubated during this time period with 0.2 mg/mL of each of the NPs and observed under TEM and fluorescent microscopy were clearly and intensively penetrated by all of these NPs tested as described by the 3 observers, and no increment of NP penetration in cells was found after this time point as it was said. In this way, an incubation period of 120 min with 0.2 mg/mL of NPs was selected as the best conditions for NP penetration into cells.

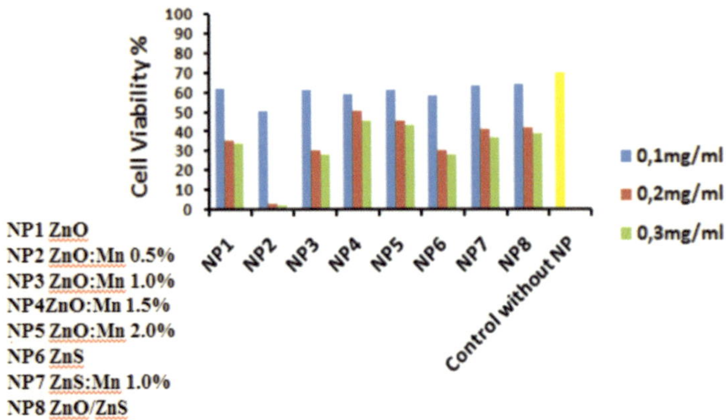

Figure 5. Effect of three different doses of each of the 8 NPs tested on the viability of B-CLL cells at 48 h of incubation after PDT. The dose 0.2 mg/mL produced the most intense killing activity. Increasing this dose up to 0.3 mg/mL did not produce further significant increase in cell mortality as seen with 0.2 mg/mL.

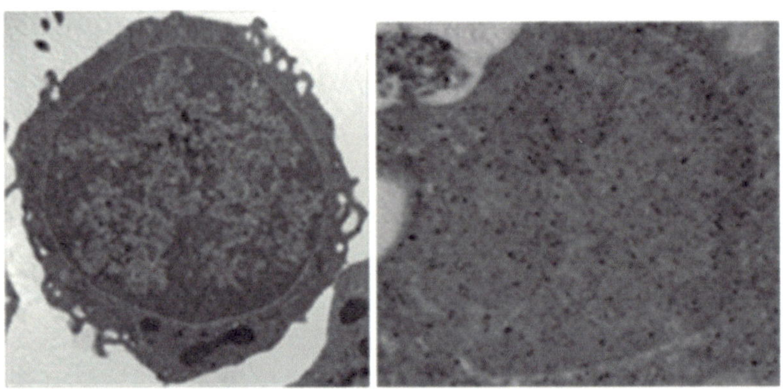

Figure 6. (a) B-CLL cell in culture with no NPs observed with TEM at time 0. Penetration degree: none. (b) B-CLL cell penetration by 0.5% Mn-doped ZnO NPs observed at 2 h by TEM. Penetration degree: intense. As panel b suggests, the NPs also penetrated the cell nucleus.

3.9. Cell viability and mortality testing

Then we evaluated the effect of those same three different doses (0.1, 0.2, and 0.3 mg/mL) of each of the 8 NPs produced on the viability of B-CLL cells at 24 and 48 h of incubation after PDT (Fig 5). In these probes, 0.2 mg/mL of each of the NPs tested again resulted in the best B-CLL cell killing activity. Normal lymphocytes also had the greatest mortality rates at this NPs concentration but were always significantly lower and mostly insignificant in relation to that observed for B-CLL cells. It was also seen that 0.1 mg/mL of each NP had almost no significant difference in the viability of B-CLL cells in relation with that of the control samples without NPs. In this way, this concentration did not seem to be the best one to be tried in further experiments. Scaling up the NPs concentration to 0.3 mg/mL did not either significantly improved the cell killing activity of those same NPs in relation to that concentration of 0.2 mg/mL. Then this concentration of 0.2 mg/mL was selected and used for all other experiments. From the 8 NPs especially designed and produced for this study, 0.5% Mn-doped ZnO NPs were chosen as the most powerful killing NPs against B-CLL cells when associated with PDT but with minimum impact on normal lymphocytes. At the mentioned concentration of 0.2 mg/mL, NPs2 (0.5% Mn-doped ZnO NPs) were the most effective NPs in relation to its killing activity of B-CLL cells (Fig 7). In this way, NP2 was selected for the performance and cytotoxicity procedures.

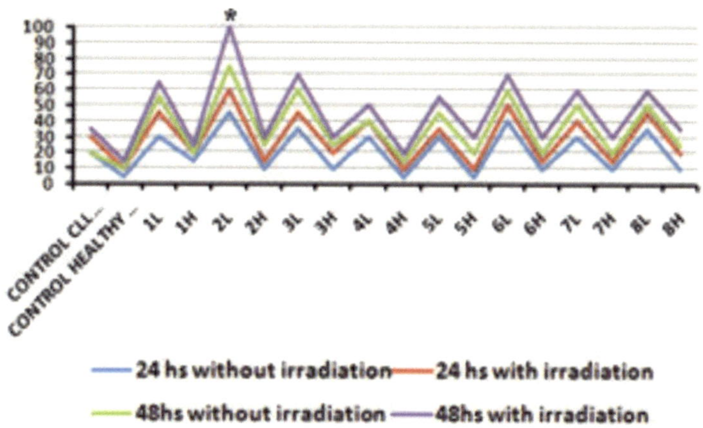

Figure 7. Cytotoxicity levels of B-CLL cells (L) from 5 patients and normal B lymphocytes (H) from 5 healthy donors for each NP at 24 and 48 h with and without laser irradiation. Clearly, the most intense mortality is observed in B-CLL cells exposed to NPs2 at 48 h and laser irradiated.

3.10. Intracellular so production determinations

Changes in the production of intracellular SO were determined in both normal and B-CLL cells after being penetrated by NPs and laser irradiated. The increase of intracellular SO was significantly higher in B-CLL cells than in normal B lymphocytes. Measurements of the intracellular SO generation quantum yield after PDT was done by fluorometry quantitative analysis of photooxidation reactions using either DPBF as the quencher or SOSG as a fluorescent probe for singlet oxygen, as previously described. B-CLL cells as well as normal B lymphocytes when incubated during 2 h with SOSG and observed under fluorescent microscopy were clearly penetrated by this fluorescent probe. The measurement of the intracellular fluorescence spectra of SOSG in the presence of 0.5% Mn-doped ZnO NPs inside B-CLL cells and normal B lymphocytes was possible by using our described method and by recording its changes every minute up to 7 min upon irradiation (Figure 8). A selective increase in the intensity of the fluorescence of SOSG especially in B-CLL cells as a result of the larger production of intracellular SO induced by the action of light when these 0.5% Mn-doped ZnO NPs have already penetrated these cells was recorded. SO quantum yields were determined with the graph of time dependent of SOSG in the presence of NPs inside cells after PDT (Figure 9). A quantitative comparison of the intracellular SO generation between normal lymphocytes and B-CLL cells, both treated with Mn 0.5%-doped ZnO NPs and PDT, using this SOSG fluorescent probe, showed a significant increase in SO generation in malignant leukemic cells rather than in normal ones (Figure 10a and b). The quantum yield was calculated using Equation (1) [91], and the values were 0.88 in B-CLL cells and 0.49 in normal lymphocytes using SOSG as a fluorescent probe for singlet oxygen, as previously described.

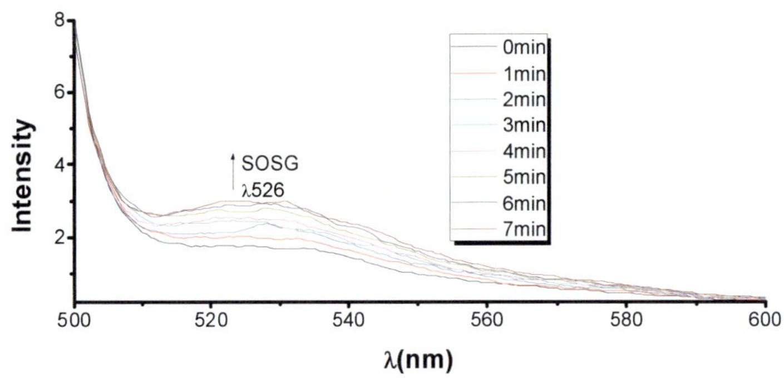

Figure 8. Intracellular PL spectra of SOSG at 5 μL/mL from B-CLL cells (4 million/2 mL PBS) penetrated by of 0.5% Mn-doped ZnO NPs at 0.2 mg/mL, while the cellular suspension was irradiated with a green laser 532 nm at a distance of 40 cm every minute up to 7 min. The excitation wavelength was 488 nm. The increase in the fluorescence intensity of SOSG as a function of time irradiation is clearly observed. There was no interference in the measurements produced by the cells.

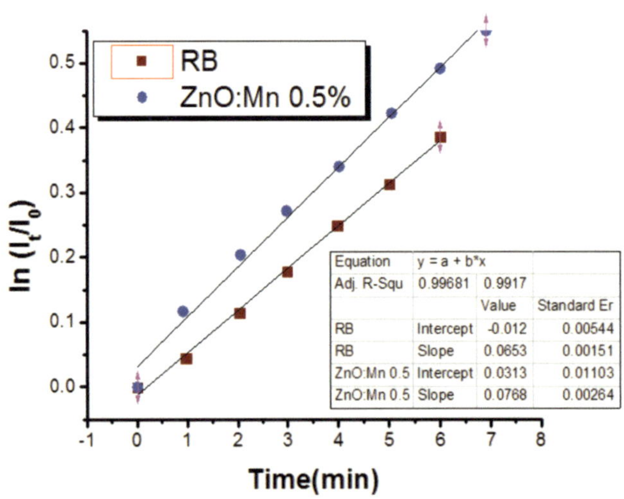

Figure 9. Time dependent of SOSG at 5 μL/mL by SO produced by 0.5% Mn-doped ZnO NPs at 0.2 mg/mL and RB at 1.0×10^{-5} M and incubated with B-CLL lymphocytic cells (4 million/2 mL PBS) while irradiating with a green laser 532 nm at a distance of 40 cm up to 7 min every 1 min.

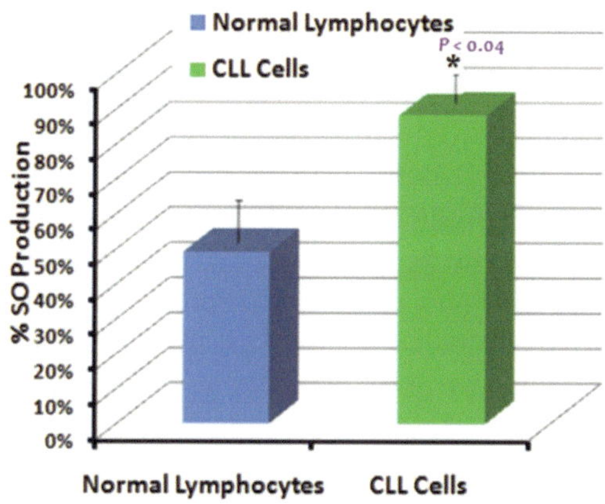

(a)

SOSG QY	Lymphocytes	B-CLL Lymphocytic cells
ZnO:Mn $^{+2}$ 0.5% doping with HSA	0.49	0.88

(b)

Figure 10. (a) Quantitative comparison of the intracellular SO generation after PDT by a fluorescent probe SOSG between normal lymphocytes and B-CLL cells from 5 healthy donors and 5 CLL patients treated with 0.5% Mn-doped ZnO NPs. (b) Singlet oxygen sensor green (SOSG) quantum yield (QY) of Mn 0.5%-doped ZnO NPs inside normal lymphocytes and B-CLL cells.

B-CLL cells as well as normal B lymphocytes when incubated during 2 h with SOSG and observed under fluorescent microscopy were clearly penetrated by this fluorescent probe. The measurement of the intracellular fluorescence spectra of SOSG in the presence of 0.5% Mn-doped ZnO NPs inside B-CLL cells and normal B lymphocytes was possible using our described method and recording its changes every minute up to 7 min upon irradiation (Figure 8). A selective increase in the intensity of fluorescence of SOSG especially in B-CLL cells as a result of the larger production of intracellular SO induced by the action of light when these 0.5% Mn-doped ZnO NPs have already penetrated these cells was recorded. SO quantum yields were determined with the graph of time dependent of SOSG in the presence of NPs inside cells after PDT (Figure 9). A quantitative comparison of the intracellular SO generation between normal lymphocytes and B-CLL cells, both treated with 0.5% Mn-doped ZnO NPs and PDT, using this SOSG fluorescent probe, showed a significant increase in SO generation in malignant leukemic cells rather than in normal ones (Figure 10a and b). The quantum yield was calculated using Equation (1) [91], and the values were 0.88 in B-CLL cells and 0.49 in normal lymphocytes using SOSG as a fluorescent probe for SO, making this difference significant ($p < 0.04$) (Figure 10a). In Equation (1), $\Phi\Delta_{sample} = \Phi\Delta_{ref} K_{sample} / K_{ref}$, where $\Phi\Delta_{ref}$ is the SO quantum yield of rose bengal (RB) and K_{sample} and K_{ref} are the slopes of the plot of the time-dependent increase of SOSG, expressed as the increase of fluorescence at 526 nm of the measured 0.5% Mn-doped ZnO NPs and the RB, respectively (Figure 9). The other method used to calculate the production of intracellular SO was that in which DPBF performed as the chemical quencher in a decomposition reaction. In the analysis of DPBF oxidation by SO, K_{sample} and K_{ref} are the slopes of the plot of the time-dependent decomposition of DPBF, expressed as the decrease of fluorescence at 453 nm of the measured 0.5% Mn-doped ZnO NPs and the RB, respectively (Figure 11). In this way, SO production was significantly higher in B-CLL cells compared to normal lymphocytes when both types of cells were treated with NPs and PDT [6, 18, 51] (Figure 12a and b). Fluorescence spectra photooxidation of DPBF in the presence of 0.5% Mn-doped ZnO NPs inside B-CLL cells showed that DPBF reacts with SO, causing a progressive decrease in the intensity of the quencher (Fig 13). This decomposition of DPBF by SO produced by the use of RB and 0.5% Mn-doped ZnO NPs in B-CLL cells was a time-dependent phenomenon, and again there was an increased production of intracellular SO much higher in B-CLL cells than in normal lymphocytes when PDT was delivered (Figure 12a and b). The quantum yield of SO for B-CLL cells was 0.21 and 0.10 for normal lymphocytes using DPBF as the chemical quencher. Then it is clear that a similar phenomenon was observed in both cases when SOSG or DPBF were used.

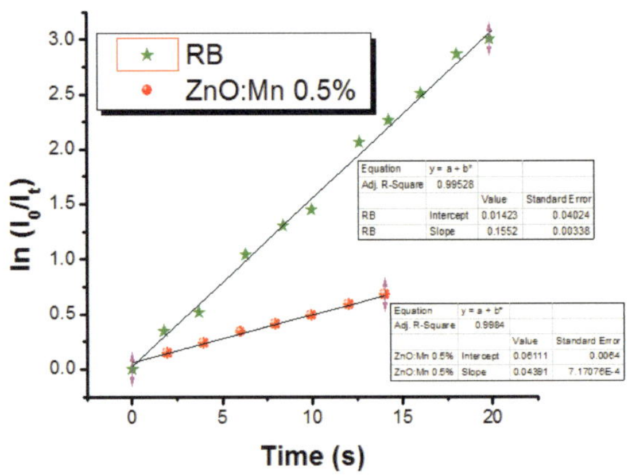

Figure 11. Time-dependent decomposition of DPBF at 6.0 × 10^{-5} M by SO produced by 0.5% Mn-doped ZnO NPs at 0.2 mg/mL and RB at 1.0 × 10^{-5} M and incubated with B-CLL cells (4 million/2 mL PBS) and irradiated with a green laser 532 nm at a distance of 40 cm up to 14 s every 2 s.

SO production was found to be increased in both normal and B-CLL cells when cultured with 0.5% Mn-doped ZnO NPs and laser irradiated, but this increase in SO production was always significantly higher in B-CLL cells compared to normal lymphocytes.

3.11. Cytotoxicity levels produced by NP treatment with and without PDT

Cytotoxicity levels produced by each of the NPs described before on B-CLL cells compared to that on normal B lymphocytes at 24 and 48 h with and without laser irradiation was in all cases significantly higher (Figure 14). At the 0.2 mg/mL concentration, NP2 (0.5% Mn-doped ZnO NPs) was the most effective NP in relation to killing activity of B-CLL cells while having a minimum effect on normal B lymphocytes. The 0.5% Mn-doped ZnO NPs effectively elimi-

http://dx.doi.org/10.5772/61796

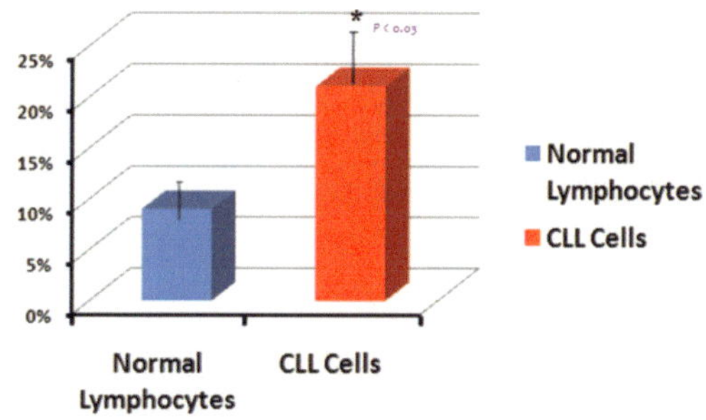

(a)

SO QY	Lymphocytes	B-CLL Lymphocytic cells
ZnO:Mn $^{+2}$ 0.5% doping with HSA (0.2mg/mL)	0.10	0.21

(b)

Figure 12. (a) Quantitative comparison of the intracellular SO generated after PDT by fluorometry quantitative analysis of photooxidation reactions using DPBF as quencher between normal lymphocytes and B-CLL cells penetrated by 0.5% Mn-doped ZnO. (b) Singlet oxygen (SO) quantum yield (QY) generated in normal lymphocytes and B-CLL cells penetrated by 0.5% Mn-doped ZnO after PDT.

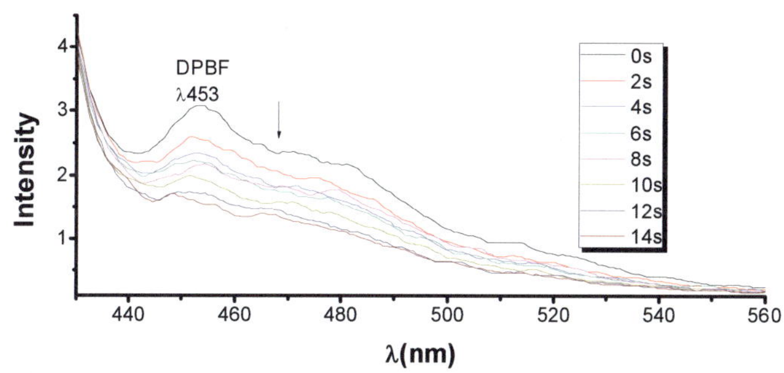

Figure 13. Intracellular PL spectra photooxidation of DPBF at 6.0 × 10^{-5} M from B-CLL (4 million/2 mL PBS) cells penetrated by 0.5% Mn-doped ZnO NPs at 0.2 mg/mL. The suspension was irradiated with a green laser 532 nm at a distance of 40 cm every 2 and up to 14 s. The excitation wavelength was 410 nm. DPBF reacts with SO, which causes a decrease in the intensity of the quencher. There was no interference in the measurements by the cells.

nated the largest amount of fludarabine-resistant B-CLL cells with almost no lost produced in the viability of normal healthy lymphocytes. The intracellular increase of SO production correlated well with cell mortality, as will be described later. After 24 h in culture, both healthy (H) and leukemia (L) cells without NPs had a spontaneous cell death of 5% and 20%, respectively (Figure 14). Cell irradiation with lasers showed no statistical difference in terms of apoptosis or mortality in both cell populations at this time, when no NPs were used. However, when cultured during the same period of time, but exposed to Zn NPs, B-CLL cells without irradiation showed an important loss of viability, especially if culturing time is prolonged to 48 h. Percentages of cytotoxicity increased significantly with PDT at 24 and 48 h in B-CLL cells cultured with NPs. The maximum increase in mortality of B-CLL cells was achieved with NPs2 at 48 h when PDT was applied. Our NPs have distinct effects on cell viability by killing B-CLL cells, but it had very few effects on normal lymphocytes. The marked differences observed in cytotoxicity between B-CLL cells and normal lymphocytes especially using the 0.5% Mn-doped NPs suggest a very exciting potential for these NPs as a novel alternative for leukemia treatment, especially when PDT was applied simultaneously. These NPs induce autophagy in B-CLL cells, which is mediated by SO. B-CLL cells are known to have elevated levels of ROS [1, 6, 56]. We aimed to test a novel ROS-mediated strategy to eliminate fludarabine-resistant B-CLL based on this redox alteration. Our study demonstrated that the Mn-doped ZnO NPs with PDT are effective in eliminating fludarabine-resistant B-CLL cells through SO mechanism with low toxicity to normal lymphocytes. Apoptosis levels for irradiated and nonirradiated cells cultured with NPs2 at 24 and 48 h detected by flow cytometric analysis (annexin V/PI double staining) were always significantly higher in B-CLL cells compared to normal lymphocytes (Figure 14). Apoptotic normal B lymphocytes and B-CLL cells at 24 h cultured with NPs2 were 14% and 49%, while these percentages moved up after laser irradiation (PDT) to 28% and 90% ($p < 0.001$), respectively (Figure 14). Comparison of the mean IC50 of 0.5% Mn-doped ZnO on B-CLL cells ($n = 5$) and normal lymphocytes ($n = 5$) clearly showed a significant difference when NPs2 were used to treat B-CLL cells. Fludarabine-resistant B-CLL cells were clearly much more sensitive to NPs2, with an IC50 value of 0.1 mg/mL, while normal lymphocytes had an IC50 value a lot above and significantly higher for that same NP2 of (Figure 15). MTT assays comparing primary B-CLL cells isolated from the blood samples of the 5 CLL patients (L), which were considered clinically fludarabine resistant with unmutated Ig VH and that of normal B lymphocytes from healthy subjects (H) sensitivity to the action of NPs, clearly showed that the dose response to NPs2 in the fludarabine-resistant B-CLL cells was significantly greater than that observed in normal lymphocytes (Figure 14). SO production was found to increase in both normal and B-CLL cells when cultured with NPs2. This increase in SO production was significantly higher in B-CLL cells compared to normal lymphocytes. This increased intracellular SO production correlated well with cell mortality (Figure 16).

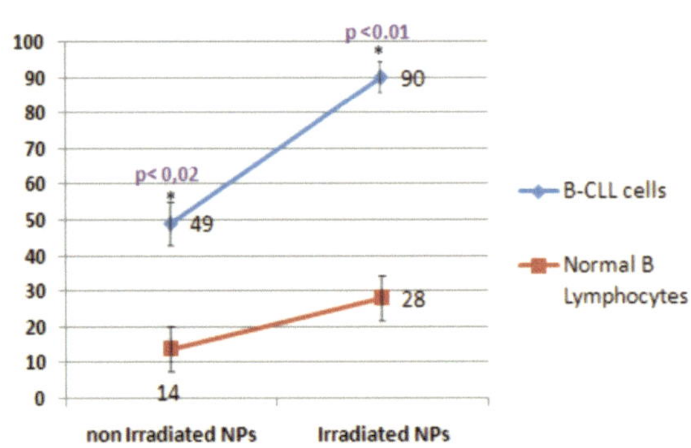

Figure 14. Apoptosis levels for irradiated and nonirradiated B-CLL cells and normal B lymphocytes cultured with 0.5% Mn-doped ZnO NPs (NPs2) at 24 h detected by flow cytometric analysis (annexin V/PI double staining)

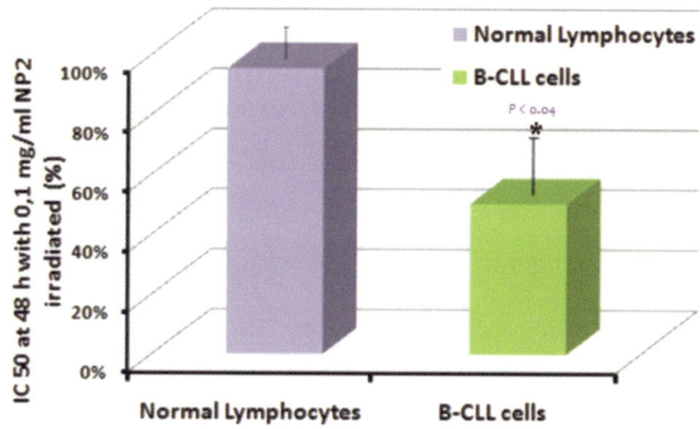

Figure 15. Comparison of the mean IC50 of 0.5% Mn-doped ZnO NPs on B-CLL cells (n = 5) and normal B lymphocytes (n = 5).

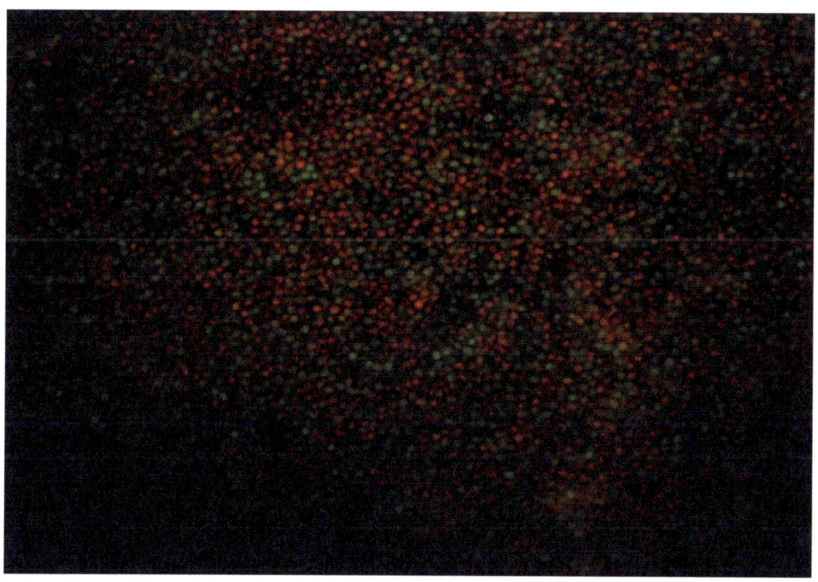

Figure 16. Mortality/viability levels of B-CLL cells incubated with 0.2 mg/mL of 0.5% Mn-doped ZnO NPs for 48 h and PDT. Observed under fluorescence microscopy with FluoroQuench (acridine orange/propidium iodine: 95% mortality).

Mortality/viability levels of B-CLL cells incubated with different NPs were tested using our FluoroQuench method as well with MTT and flow cytometry techniques, as explained before. The results were similar no matter the technique used; the incubation of B-CLL cells with 0.2 mg/mL of 0.5% Mn-doped ZnO NPs for 48 h and PDT produced the highest level of cell mortality (Figure 16). Also, as it has been described in Chapter 4.1.10, in every case, cells were used for cell viability testing normal and B-CLL cells without NPs were always used as blanks or controls samples.

3.12. Measurement of free ion Zn after incubation of cells with NPs

No dosable free ion Zn was measured in the ultrapure water with NPs2 after 72 h of incubation. Tests of cytotoxicity with the possible amount of free ion Zn that could have been determined in these measurements were not further necessary as no free Zn was detected at all in the analyzed ultrapure water.

3.13. Morphological cell changes after treatment with NPs with or without PDT

As observed by optical and fluorescent microscopy, but especially by TEM, and photographed (Figure 17), both types of cells could undergo a process of cell death after 0.5% Mn-doped ZnO NP treatment with or without PDT, corresponding to features of autophagy, but this phenomenon was always stronger when PDT was applied. This autophagic cell death was especially pronounced, much more advanced, massive, and faster on B-CLL cells, affecting almost all of them treated in this way (Fig 17). In the other hand, normal B lymphocytes only suffered autophagic changes in a very lesser degree and basically in the form of an isolated pattern in which only few cells went through this dying pathway besides being treated in the same way and during the same period of time. In this scenario of autophagy, the formation of double membrane-bound organelles predominated in B-CLL cells when treated with 0.5% Mn-doped ZnO NPs alone but predominantly when PDT was simultaneously applied. These organelles were clearly autophagosomes, and by this specific detail, the observed dying process can undoubtedly be considered as autophagy (Figure 17), which denotes any cellular pathway involving the delivery of cytoplasmic material to the lysosome for degradation [109, 110, 111].

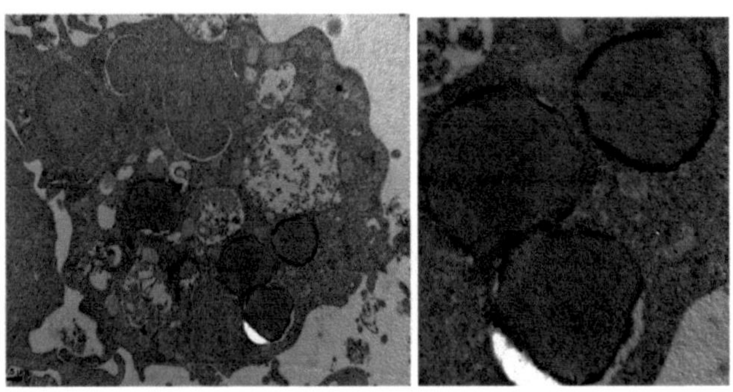

Figure 17. Thin-section TEM images of formation of double membrane-bound organelles in a B-CLL cells when treated with 0.5% manganese-doped ZnO NPs and PDT. These organelles are autophagosomes, and the cell dying process is undoubtedly autophagy

4. General conclusions

In this study, light parameters were primarily evaluated (e.g., intensity of light, broad vs. specific wavelength, and coherent vs. noncoherent nature of light source) for the PSs and quenchers selected to enhance their effect on SO production. The indirect method using DPBF and DPF as quenchers of SO was tested with different light sources incorporating variations in their intensity. Different coherent and noncoherent light emissions with broad and specific wavelength characteristics were used, finding useful and reliable correlations with enhanced generation of SO species in methanol and water. All this information was of great importance for the in vitro studies later on performed as the corresponding SO quantum yields in each case were elucidated and confirmed. Our results clearly suggest the strong influence of the LED lasers and light power intensities on the quantum yield of SO in the presence of different PS–quencher photooxidation pairs under simultaneous aeration in methanol and water. The best results in these circumstances were obtained with specific wavelength LED lasers, which allowed the exact selection of wavelengths and the precise application of light in contrast to lamps, LED flashlight, and fluorescent light bulbs. Considering that PDT depends largely on the light source, the choice of the emission wavelength could usually range from 350 to 1100 nm, depending on the area of the tumor to be treated. In our case, after performing many systematic experiments on the effects of LED lasers of different intensities as excitation sources on SO quantum yields, we choose a laser on a wavelength of 532 nm because at this wavelength are excited nanoparticles to trigger photochemical reactions, which produced reactive SO that killed BCLL by autophagy. Important data between fundamental physical properties of light sources and enhanced SO production using standard sensitizers and inorganic NPs have also been found and analyzed in order to characterize for the reliable, precise, and reproducible measurement and employment of SO in cancer treatment, especially B-CLL. The quantum yield of SO production via sensitization may be given by the sum of contributions due to O_2 quenching of S1 and T1, the lowest excited singlet and triplet states of the PS. Values of $\phi\Delta$ depend on solvent, reaction conditions, light source, measurement technique, and concentration of O_2. Values obtained here are very consistent with the literature for RB and MB using different quenchers or scavengers. We obtained very good results in agreement with the literature, where the QYs of SO were 0.75 for RB and 0.5 for MB using RNO with L-histidine or imidazole as chemical scavengers in both cases. SO reacts with L-histidine or imidazole via a Type II mechanism, in which SO is generated via an energy transfer process. As a very interesting and novel contribution, NPs were found to be able to participate in the actual mechanisms of PDT, mainly by acting as photosensitizers themselves and clearly enhancing SO generation extra- and intracellularly. We produced and tested a variety of metal Zn NPs with good properties for SO generation, of which one made of 0.5% Mn-doped ZnO (0.5% Mn-doped ZnO) had the best killing activity in fludarabine-resistant and unmutated Ig VH B-CLL cells, especially when combined with PDT. Some nanomaterials like this last one can generate and enhance SO inside and outside the cells, with and without PDT, but especially if it is used. Although this area has not received as much attention as the application of nanomaterials to electronics or catalysis, it represents a promising route to overcoming many of the difficulties associated with traditional PDT. Quantum dots meet the first five criteria for good PSs: they are compounds with constant composition, are not cytotoxic in the absence of light, but have a potential to induce cytotoxicity with and even without UV irradiation. The intracellular delivery of QDs can be facilitated by surface coatings, and they can be functionalized to be both water soluble and biocompatible. The synthesis of different immunocompatible QD bioconjugates (e.g., QD-cluster-of-differentiation (CD) antibodies) can guarantee their specific localization into target tissues. One benefit of their unique optical properties is that they can be precisely tuned from the UV to the infrared (IR) region of the spectrum by changing their size and composition. Their emission properties result from quantum-confinement effects and can be tuned to emit into the near-IR region in contrast to the visible emission of the most conventional PSs. Furthermore, because of their large transition dipole moment, QDs are strong absorbers, making them potential candidates for application in photodynamic processes, which has been clearly demonstrated in our B-CLL cell tests, also specifically inducing the autophagic cell death of these malignant cells especially when PDT is delivered simultaneously. NPs seem to offer the best hope for extending the reach of this promising therapy to regions deep in the body or even the blood in patients with B-CLL. It is clear now that NPs could provide many advantages over those of traditional PS such as RB. These PS have limits, especially in their clinical applications, derived from a very low lipid solubility as well as by their possible intrinsic toxicity due to a high polarity. Then metal NPs, like the ones described here, could be an optional effective treatment for drug-resistant forms of B-CLL and may also be for many other types of malignant tumors like lymphomas. As shown in our results, we measured the generation of SO in all our cell experiments using NPs with and without laser irradiation at a wavelength of 532 nm by three different analytical methods: spectrophotometry and fluorometry analysis of DPBF oxidation as well as by the use of a fluorescent probe: singlet oxygen sensor green (SOSG). A standard photosensitizer, RB, of a known SO quantum yield was used to calculate de SO QY of the NPs. The singlet oxygen quantum yield of rose bengal was always significantly higher compared with the QY of any of the NPs. Anyway, as NPs could have several advantages, compared to PSs such as RB, our results are surely of great importance especially in the translational use of these new technologies. It was clearly demonstrated that there was a significant higher generation of SO when 0.5% Mn-doped ZNO NPs were used, and these results seem to indicate that this kind of NP could be the most appropriate to use in living models when SO generation could be needed as a therapeutic strategy. Then the most interesting sample tested in order to use in further experiments with living cells, animal models, or even patients as a potential intracellular SO generator should be 0.5% Mn-doped ZnO NPs, which generated the highest amounts of SO compared to the other Mn-doped samples at 1%, 1.5%, and 2%. These features make 0.5% Mn-doped ZnO nanoparticles potential potent photosensitizers for a combine treatment with PDT (photodynamic therapy). One important aspect that we consider fundamental at the moment of characterization and in vitro cell testing of NPs of these kinds is its degree of sample agglomeration. For investigations of the in vivo effects of ZnO NPs in the circulation as well as for measuring their effects in vitro, on different cell types, NPs have to be dispersed and deagglomerated well in physiological solutions. However, particles in solutions with physiological salt concentrations and pH values usually form greater-sized coarse agglomerates. Coarse agglomerates of NPs have been shown to exert different biological effects as compared to well-dispersed NPs and could change some of the characterization parameters. Therefore, investigating the biological effects of nanoscaled particles with dispersions containing coarse agglomerates is not appropriate. Previously, different methods have been published on ways to avoid the formation of these coarse agglomerates of NPs dispersed in physiological solutions. The importance of the correct ultrasound energy as well as the use of dispersion stabilizers should always be emphasized for the optimal deagglomeration of NPs. We tried several procedures described previously in the literature, making human albumin with strong sonication as the most effective for this purpose. As agglomeration could be a crucial point at the moment to perform NPs characterization as well as in vivo cellular probes and its clinical introduction in living organisms, we suggest to take this point in account very seriously in order to not interfere with the results. When NPs are delivered into the circulation of living organisms, they first get in contact with albumin and other serum proteins. These proteins cover the nanoparticles. Our procedure of deagglomeration uses also albumin; thus, NPs dispersed with this method are covered with the same proteins NPs encounter in the circulation. TEM and SEM confirmed our findings as preparation with this optimized method resulted in an improved dispersion and deagglomeration with any of the NPs studied. Doping at 0.5% with Mn^{+2} increases the production of SO, which was attributed to the optical properties of NPs that were changed, and this fact was closely related to the actions of Mn within the doped NPs. The surface traps of these NPs were eventually quenched by the incorporation of Mn and was confirmed by PL emission, a phenomenon that correlated well with the reduction in the surface traps. At higher concentrations of Mn^{+2} than 0.5%, the generation of SO was lower due the greatest loss of fluorescence of the NPs, inducing higher density of defects not favoring energy transfer processes that enter the NPs and oxygen needed in the SO production. When a dopant is introduced into a nanoparticle like the ones presented here, a range of percent doping may be most effective in a specific desire clinical action like anticancer selective activity. Additionally, it may be the case that the most effective percent range depends on the nanoparticle composition and the dopant composition. In our case, 0.5% Mn^{+2}-doped NPs had the highest effectiveness in the production of SO. This may be explained in terms of their optical properties with the presence of this doping, higher fluorescence in the visible region as compared to those Mn^{+2}-doped NPs at 1.0%, 1.5%, and 2.0%. At this percentage, the optical and electronic properties of the NPs were favorable for PDT. Mn-doped ZnO NPs have distinct effects on cell viability by killing B-CLL cells with low toxicity to normal lymphocytes. These NPs induced a predominant process of autophagy, leading to the massive death of B-CLL cells related to a higher production of SO. This type of NPs could selectively and rapidly increase, just by themselves, the intracellular levels of SO in B-CLL cells conducting them to an autophagic death program that could irreversibly kill them easily but very strongly when delivered with PDT. Using this kind of treatment, B lymphocytes persist mostly alive and not harmed at all by these NPs, PDT, or its combination, as it has been proven here. We have seen that very small variations of intracellular SO concentrations in therapy-resistant leukemic cells could execute and accelerate these deadly pathways, being these mechanisms potentiated and increased by the concomitant delivery of PDT, rendering normal cells almost untouched. An interesting and rapid dying process of the B-CLL cells when incubated with these 0.5% Mn^{+2}-doped ZnO NPs clearly corresponding to autophagy always occurred. There was double membrane-bound organelles cell formation known as autophagosomes, seen under transmission electronic microscopy (TEM) and correlating well with those intracellular increases of SO, that we have measured by a novel method first described by us, which was again more intense when PDT was applied. SO is believed to be the major cytotoxic agent involved in PDT. B-CLL cells are known to have elevated levels of ROS. We aimed to test a novel ROS-mediated strategy to eliminate fludarabine-resistant B-CLL based on this redox alteration. The measurement of SO in biological environments has been a major task, especially when intracellular values, without interferences from the external medium, are required. Near-infrared (NIR) luminescence at 1270 nm in cell environments is confounded by the strongly reduced SO lifetime and probably had never been achieved until a research group developed an NIR-sensitive photomultiplier tube probe that allowed to clearly identify and measure a true intracellular component of SO signal. However, these few described methods are expensive and required of a complex technology to be performed. We developed a comparative extensive study with 3 different analytical methods: spectrophotometry, fluorometry analysis of DPBF oxidation, and analysis of fluorescent probe: singlet oxygen sensor green (SOSG), using a novel method first described by us, which measured the efficiency of the intracellular production of SO by the use of the different NPs with and without PDT. There is no current scientific literature of this kind doing comparative studies of the intracellular production of SO, making our group the pioneers worldwide. We synthesized a series of ZnO nanoparticles with varying concentrations of Mn dopant. Each of the nanoparticles were tested for cytotoxic effects in B-CLL cells as assayed by flow cytometry and propidium iodide/acridine orange staining as well as MTT assays. It is clear by the results of our experiments that the lowest concentration of Mn doping (0.5%) could play the most important role in enhancing the cytotoxic effects of our nanoparticles of the present research. Our intracellular SO measurement method proved to be good enough, inexpensive, and quite simple that it could easily soon be introduced as a routine but very important diagnostic tool. PDT is a clinically tested promising technique to treat cancer and can be associated therapeutically with NPs. Visible emission processes should involve transitions in which the photogenerated holes at the surface of NPs could be trapped by O_2 ions as they are responsible of this phenomenon. Doping with Mn could increase these surface defects of NPs and improve the processes of PDT. The 0.5% Mn^{+2}-doped ZnO NPs2 were able to produce the highest level of cytotoxicity and apoptosis in unmutated B-CLL cells as compared to normal lymphocytes that were quite resistant to this type of therapy, especially after being irradiated with a green laser ($p < 0.01$). This differential effect could be due to changes observed by several authors in the redox state of leukemic and other neoplastic cells respect to normal ones. The fact that unmutated B-CLL cells responded strongly to the cytotoxic effect of these 0.5% Mn-doped ZnO NPs after PDT is also very important, suggesting that this novel therapy with modifications could be used may be soon, as an alternative effective treatment especially under the occurrence of B-CLL-resistant phenotypes. The 0.5% Mn-doped ZnO NPs combined with PDT show much promise as a new anticancer therapy, given the specific autophagic responses triggered in these leukemia cells. It is also interesting to mention the fact that the best killing results were obtained with the lowest Mn doping concentrations. This fact could open the door to future studies with even lowest amounts of this doping agent in the search of the best NP design. NPDT uses light to activate light-sensitive drugs (photosensitizers) to produce short-lived cytotoxic species such as SO to destroy malignant cells. We investigated the mechanisms of cell death during PDT using fluorescence microscopy and imaging and performing fluorometric measurements to help design the better treatments for resistant forms of B-CLL. We can envision external devices for blood irradiation by PDT after NP treatments, although "intelligent" ZnO NPs with self-assemblies for energy discharge and light emission from their same structure or "hybrids" of biodegradable shell nanoparticles coated with specific monoclonal antibodies are being loaded in their core with Zn nanoparticles. As this therapy seems to be very specific to fludarabine-resistant B-CLL cells, without much or any damage made at all to normal lymphocytes, it could contribute as a new innovative targeted strategy in the near future to be delivered in the clinical setting for the definitive benefit of these bad prognostic patients. As normal B lymphocytes are much more resistant than B-CLL cells to the cytotoxic effect of NPs with PDT, we could call this new therapeutic approach as a very specific one with very low toxicity for nonleukemic cells and probably very useful not only for B-CLL but also for all the other indolent lymphomas as well as for all types of cancer.

Author details

Sandra Loydover Peña Luengas[1*], Gustavo H. Marin[2], Luis Rivera[1], Adrian Tarditti[2], Gustavo Roque[2] and Eduardo Mansilla[2]

*Address all correspondence to: sandraluengas@yahoo.es

1 Chemistry Department, University of Puerto Rico at Mayaguez Campus, Puerto Rico, USA

2 Tissue Engineering, Regenerative Medicine and Cell Therapies Laboratory, CUCAIBA, Ministry of Health, Province of Buenos Aires, Argentina

References

[1] M. Palma, P. Kokhaei, J. Lundin, a Choudhury, H. Mellstedt, and a Osterborg, "The biology and treatment of chronic lymphocytic leukemia," *Ann. Oncol.*, vol. 17 Suppl 1, pp. x144–54, Sep. 2006.

[2] C. SHERR, "Principles of tumor suppression," *Cell*, vol. 116, no. 2, pp. 235–246, Jan. 2004.

[3] K. Fischer, P. Cramer, R. Busch, S. Stilgenbauer, J. Bahlo, C. D. Schweighofer, S. Böttcher, P. Staib, M. Kiehl, M. J. Eckart, G. Kranz, V. Goede, T. Elter, A. Bühler, D. Winkler, M. Kneba, H. Döhner, B. F. Eichhorst, M. Hallek, and C.-M. Wendtner, "Bendamustine combined with rituximab in patients with relapsed and/or refractory chronic lymphocytic leukemia: a multicenter phase II trial of the German Chronic Lymphocytic Leukemia Study Group," *J. Clin. Oncol.*, vol. 29, no. 26, pp. 3559–66, Sep. 2011.

[4] B. Turgut, O. Vural, F. S. Pala, G. E. Pamuk, K. Tabakcioglu, M. Demir, S. Ongören, T. Soysal, and C. Algünes, "17p deletion is associated with resistance of B-cell chron-

ic lymphocytic leukemia cells to in vitro fludarabine-induced apoptosis.," *Leuk. Lymphoma*, vol. 48, pp. 311–20, 2007.

[5] L. R. Martins, P. Lúcio, A. Melão, I. Antunes, B. A. Cardoso, R. Stansfield, M. T. S. Bertilaccio, P. Ghia, D. Drygin, M. G. Silva, and J. T. Barata, "Activity of the clinical-stage CK2-specific inhibitor CX-4945 against chronic lymphocytic leukemia," *Leukemia*, vol. 28, no. 1, pp. 179–82, Jan. 2014.

[6] E. Y. O. and S. A. R. Marina A. Orlova, "Effect of 67Zn-nanoparticles on leukemic cells and normal lymphocytes," *Br. J. Med. Med. Res.*, vol. 2, pp. 21–30, 2012.

[7] D. Trachootham, H. Zhang, W. Zhang, L. Feng, M. Du, Y. Zhou, Z. Chen, H. Pelicano, W. Plunkett, W. G. Wierda, M. J. Keating, and P. Huang, "Effective elimination of fludarabine-resistant CLL cells by PEITC through a redox-mediated mechanism," *Blood*, vol. 112, no. 5, pp. 1912–22, Sep. 2008.

[8] M. R. Grever, D. M. Lucas, G. W. Dewald, D. S. Neuberg, J. C. Reed, S. Kitada, I. W. Flinn, M. S. Tallman, F. R. Appelbaum, R. a Larson, E. Paietta, D. F. Jelinek, J. G. Gribben, and J. C. Byrd, "Comprehensive assessment of genetic and molecular features predicting outcome in patients with chronic lymphocytic leukemia: results from the US Intergroup Phase III Trial E2997," *J. Clin. Oncol.*, vol. 25, no. 7, pp. 799–804, Mar. 2007.

[9] S. a Parikh, K. G. Rabe, N. E. Kay, T. G. Call, W. Ding, S. M. Schwager, D. a Bowen, M. Conte, D. F. Jelinek, S. L. Slager, and T. D. Shanafelt, "Chronic lymphocytic leukemia in young (≤55 years) patients: a comprehensive analysis of prognostic factors and outcomes," *Haematologica*, vol. 99, no. 1, pp. 140–7, Jan. 2014.

[10] T. S. Lin, M. Moran, M. Lucas, S. Waymer, S. Jefferson, D. B. Fischer, M. R. Grever, and J. C. Byrd, "Antibody therapy for chronic lymphocytic leukemia: a promising new modality," *Hematol. Oncol. Clin. North Am.*, vol. 18, no. 4, pp. 895–913, ix–x, Aug. 2004.

[11] M. Hirose, E. Hosoi, S. Humano, and A. Jalili, "Multidrug resistance in hematological malignancy," *J. Med. Invest.*, vol. 50, no. 3–4, pp. 126–35, 2003.

[12] V. Jonsson, C. Gemmell, and A. Wiik, "Emerging concepts in the management of the malignant haematological disorders," *Expert. Opin. Pharmacother.*, vol. 1, no. 4, pp. 713–735, 2000.

[13] P. Piccaluga, G. Martinelli, and M. Baccarani, "Advances in the treatment for haematological malignancies," *Expert. Opin. Pharmacother.*, vol. 7, no. 6, pp. 721–732, 2006.

[14] M. A. Albrecht, C. W. Evans, and C. L. Raston, "Green chemistry and the health implications of nanoparticles," *Green Chem.*, vol. 8, no. 5, p. 417, May 2006.

[15] H. Hahn, "Unique features and properties of nanostructured materials," *Adv. Eng. Mater.*, vol. 5, no. 5, pp. 277–284, May 2003.

[16] A. Henglein, "Small-particle research: physicochemical properties of extremely small colloidal metal and semiconductor particles," *Chem. Rev.*, vol. 89, no. 8, pp. 1861–1873, Dec. 1989.

[17] K. Cho, X. Wang, S. Nie, Z. G. Chen, and D. M. Shin, "Therapeutic nanoparticles for drug delivery in cancer," *Clin. Cancer Res.*, vol. 14, no. 5, pp. 1310–6, Mar. 2008.

[18] M. Ferrari, "Cancer nanotechnology: opportunities and challenges," *Nat. Rev. Cancer*, vol. 5, no. 3, pp. 161–71, Mar. 2005.

[19] J. M. Koziara, P. R. Lockman, D. D. Allen, and R. J. Mumper, "In situ blood–brain barrier transport of nanoparticles," *Pharm. Res.*, vol. 20, no. 11, pp. 1772–8, Nov. 2003.

[20] M.-D. Cheng, "Effects of nanophase materials (< or = 20 nm) on biological responses," *J. Environ. Sci. Health. A. Tox. Hazard. Subst. Environ. Eng.*, vol. 39, no. 10, pp. 2691–705, Jan. 2004.

[21] K. Bogunia-Kubik and M. Sugisaka, "From molecular biology to nanotechnology and nanomedicine," *Biosystems.*, vol. 65, no. 2–3, pp. 123–38.

[22] S. M. Moghimi, A. C. Hunter, and J. C. Murray, "Nanomedicine: current status and future prospects," *FASEB J.*, vol. 19, no. 3, pp. 311–30, Mar. 2005.

[23] W. E. Bawarski, E. Chidlowsky, D. J. Bharali, and S. a Mousa, "Emerging nanopharmaceuticals," *Nanomedicine*, vol. 4, no. 4, pp. 273–82, Dec. 2008.

[24] N. Ashammakhi, "Nanosize, mega-impact, potential for medical applications of nanotechnology," *J. Craniofac. Surg.*, vol. 17, no. 1, pp. 3–7, Jan. 2006.

[25] S. Auvinen, M. Alatalo, H. Haario, J.-P. Jalava, and R.-J. Lamminmaki, "Size and Shape Dependence of the Electronic and Spectral Properties in TiO 2 Nanoparticles," *J. Phys. Chem. C*, vol. 115, no. 17, pp. 8484–8493, May 2011.

[26] X. He, W. Zhong, C.-T. Au, and Y. Du, "Size dependence of the magnetic properties of Ni nanoparticles prepared by thermal decomposition method," *Nanoscale Res. Lett.*, vol. 8, no. 1, p. 446, Jan. 2013.

[27] O. Aktsipetrov, P. Elyutin, A. Nikulin, and E. Ostrovskaya, "Size effects in optical second-harmonic generation by metallic nanocrystals and semiconductor quantum dots: the role of quantum chaotic dynamics," *Phys. Rev. B. Condens. Matter*, vol. 51, no. 24, pp. 17591–17599, Jun. 1995.

[28] R. Bakalova, H. Ohba, Z. Zhelev, M. Ishikawa, and Y. Baba, "Quantum dots as photosensitizers?," *Nat. Biotechnol.*, vol. 22, no. 11, pp. 1360–1, Nov. 2004.

[29] H. Zhang, B. Chen, and J. F. Banfield, "Particle Size and pH Effects on Nanoparticle Dissolution," *J. Phys. Chem. C*, vol. 114, no. 35, pp. 14876–14884, Sep. 2010.

[30] A. M. Schrand, M. F. Rahman, S. M. Hussain, J. J. Schlager, D. A. Smith, and A. F. Syed, "Metal-based nanoparticles and their toxicity assessment," *Wiley Interdiscip. Rev. Nanomed. Nanobiotechnol.*, vol. 2, no. 5, pp. 544–68.

[31] A. Nel, T. Xia, L. Mädler, and N. Li, "Toxic potential of materials at the nanolevel," *Science*, vol. 311, no. 5761, pp. 622–7, Feb. 2006.

[32] S. Nair, A. Sasidharan, V. V Divya Rani, D. Menon, S. Nair, K. Manzoor, and S. Raina, "Role of size scale of ZnO nanoparticles and microparticles on toxicity toward bacteria and osteoblast cancer cells," *J. Mater. Sci. Mater. Med.*, vol. 20 Suppl 1, pp. S235–41, Dec. 2009.

[33] A. C. S. Samia, X. Chen, and C. Burda, "Semiconductor quantum dots for photodynamic therapy," *J. Am. Chem. Soc.*, vol. 125, no. 51, pp. 15736–7, Dec. 2003.

[34] I. L. Medintz, H. T. Uyeda, E. R. Goldman, and H. Mattoussi, "Quantum dot bioconjugates for imaging, labelling and sensing," *Nat. Mater.*, vol. 4, no. 6, pp. 435–46, Jun. 2005.

[35] A. A. B. Vladimir A Fonoberov, "ZnO quantum dots: physical properties and optoelectronic applications," *J. Nanoelectron. Optoelectron.*, vol. 1, 2006.

[36] K. M. Reddy, K. Feris, J. Bell, D. G. Wingett, C. Hanley, and A. Punnoose, "Selective toxicity of zinc oxide nanoparticles to prokaryotic and eukaryotic systems," *Appl. Phys. Lett.*, vol. 90, no. 213902. pp. 2139021–2139023, 24-May-2007.

[37] G. Oberdörster, E. Oberdörster, and J. Oberdörster, "Nanotoxicology: an emerging discipline evolving from studies of ultrafine particles," *Environ. Health Perspect.*, vol. 113, no. 7, pp. 823–39, Jul. 2005.

[38] N. C. Mueller and B. Nowack, "Exposure modeling of engineered nanoparticles in the environment," *Environ. Sci. Technol.*, vol. 42, no. 12, pp. 4447–4453, Jun. 2008.

[39] S. Singh and H. S. Nalwa, "Nanotechnology and health safety—toxicity and risk assessments of nanostructured materials on human health," *J. Nanosci. Nanotechnol.*, vol. 7, no. 9, pp. 3048–70, Sep. 2007.

[40] C. Sinico and A. Fadda, "Vesicular carriers for dermal drug delivery," *Expert. Opin. Drug Deliv.*, vol. 6, no. 8, pp. 813–825, 2009.

[41] T. Islam and L. Josephson, "Current state and future applications of active targeting in malignancies using superparamagnetic iron oxide nanoparticles," *Cancer Biomark.*, vol. 5, no. 2, pp. 99–107, 2009.

[42] D. Rao, M. Forrest, A. Alani, G. Kwon, and J. Robinson, "Biodegradable PLGA based nanoparticles for sustained regional lymphatic drug delivery," *J. Pharm. Sci.*, vol. 99, no. 4, pp. 2018–31, 2010.

[43] L. Guopei, Y. Xianjun, J. Chen, Y. Feng, F. Deliang, and L. Weiyue, "LyP-1-conjugated nanoparticles for targeting drug delivery to lymphatic metastatic tumors," *Int. J. Pharm.*, vol. 385, no. 1–2, pp. 150–156, 2010.

[44] J. Arias, L. Reddy, and P. Couvreur, "Polymeric nanoparticulate system augmented the anticancer therapeutic efficacy of gemcitabine," *J. Drug Target.*, vol. 17, no. 8, pp. 586–98, 2009.

[45] Y. Matsumura, "Polymeric micellar delivery systems in oncology," *Jpn. J. Clin. Oncol.*, vol. 38, no. 12, pp. 793–802, 2008.

[46] J. Enbäck and P. Laakkonen, "Tumour-homing peptides—tools for targeting, imaging and destruction," *Biochem. Soc. Trans.*, vol. 35, no. Pt 4, pp. 780–3, 2007.

[47] E. Mansilla, G. H. Marin, L. Nuñez, H. Drago, F. Sturla, C. Mertz, L. Rivera, T. Ichim, N. Riordan, and C. Raimondi, "The lysosomotropic agent, hydroxychloroquine, delivered in a biodegradable nanoparticle system, overcomes drug resistance of B-chronic lymphocytic leukemia cells in vitro," *Cancer Biother. Radiopharm.*, vol. 25, no. 1, pp. 97–103, Feb. 2010.

[48] D. K. Chatterjee, L. S. Fong, and Y. Zhang, "Nanoparticles in photodynamic therapy: an emerging paradigm," *Adv. Drug Deliv. Rev.*, vol. 60, no. 15, pp. 1627–37, Dec. 2008.

[49] E. Ricci-Júnior and J. M. Marchetti, "Zinc(II) phthalocyanine loaded PLGA nanoparticles for photodynamic therapy use," *Int. J. Pharm.*, vol. 310, no. 1–2, pp. 187–95, Mar. 2006.

[50] E. Mansilla, G. Marin, and L. Núñez, "Present and future application of nanoparticle based therapies in B-chronic lymphocytic leukemia (B-CLL)," in *intechopen.com*, no. 3, 2012, pp. 431–448.

[51] S. Ostrovsky, G. Kazimirsky, A. Gedanken, and C. Brodie, "Selective cytotoxic effect of ZnO nanoparticles on glioma cells," *Nano Res.*, vol. 2, no. 11, pp. 882–890, Nov. 2009.

[52] Y.-N. Wu, D.-H. Chen, X.-Y. Shi, C.-C. Lian, T.-Y. Wang, C.-S. Yeh, K. R. Ratinac, P. Thordarson, F. Braet, and D.-B. Shieh, "Cancer-cell-specific cytotoxicity of non-oxidized iron elements in iron core-gold shell NPs," *Nanomedicine*, vol. 7, no. 4, pp. 420–7, Aug. 2011.

[53] R. Ullah and J. Dutta, "Photocatalytic degradation of organic dyes with manganese-doped ZnO nanoparticles," *J. Hazard. Mater.*, vol. 156, no. 1–3, pp. 194–200, Aug. 2008.

[54] L. Jing, K. Ding, S. Kalytchuk, Y. Wang, R. Qiao, S. V. Kershaw, A. L. Rogach, and M. Gao, "Aqueous manganese-doped core/shell CdTe/ZnS quantum dots with strong fluorescence and high relaxivity," *J. Phys. Chem. C*, vol. 117, no. 36, pp. 18752–18761, Sep. 2013.

[55] R. Bhargava, D. Gallagher, X. Hong, and A. Nurmikko, "Optical properties of manganese-doped nanocrystals of ZnS," *Phys. Rev. Lett.*, vol. 72, no. 3, pp. 416–419, Jan. 1994.

[56] P. T. Schumacker, "Reactive oxygen species in cancer cells: live by the sword, die by the sword," *Cancer Cell*, vol. 10, no. 3, pp. 175–6, Sep. 2006.

[57] J. C. Byrd, T. S. Lin, and M. R. Grever, "Treatment of relapsed chronic lymphocytic leukemia: old and new therapies," *Seminars in oncology*, vol. 33, no. 2. pp. 210–9, Apr-2006.

[58] M. J. Akhtar, M. Ahamed, S. Kumar, M. M. Khan, J. Ahmad, and S. a Alrokayan, "Zinc oxide nanoparticles selectively induce apoptosis in human cancer cells through reactive oxygen species," *Int. J. Nanomedicine*, vol. 7, pp. 845–57, Jan. 2012.

[59] C. Hanley, J. Layne, A. Punnoose, K. M. Reddy, I. Coombs, A. Coombs, K. Feris, and D. Wingett, "Preferential killing of cancer cells and activated human T cells using ZnO nanoparticles," *Nanotechnology*, vol. 19, no. 29. p. 295103, 23-Jul-2008.

[60] D. Bechet, P. Couleaud, C. Frochot, M.-L. Viriot, F. Guillemin, and M. Barberi-Heyob, "Nanoparticles as vehicles for delivery of photodynamic therapy agents," *Trends Biotechnol.*, vol. 26, no. 11, pp. 612–21, Dec. 2008.

[61] P. Juzenas, R. Generalov, N. Generalova, and I. Christensen, "Quantum dots and nanoparticles for photodynamic and radiation therapies of cancer," *Adv. Drug Deliv. Rev.*, vol. 60, no. 15, pp. 1600–14, 2008.

[62] Z. L. Wang, X. Y. Kong, Y. Ding, P. Gao, W. L. Hughes, R. Yang, and Y. Zhang, "Semiconducting and Piezoelectric Oxide Nanostructures Induced by Polar Surfaces," *Adv. Funct. Mater.*, vol. 14, no. 10, pp. 943–956, Oct. 2004.

[63] J. Zhou, N. S. Xu, and Z. L. Wang, "Dissolving behavior and stability of ZnO wires in biofluids: a study on biodegradability and biocompatibility of ZnO nanostructures," *Adv. Mater.*, vol. 18, no. 18, pp. 2432–2435, Sep. 2006.

[64] "Chemical and thermal stability of the characteristics of filtered vacuum arc deposited ZnO, SnO2 and zinc stannate thin films—abstract," *J. Phys. D. Appl. Phys.*, vol. 40, no. 17, pp. 1088–99, 2007.

[65] U. Ozgur, Y. I. Alivov, C. Liu, A. Teke, M. A. Reshchikov, S. Dogan, V. Avrutin, S.-J. Cho, and H. Morkoc, "A comprehensive review of ZnO materials and devices," *J. Appl. Phys.*, vol. 98, no. 4, p. 041301, Aug. 2005.

[66] A. H. Mokdad, J. S. Marks, D. F. Stroup, and J. L. Gerberding, "Actual causes of death in the United States, 2000," *JAMA*, vol. 291, no. 10, pp. 1238–45, Mar. 2004.

[67] G. Danaei, S. Vander Hoorn, A. D. Lopez, C. J. L. Murray, and M. Ezzati, "Causes of cancer in the world: comparative risk assessment of nine behavioural and environmental risk factors," *Lancet*, vol. 366, no. 9499, pp. 1784–93, Nov. 2005.

[68] Z. Huang, "A review of progress in clinical photodynamic therapy," *Technol. Cancer Res. Treat.*, vol. 4, no. 3, pp. 283–93, Jun. 2005.

[69] M. E. B. Tamesis and J. G. Morelli, "Vitiligo treatment in childhood: a state of the art review," *Pediatr. Dermatol.*, vol. 27, no. 5, pp. 437–45.

[70] J. N. Silva, P. Filipe, P. Morlière, J.-C. Mazière, J. P. Freitas, J. L. Cirne de Castro, and R. Santus, "Photodynamic therapies: principles and present medical applications," *Biomed. Mater. Eng.*, vol. 16, no. 4 Suppl, pp. S147–54, Jan. 2006.

[71] W. W. Yu, E. Chang, R. Drezek, and V. L. Colvin, "Water-soluble quantum dots for biomedical applications," *Biochem. Biophys. Res. Commun.*, vol. 348, no. 3, pp. 781–6, Sep. 2006.

[72] F. Wilkinson, W. Helman, and A. Ross, "Quantum yields for the photosensitized formation of the lowest electronically excited singlet state of molecular oxygen in solution," *J. Phys.*, pp. 1–29, 1993.

[73] R. C. DeRosa, M, "Photosensitized singlet oxygen and its applications," *Coord. Chem. Rev.*, vol. 233–234, no. null, pp. 351–371, Nov. 2002.

[74] J. P. Tardivo, A. Del Giglio, C. S. de Oliveira, D. S. Gabrielli, H. C. Junqueira, D. B. Tada, D. Severino, R. de Fátima Turchiello, and M. S. Baptista, "Methylene blue in photodynamic therapy: from basic mechanisms to clinical applications," *Photodiagnosis Photodyn. Ther.*, vol. 2, no. 3, pp. 175–191, Sep. 2005.

[75] D. Tada, L. Vono, E. Duarte, and R. Itri, "Methylene blue-containing silica-coated magnetic particles: a potential magnetic carrier for photodynamic therapy," *Langmuir*, no. 21, pp. 8194–8199, 2007.

[76] K. Takahashi, A. Yoshikawa, and A. Sandu, *Wide Bandgap Semiconductors: Fundamental Properties and Modern Photonic and Electronic Devices*. 2007, p. 357.

[77] L. Pugazhenthy, *Zinc Handbook: Properties, Processing, and Use in Design*. 1991, p. 619.

[78] X. Wang, J. Song, C. J. Summers, J. H. Ryou, P. Li, R. D. Dupuis, and Z. L. Wang, "Density-controlled growth of aligned ZnO nanowires sharing a common contact: a simple, low-cost, and mask-free technique for large-scale applications," *J. Phys. Chem. B*, vol. 110, no. 15, pp. 7720–4, Apr. 2006.

[79] A. Mang, K. Reimann, and S. Rübenacke, "Band gaps, crystal-field splitting, spin-orbit coupling, and exciton binding energies in ZnO under hydrostatic pressure," *Solid State Commun.*, vol. 94, no. 4, pp. 251–254, Apr. 1995.

[80] O. Dulub, U. Diebold, and G. Kresse, "Novel stabilization mechanism on polar surfaces: ZnO(0001)-Zn," *Phys. Rev. Lett.*, vol. 90, no. 1, p. 016102, Jan. 2003.

[81] H. S. Mansur, "Quantum dots and nanocomposites," *Wiley Interdiscip. Rev. Nanomed. Nanobiotechnol.*, vol. 2, no. 2, pp. 113–29.

[82] Y. R. Ryu, T. S. Lee, and H. W. White, "Properties of arsenic-doped p-type ZnO grown by hybrid beam deposition," *Appl. Phys. Lett.*, vol. 83, no. 1, p. 87, Jul. 2003.

[83] C. Ye, T. Tamagawa, and D. L. Polla, "Experimental studies on primary and secondary pyroelectric effects in Pb(ZrxTi1−x)O3, PbTiO3, and ZnO thin films," *J. Appl. Phys.*, vol. 70, no. 10, p. 5538, Nov. 1991.

[84] J. D. Albrecht, P. P. Ruden, S. Limpijumnong, W. R. L. Lambrecht, and K. F. Brennan, "High field electron transport properties of bulk ZnO," *J. Appl. Phys.*, vol. 86, no. 12, p. 6864, Dec. 1999.

[85] S. Jana, B. B. Srivastava, and N. Pradhan, "Correlation of dopant states and host bandgap in dual-doped semiconductor nanocrystals," *J. Phys. Chem. Lett.*, vol. 2, no. 14, pp. 1747–1752, Jul. 2011.

[86] B. B. Srivastava, S. Jana, N. S. Karan, S. Paria, N. R. Jana, D. D. Sarma, and N. Pradhan, "Highly luminescent Mn-doped ZnS nanocrystals: gram-scale synthesis," *J. Phys. Chem. Lett.*, vol. 1, no. 9, pp. 1454–1458, May 2010.

[87] M. W. Porambo, H. R. Howard, and A. L. Marsh, "Dopant effects on the photocatalytic activity of colloidal zinc sulfide semiconductor nanocrystals for the oxidation of 2-chlorophenol," *J. Phys. Chem. C*, vol. 114, no. 3, pp. 1580–1585, Jan. 2010.

[88] M. Geszke, M. Murias, L. Balan, G. Medjahdi, J. Korczynski, M. Moritz, J. Lulek, and R. Schneider, "Folic acid-conjugated core/shell ZnS:Mn/ZnS quantum dots as targeted probes for two photon fluorescence imaging of cancer cells," *Acta Biomater.*, vol. 7, no. 3, pp. 1327–38, Mar. 2011.

[89] T. K. Kundu, N. Karak, O. Barik, and S. Saha, "Optical properties of Zno nanoparticles prepared by chemical method using poly (VinylAlcohol) (PVA) as capping agent," *Int. J. Soft Comput. Eng.*

[90] S. Dumas, J.-C. Leprêtre, a. Lepellec, a. Darmanyan, and P. Jardon, "Reactivity of the photo excited forms of Hypericin, Hypocrellin A, Hypocrellin B and methylated Hypericin towards molecular oxygen," *J. Photochem. Photobiol. A. Chem.*, vol. 163, no. 3, pp. 297–306, May 2004.

[91] M. Kostka, P. Zimcik, M. Miletin, P. Klemera, K. Kopecky, and Z. Musil, "Comparison of aggregation properties and photodynamic activity of phthalocyanines and azaphthalocyanines," *J. Photochem. Photobiol. A. Chem.*, vol. 178, no. 1, pp. 16–25, Feb. 2006.

[92] A. G. Ali, F. B. Dejene, and H. C. Swart, "Effect of Mn doping on the structural and optical properties of sol-gel derived ZnO nanoparticles," *Cent. Eur. J. Phys.*, vol. 10, no. 2, pp. 478–484, Dec. 2011.

[93] Y. Abdollahi, A. H. Abdullah, Z. Zainal, and N. A. Yusof, "Synthesis and characterization of manganese doped ZnO nanoparticles," *Int. J. Basic Appl. Sci. IJBAS-IJENS.*, vol. 11, pp. 62–69, 2011.

[94] U. O. A. N. Ezema, F I, "Effect of concentration of Mn dopant ions on the structural and optical properties of zinc oxide crystals," *Dig. J. Nanomater. Biostruct.*, vol. 6, no. 1, pp. 271–278, 2011.

[95] S. Nagarajan and K. Arumugam Kuppusamy, "Extracellular synthesis of zinc oxide nanoparticle using seaweeds of gulf of Mannar, India," *J. Nanobiotechnology*, vol. 11, no. 1, pp. 2–11, Jan. 2013.

[96] A. Menon, N. Kalarikkal, and S. Thomas, "Studies on structural and optical properties of ZnO and Mn doped ZnO nanopowders," *Indian J. Nanosci.*, vol. 1, no. 2, pp. 16–24, 2013.

[97] Z. M. Gibbs, A. LaLonde, and G. J. Snyder, "Optical band gap and the Burstein–Moss effect in iodine doped PbTe using diffuse reflectance infrared Fourier transform spectroscopy," *New J. Phys.*, vol. 15, no. 7, p. 075020, Jul. 2013.

[98] V. Mote, J. Dargad, and B. Dole, "Effect of Mn Doping Concentration on Structural, Morphological and Optical Studies of ZnO Nano-particles," *Nanosci. Nanoeng.*, vol. 1, no. 2, pp. 116–122, 2013.

[99] P. Bihari, M. Vippola, S. Schultes, M. Praetner, A. G. Khandoga, C. a Reichel, C. Coester, T. Tuomi, M. Rehberg, and F. Krombach, "Optimized dispersion of nanoparticles for biological in vitro and in vivo studies," *Part. Fibre Toxicol.*, vol. 5, p. 14, Jan. 2008.

[100] S. H. Lila A Alkhtaby, "Structural and optical properties of Mn doped ZnO nanoparticles," *Asian J. Chem.*, vol. 23, no. 12, pp. 5605–5607, 2011.

[101] K. Donaldson, "Resolving the nanoparticles paradox," *Nanomedicine (Lond).*, vol. 1, no. 2, pp. 229–34, Aug. 2006.

[102] R. T. M. Boudreau, D. M. Conrad, and D. W. Hoskin, "Differential involvement of reactive oxygen species in apoptosis caused by the inhibition of protein phosphatase 2A in Jurkat and CCRF-CEM human T-leukemia cells," *Exp. Mol. Pathol.*, vol. 83, no. 3, pp. 347–56, Dec. 2007.

[103] H. Pelicano, L. Feng, Y. Zhou, J. S. Carew, E. O. Hileman, W. Plunkett, M. J. Keating, and P. Huang, "Inhibition of mitochondrial respiration: a novel strategy to enhance drug-induced apoptosis in human leukemia cells by a reactive oxygen species-mediated mechanism," *J. Biol. Chem.*, vol. 278, no. 39, pp. 37832–9, Sep. 2003.

[104] A. Manke, L. Wang, and Y. Rojanasakul, "Mechanisms of nanoparticle-induced oxidative stress and toxicity," *Biomed Res. Int.*, vol. 2013, p. 942916, Jan. 2013.

[105] W. Lin, Y. Xu, C.-C. Huang, Y. Ma, K. B. Shannon, D.-R. Chen, and Y.-W. Huang, "Toxicity of nano- and micro-sized ZnO particles in human lung epithelial cells," *J. Nanoparticle Res.*, vol. 11, no. 1, pp. 25–39, Jun. 2008.

[106] L. S. E. Fong, D. K. Chatterjee, and Y. Zhang, "Use of upconverting nanoparticles in photodynamic therapy."

[107] A. P. Castano, P. Mroz, and M. R. Hamblin, "Photodynamic therapy and anti-tumour immunity," *Nat. Rev. Cancer*, vol. 6, no. 7, pp. 535–45, Jul. 2006.

[108] D. J. Norris, A. L. Efros, and S. C. Erwin, "Doped nanocrystals," *Science*, vol. 319, no. 5871, pp. 1776–9, Mar. 2008.

[109] D. Glick, S. Barth, and K. F. Macleod, "Autophagy: cellular and molecular mechanisms," *J. Pathol.*, vol. 221, no. 1. pp. 3–12, May-2010.

[110] Y. Chen, E. McMillan-Ward, J. Kong, S. J. Israels, and S. B. Gibson, "Oxidative stress induces autophagic cell death independent of apoptosis in transformed and cancer cells," *Cell Death Differ.*, vol. 15, no. 1, pp. 171–82, Jan. 2008.

[111] S. Hackenberg, A. Scherzed, A. Gohla, A. Technau, K. Froelich, C. Ginzkey, C. Koehler, M. Burghartz, R. Hagen, and N. Kleinsasser, "Nanoparticle-induced photocatalytic head and neck squamous cell carcinoma cell death is associated with autophagy," *Nanomedicine (Lond).*, vol. 9, no. 1, pp. 21–33, Jan. 2014.

Chapter 11

Update on Leukemia in Pregnancy

Khalid Ahmed Al-Anazi

Additional information is available at the end of the chapter

http://dx.doi.org/10.5772/61290

Abstract

Leukemia is a rare event in pregnancy. Acute leukemia represents 90% of leukemias occurring during pregnancy with AML accounting for two thirds of these cases. During the first trimester of pregnancy, standard chemotherapy has a teratogenicity rate of up to 20% depending on the specific agent employed. Exposure to cytotoxic agents during the second and third trimesters is not teratogenic but may predispose the fetus to growth retardation, premature delivery and bone marrow suppression. Additionally, the mother and the fetus are at risk of thromboembolism and sepsis. Only absolutely necessary radiologic work-up is justified during the first trimester of pregnancy as exposure to radiation during the first 2 weeks of pregnancy is usually lethal. Thereafter, radiation predisposes to congenital malformations, growth retardation and malignancy in the newborn. Although most infants exposed to multi-agent chemotherapy seem to suffer no long-term detrimental consequences, studies have shown that: (1) cytotoxic chemotherapy can cross the placenta and cause teratogenicity, (2) there is a potential risk of adult cancer after intrauterine exposure to radiation, and (3) cytotoxic chemotherapy and radiotherapy increase genetic defects in germ cells. In the first trimester, the termination of pregnancy should seriously be considered if the disease is aggressive and if intensive chemotherapy is needed. In the second and third trimesters, standard chemotherapy can safely be administered without resorting to pregnancy termination. The choice of specific regimens depends upon several factors that include: the gestational age, the clinical status of the patient, the specific type of leukemia and the anticipated toxicity of the cytotoxic agents employed. The decision is often difficult and confounded by several concerns, but the management of each pregnant patient with leukemia has to be individualized and should have a multidisciplinary approach. Vaginal delivery is preferable while caesarean section is reserved for certain obstetric complications. It is preferable to time delivery between 32 and 36 weeks of gestation to ensure optimal fetal maturation and it is recommended to avoid maternal bone marrow suppression prior to delivery.

The management of chronic leukemia in pregnancy is generally easier than that of acute leukemia. However, certain precautions should be taken as some targeted therapies need to be avoided and they may need to be replaced by alternative therapies that are less effective in controlling chronic leukemia. Pregnancy in patients with chronic myeloid leukemia on tyrosine kinase inhibitors requires proper planning as it is essential to have optimal control of the disease for 2 to 3 years prior to having pregnancy in order to avoid acceleration of the disease during pregnancy.

Leukemia diagnosed during pregnancy can be considered a poor clinical prognostic factor owing to the less than average long-term disease-free survival due to high relapse rates and high incidence of refractoriness to chemotherapy. Countries should have registries for mothers and children exposed to chemotherapy and radiotherapy and it is essential to have guidelines on the management of various types of leukemia during pregnancy.

Keywords: Acute leukemia, pregnancy, cytotoxic chemotherapy, chronic leukemia, abortion, teratogenicity

1. Introduction

During pregnancy, the body of the mother undergoes certain physiological changes that may make the diagnosis of leukemia more challenging. Thus the diagnosis of leukemia may be delayed as non-specific manifestations of leukemia such as fatigue, weakness and dyspnea may be attributed to gestation. Additionally, pregnancy itself may be associated with anemia and leukocytosis which are also common laboratory findings in patients with leukemia [1].

The diagnosis of leukemia requires morphologic, immunophenotypic and cytogenetic examination of bone marrow samples. However, bone marrow biopsies can be safely performed under local anesthesia in pregnant females without any harm to the fetus [1]. Leukemia itself often presents as a medical emergency that requires prompt initiation of appropriate therapy. Also, the diagnosis of leukemia in pregnancy is a rather exceptional event that can generate complex ethical and therapeutic dilemmas. Therefore a multidisciplinary team that includes hematologists, obstetricians, neonatologists, psychologists and social workers in addition to the patient should all be involved in making therapeutic decisions [2].

The decision to initiate chemotherapy during pregnancy must be weighed against the consequences of delaying treatment on maternal survival. In general, therapeutic decisions must be made on data obtained from prospective clinical trials, but unfortunately the available data in the literature on the management of most leukemias diagnosed during pregnancy are derived from retrospective case reports, case series and few meta-analyses [1].

This literature review will cover the following: the consequences of maternal and fetal exposures to cytotoxic chemotherapy, radiotherapy and targeted therapies; the detailed description of coexistence between various types of leukemia and pregnancy; and the specific data obtained from the major studies and the important case reports on pregnancy in different types of leukemia.

2. Physiological and hematological alterations in pregnancy

Pregnancy is associated with the following physiological changes that may alter drug metabolism: (1) slow gastric emptying, (2) increase in plasma volume by 50%, (3) increase in plasma proteins and decrease in serum albumin, (4) enhanced hepatic oxidation, and (5) increase in glomerular filtration and renal plasma flow [3]. Also, pregnancy is associated with several hematological complications that include: (1) anemia with iron deficiency, due to blood loss and nutritional causes, being the commonest hematological disorder; (2) thrombocytopenia which can be: gestational, due to idiopathic thrombocytopenic purpura, microangiopathic hemolytic anemia, pre-eclampsia, antiphospholipid antibody syndrome or systemic lupus erythromatosis evolving during pregnancy; (3) pancytopenia due to: acute fatty degeneration of the liver, bone marrow failure caused by aplastic anemia or congenital causes, leukemia, lymphoma or metastatic cancer evolving during pregnancy; (4) inherited or acquired bleeding disorders such as von Willebrand disease; and (5) venous thromboembolism [4-6].

3. Maternal exposures during pregnancy

Maternal exposure to the following agents during pregnancy may increase the risk of leukemia in the newborn infants: alcohol intake by the mother, cigarette smoking, antibiotic use, benzene exposure, exposure to estrogens, diethylstilbestrol and other hormones, bacterial infections, food-related or respiratory maternal IgE and *Helicobacter pylori* immunoglobulin G [7-14]. However, intake of the following by pregnant women may have protective effect against the development of leukemia in the newborn: vitamin supplements, folate supplements and diet rich in vegetables [15-17].

4. Exposure to diagnostic and therapeutic radiation

The association between in utero irradiation and the increased risk of childhood malignancies has been studied since the 1950s [18]. The potential deleterious consequences of ionizing radiation on the fetus include the following: (1) pregnancy loss; stillbirth or miscarriage, (2) congenital malformations, (3) disturbances in growth or development; growth and mental retardation, and (4) mutagenic and carcinogenic effects [19]. Radiotherapy given during the first trimester is associated with teratogenic effects and an increase in the risk of childhood malignancy [20]. Radiotherapy given during the second and third trimesters of pregnancy is associated with: (1) an increased risk for the development of leukemia and solid tumors within the first decade of life, and (2) an increased risk of neurodevelopmental delay [20].

Diagnostic irradiation of the mother during pregnancy increases the risk of childhood acute lymphoblastic leukemia (ALL). Also, there is some evidence that exposure of the father to abdominal X-rays or intravenous pyelograms, prior to conception, increases the incidence of ALL in the offspring [21]. Prenatal X-ray exposure is associated with 40-80% increase in childhood cancers [22]. Prenatal exposure to ionizing radiation has been associated with a statistically significant increase in the incidence of all cancers and specifically leukemia in newborn infants [18]. However, the average radiation dose from individual diagnostic and therapeutic procedures has historically declined owing to the improvements in technology and equipment safeguards [18]. Postnatal X-ray exposure is also linked to a small elevation in the risk of all cancers in childhood [22]. At doses < 0.05 Gy there is no evidence of increased risk of: intellectual disability, fetal anomalies, loss of pregnancy or growth retardation [19]. During the first 14 days after fertilization: intact survival or death is the most likely outcome of radiation exposure ≥ 0.05 Gy (5 Rads). A conservative estimate of the threshold for intrauterine fetal death is > 1 Gy (10 Rads) [19]. After the first 14 days of gestation, radiation exposure ≥ 0.5 Gy may be associated with increased risks of congenital malformations, growth retardation and intellectual disability [19]. A total of 10-20 Gy of radiation, when given during organogenesis is considered to be the threshold dose for severe congenital malformations [20].

There are no reports of adverse fetal effects from diagnostic doses of radioactive iodine. However, radioactive iodine should not be administered to pregnant women because there is a concern that it may induce thyroid cancer in the offspring [19]. Antenatal ultrasound exposure is not associated with an increase in the risk of childhood cancer, so it is safe during all stages of pregnancy [19,22,23]. Magnetic resonance imaging (MRI) is generally preferred to other imaging modalities that involve ionizing radiation. However, gadolinium is not recommended for use in pregnant women [19]. Computed axial and positron emission scans are contraindicated during pregnancy, particularly in the first two trimesters. Both procedures can be performed after delivery but caution should be taken in breast-feeding women [23].

5. Exposure to cytotoxic chemotherapy in utero

The effects of cytotoxic chemotherapy on the developing fetus are dependent on the time of gestation at which such treatment is administered. In the pre-embryonic phase that extends from fertilization till 17 days after conception, significant damage to the conceptus cells results in miscarriage [24]. In the embryonic or organogenesis phase which occurs between 2 to 8 weeks following conception, chemotherapy may cause irreversible damage to the newly formed fetal body organs, while in the fetal phase which extends between the 8th and the 38th weeks after conception the gastrointestinal and renal tracts as well as cerebral cortex remain susceptible to chemotherapy-induced toxicity [24].

In a retrospective study that included 84 mothers with various hematological malignancies who had received cytotoxic chemotherapy during gestation, 38 fetuses were exposed to cytotoxic chemotherapy in utero during the first trimester of pregnancy [25]. The delivered children were followed up for a median time of 18.7 years (range 6-29 years). No cancer or acute leukemia was reported in the children who had been exposed to chemotherapy in utero so pregnant females having aggressive hematological malignancies including leukemia can receive cytotoxic chemotherapy at full doses even during the first trimester of pregnancies [25]. In another retrospective study that included 21 pregnancies in 18 patients with hematological malignancies, 8 babies were exposed to cytotoxic chemotherapy in utero [26]. Out of the 4 babies exposed to chemotherapy during the first trimester of gestation, 3 had low birth weight and one was born healthy but died three months later because of gastroenteritis. The fourth baby had been exposed to chemotherapy during the 3 trimesters of pregnancy, the baby was born prematurely and subsequently died of intracranial hemorrhage. Out of the 3 babies exposed to chemotherapy during the second and third trimesters of pregnancy: one died in utero, one had low birth weight and one was born alive but died of pulmonary hemorrhage later on. [26]. The adverse effects of cytotoxic and targeted therapies in pregnant females and newborn infants are summarized in Table 1 [3,27-30]. The adverse effects of cytotoxic chemotherapy and radiotherapy in pregnant mothers and fetuses are included in Table 2 [30]. The genotoxic and teratogenic effects of various cytotoxic agents are shown in Table 3 [31-33]. The recommended therapies that are relatively safe in treating pregnant females with leukemia are summarized in Table 4 [1,2,20,23,34-39].

Drug (class)	Common adverse effects in pregnant mothers	Common adverse effects in newborn infants	Teratogenic effects
Cytarabine (pyrimidine analogue)	- Myelosuppression - Diarrhea - Skin rashes - Fever - Hepatotoxicity	- Myelosuppression - Infections - Hepatopathy - Meningeal hemorrhage - Respiratory distress symptoms -Chromosomal abnormalities: Down's syndrome and inversion of chromosome 9. - Growth defects and congenital malformations.	- Teratoginic in animals. - Expected to penetrate the blood placental barrier. - No measurements performed in human placenta.
Daunorubicin (anthracycline)	- Myelosuppression - Acute and chronic cardiotoxicity - Mucositis - Alopecia - Nausea and vomiting	- Myelosuppression; pancytopenia and anemia. - Hepatopathy and elevated CK level - Seizures and respiratory tract infections	- Teratogenic in mice - Less teratogenic than doxorubicin

Drug (class)	Common adverse effects in pregnant mothers	Common adverse effects in newborn infants	Teratogenic effects
		- Spontaneous abortions, premature delivery and still birth. -Chromosomal abnormalities and congenital malformations	
Idarubicin (anthracycline)	- Myelosuppression - Acute and chronic cardiotoxicity - Mucositis - Alopecia - Nausea and vomiting	- Myelosuppression - Cardiomyopathy - Hepatopathy and elevated CK level - Acrocyanosis and hyperbilirubinemia - Intrauterine fetal death and growth retardation - Congenital malformations: short limbs and macrognathia	- Idarubicin is more lipophilic than other anthracyclines so it may increase the concentration crossing the placenta
Doxorubicin (anthracycline)	- Myelosuppression - Cardiotoxicity - Mucositis and alopecia - Nausea and vomiting	- No major side effects. - Transient myelosuppression - Hyaline membrane disease - Meningeal hemorrhage - Premature delivery & fetal distress - Imperforate anus and rectovaginal fistula	- Crosses the placenta - Can distribute into fetal tissues including liver, lung and kidneys.
Etoposide (topoisomerase inhibitor)	- Myelosuppression - Prolongation of PT and INR - Hypotension - Fever and alopecia	- Transient pancytopenia - Leucopenia - Hearing loss	- Decreased serum albumin level - Potential of elevated free drug levels and increase in drug toxicity.
Mitoxantrone (anthracenedione)	- Cardiotoxicity - Hepatoxicity - Alopecia	- No major adverse effects reported - Pancytopenia	- Teratogenic in animals: fetal growth retardation and premature delivery.
Fludarabine (purine analogue)	- Myelosuppression - Autoimmune effects - JC virus-induced progressive multifocal leukoencephalopathy.	- No fetal adverse effects reported	- Teratogenic in rats and rabbits. - Increased incidence of skeletal malformations in rats.
Cyclophosphamide (alkylating agent)	- Hemorrhagic cystitis - Cardiotoxicity - Myelosuppression	- Myelosuppression - Low birth weight, still birth and growth retardation	- Teratogenic in animals - May cross placenta in mice

http://dx.doi.org/10.5772/61290

Drug (class)	Common adverse effects in pregnant mothers	Common adverse effects in newborn infants	Teratogenic effects
	- Alopecia, nausea and vomiting	- Imperforate anus and rectovaginal fistula, facial abnormalities, single left coronary artery and hernias.	-Teratogenic in mice, rats and rabbits.
Vincristine (vinca alkaloid)	- Neurotoxicity - Alopecia - SIADH	- Anemia and severe pancytopenia - Left shift in leukocytes and mild infections - Hyaline membrane disease - Low birth weight, spontaneous abortions, hydrocephalus and cleft lip	- Vincristine is highly protein bound. - Penetration into barriers such as blood placental barrier may be limited.
Hydroxyurea (antimetabolite)	- Myelosuppression	- Still birth without gross abnormalities - Premature delivery without congenital defects - Intrauterine fetal death and growth retardation	- None reported
Methotrexate (antimetabolite)	- Myelosuppression - Acute renal failure	- Spontaneous abortions low birth weight - Pancytopenia - Aminopterine-type syndrome	- None reported
ATRA (PML-RARA targeted therapy)	- Hemorrhage - Differentiation syndrome - DIC - Fever	- Miscarriage and fetal death - Pulmonary hyperplasia and respiratory distress - Thrombocytopenia - Intrauterine growth retardation	- When give during first trimester: severe neurological and cardiovascular complications. - Teratogenicity risk: 85%
Interferon alpha	- Fatigue - Flu-like illness - Intertility	- Fetal malformations in 1 case out of 8 patients reported (concurrent with use of hydroxyurea).	--
Imatinib (TKI; first generation)	- Fatigue - Fluid retention	- Elective abortions done due to congenital malformations. - Exophthalmos and brain abnormalities - Cardiac and renal anomalies - Hypospadias and bone abnormalities	- Teratogenic in animals: exencephaly, encephalocele, absent or reduced frontal or parietal bones
Dasatinib	- Fluid retention	- Spontaneous abortions	--

Drug (class)	Common adverse effects in pregnant mothers	Common adverse effects in newborn infants	Teratogenic effects
(second generation TKI)		- Elective abortions	
Rituximab (Anti-CD20 monoclonal antibody)	- Infusion related reactions - Myelosuppression	- Few reports show safety in all trimester of pregnancy - Transient β-cell depletion has been reported	--

Table 1. shows adverse effects of cytotoxic and targeted therapies reported in pregnant females and newborn infants

(A) cytotoxic chemotherapy given during the first trimester of pregnancy		
Drug		**Estimated risk of congenital malformations**
Cytosine arabinoside		1:8
Cyclophosphamide		1:6
Methotrexate		1:4
Chlorambucil		1:2
Busulfan		1:9
(B) effects of radiation on pregnancy and fetus		
Dose of radiation		**Effects on the fetus**
Gy	**Rad**	
< 0.1	< 10	No major effect
0.1-0.15	10-15	Increased risk
2.5	250	Malformations in most cases
> 30	> 300	Abortion
(C) adverse effects of radiation in relation to gestational age		
Gestational age		**Adverse effects**
Conception till day 10		Lethal
2 to 6 weeks		Teratogenesis and growth retardation
12 to 16 weeks		Microcephaly, mental and growth retardation
20 weeks till delivery		Sterility, malignancy and genetic defects

Table 2. Adverse effects of chemotherapy and radiation on pregnancy and fetus

High risk [> 80%]	Intermediate risk [20% - 80%]	Low risk [< 20%]	Unknown risk
- Therapeutic radiation to ovaries	- Anthracyclines	- Methotrexate	- Tyrosine kinase inhibitors

High risk [> 80%]	**Intermediate risk** [20% - 80%]	**Low risk** [< 20%]	**Unknown risk**
- Alcohol	- Cytosine arabinoside	- 5 flurouracil	- Monoclonal antibodies
- Retinoic acid	- Cisplatinum	- 6 mercaptopurine	- Taxanes
- Valproic acid	- Carboplatin	- Etoposide	- Bleomycin
- Cyclophosphamide and ifosfamide		- Fludarabine	
- Thalidomide		- Vinca alkaloids	
- Busulfan		- Actionomycin D	
- Melphalan			
- Chlorambucil			
- Decarbazine and procarbazine			
- Thiotepa			
- Stem cell transplantation			
- Doxorubicin			

Table 3. Genotoxic and teratogenic agents in human classified according to the risk levels

Type of leukemia	**First trimester**	**Second trimester**	**Third trimester**
Non-M 3 Acute myeloid leukemia	- Termination of pregnancy	- Cytarabine + doxorubicin - High dose cytarabine - Cytarabine + daunorubicin	- Cytarabine + doxorubicin - High dose cytarabine - Cytarabine + daunorubicin
Acute promyelocytic leukemia	- Termination of pregnancy	- ATRA + anthracyclines: daunorubicin, idarubicin or doxorubicin	- ATRA + anthracyclines: daunorubicin, idarubicin or doxorubicin
Acute lymphoblastic leukemia	- Termination of pregnancy - Corticosteroids	- Modified ALL-induction regimens of chemotherapy including methotrexate and corticosteroids.	- Standard induction regimens of chemotherapy.
Chronic myeloid leukemia	- Interferon - α - Hydroxyurea - Leukapheresis	- Interferon - α - Hydroxyurea - Leukapheresis - TKIs such as imatinib	- Interferon - α - Hydroxyurea - Leukapheresis -TKIs such as imatinib
Chronic lymphocytic leukemia	- Leukapheresis - Corticosteroids	- Leukapheresis - Corticosteroids - Chlorambucil - Cyclophosphamide - Rituximab	- Leukapheresis - Corticosteroids - Chlorambucil - Cyclophosphamide - Rituximab

Type of leukemia	First trimester	Second trimester	Third trimester
Hairy cell leukemia	- Splenectomy - Interferon	- Splenectomy - Interferon - Cladrabine - Rituximab	- Splenectomy - Interferon - Cladrabine - Rituximab

Table 4. Recommended therapies and relatively safe medications during pregnancy

6. Leukemia in pregnancy

The annual incidence of leukemia in pregnancy is approximately 1:100,000 pregnancies. This low incidence can be explained by the fact that leukemia usually spares childbearing ages as follows: (1) ALL occurs predominantly in childhood and acute myeloid leukemia (AML) occurs most frequently in late adulthood, and (2) chronic myeloid leukemia (CML) and chronic lymphocytic leukemia (CLL) predominantly affect individuals belonging to age groups older than childbearing age [2]. The majority of cases of leukemia in pregnancy are acute leukemia with AML representing two thirds of cases and the vast majority of chronic leukemias diagnosed during pregnancy are CML [1,2].

Virtually all cytotoxic agents can cross the placenta and reach the fetus and almost all chemotherapeutic agents have been reported to be associated with congenital malformations in animal models [1,2]. In humans, chemotherapy administered during the first trimester of pregnancy in humans may increase the risk of spontaneous abortion, fetal death and major malformations, but the risk of teratogenesis following cancer therapy appears to be lower in humans than in animals [1,2]. Exposure to chemotherapy during the first trimester of pregnancy is associated with 10-20% risk of major malformations, but this risk is usually lower when single agent chemotherapy is administered and when antimetabolites are excluded. Hence, if the administration of cytotoxic chemotherapy during the first trimester of pregnancy is essential, therapeutic abortion will become strongly recommended [1,2]. The administration of chemotherapy during the second and third trimesters of pregnancy is not associated with congenital malformations, but increases the risk of intrauterine fetal death, growth retardation and low birth weight. Delivery should be planned to occur 2-3 weeks after the last session of chemotherapy to allow bone marrow recovery [1,2]. Pregnant females or mothers with terminated pregnancies receiving cytotoxic chemotherapy require supportive care with: fluids for hydration and nutritional supplements, safe antimicrobials to treat various infectious complications, growth factors to shorten the periods of neutropenia, and blood product transfusions as needed [1].

The data and results of 2 major studies on leukemia in pregnancy are described below [40,41]. At King Faisal Specialist Hospital and Research Center in Riyadh, 32 patients who had developed leukemia during pregnancy were reported and their long-term follow up was provided [40]. The primary hematological malignancies were as follows: CML (11 patients), 5 patients with acute promyelocytic leukemia (APL), and non-M3 AML (8 patients). Spontaneous abortions occurred in 14 patients, therapeutic abortions were performed in 2 patients and 16 live births were delivered at 30-41 weeks of gestation [40]. At the end of the study, the outcomes of mothers were as follows: 19 patients (59.4%) were dead, 7 patients (21.9%) lost follow up and only 6 patients (18.8%) were alive. Five of the living patients had already received HSCT. Out of the 32 patients included in the study, 19 patients (59.4) were subjected to HSCT to control their primary hematological malignancies [40]. On long-term follow up, 14 transplanted patients (73.7%) were dead and only 5 transplanted patients (26.3%) were alive. The conclusion that can be drawn from this study is that the long term prognosis of pregnant females having leukemia is poor even if HSCT is performed for high-risk patients [40]. In another retrospective study from Japan, 16 patients with leukemia in pregnancy were reported between 2001 and 2011 [41]. Out of the 16 patients reported: 9 (56.3%) had CML, 5 (31.3%) had ALL and 2 patients (12.5%) had AML. Out of the 9 patients with CML, 4 received imatinib therapy which was subsequently interrupted (3 in the first trimester and 1 in the second trimester). Out the 9 CML patients, 6 patients required treatment with hydroxyurea and/or interferon while the remaining 3 patients required no treatment after stopping imatinib [41]. Anemia developed in 4 patients and thrombocytopenia was reported in 1 patient. Regarding fetal outcomes, no perinatal deaths or fetal abnormalities were reported. The diagnoses of acute leukemia in the 7 patients reported were made in 2 patients during the first trimester, in 2 patients during the second and in 3 patients during the third trimester of pregnancy [41]. Therapeutic abortion was performed in 2 patients with ALL. Chemotherapy was administered during the second trimester in 4 patients and 1 patient with ALL received chemotherapy after delivery. All patients with acute leukemia developed thrombocytopenia and 4 patients developed febrile neutropenia. Mean gestational age at delivery was 32 weeks and 2 perinatal deaths were reported [41]. The authors concluded that: (1) maternal and fetal morbidity is high in pregnancies complicated by acute leukemia, and (2) in pregnancies complicated by chronic leukemia, fetal and maternal prognoses appear to be more favorable and management of complications is easier compared to acute leukemia [41].

7. Acute leukemia in pregnancy

Virchow described the first case of leukemia in a pregnant woman in the year 1856 [2]. Between 1856 and 1995, more than 500 cases of leukemia in pregnancy were reported [1]. It is estimated that 23% of acute leukemias are diagnosed during the first trimester, 37% during the second trimester and 40% during the third trimester of pregnancy [2]. The majority of leukemias diagnosed in pregnancy are acute and predominantly myeloid as the incidence of ALL is more common in childhood and adolescence [1,2,24]. The presentation of acute leukemia in pregnancy is broadly similar to that in nonpregnant females although pregnancy may obscure the diagnosis of leukemia as pregnant ladies often describe nonspecific symptoms such as fatigue and tiredness [1,24]. Pregnant females with leukemia particularly acute leukemia present with anemia, thrombocytopenia and neutropenia in addition to recurrent infections due to bone marrow failure caused by the aggressive malignancy [2]. The diagnostic work up of pregnant females should be the same as their nonpregnant counterparts apart from the avoidance of certain radiological procedures due to their adverse effects on the fetus [2]. Although a bone marrow aspirate and a trephine biopsy may be performed safely in pregnancy, these can be avoided if confirmation is clear possibly by means of peripheral blood microscopy, flow cytometry and molecular analysis [24].

If the disease is left untreated, it will likely result in maternal and fetal mortality. A decision to delay initiation of induction chemotherapy negatively impacts on the likelihood of remission [24]. There are no prospective studies that compare the outcome of pregnant ladies with their nonpregnant counterparts [2]. However, data suggest that maternal outcomes for AML following chemotherapy are analogous to nonpregnant females and consequently delay in commencing chemotherapy is to be avoided. The therapeutic approach to the management of acute leukemia in pregnancy, regardless the subtype, is generally similar [24].

Vertical transmission of leukemia to the fetus is exceptionally rare due to the placental barrier and the fetal immune system [2]. Cytotoxic agents have a relatively low molecular weight and most of them can cross placental barrier and reach the fetus [2]. When treating a pregnant woman with chemotherapy, it is essential to consider many gestational physiological changes that can potentially alter the effectiveness of chemotherapeutic agents by changing their metabolism and clearance [2]. During pregnancy, plasma volume is increased leading to enhancement of renal clearance and hepatic oxidation of drugs. Lower plasma drug exposures to doxorubicin, epirubicin and carboplatin have been described during pregnancy [2]. However, the physiological changes in pregnancy have their effects on drug exposure, drug effectiveness and drug toxicity and all these factors make management of acute leukemia in pregnancy a rather difficult task [2].

The data and the results of 5 major studies on acute leukemia in pregnancy are summarized below [42-46]. In March 1993, a questionnaire was sent to 362 gynecology and obstetrics centers in Japan and answers were obtained from 260 centers [42]. A total of 103 patients with acute leukemia in pregnancy were reported in that study, 39 of them were obtained from the questionnaire survey and 64 patients were reported from literature review [42]. The following conclusions and results were made: (1) maternal survival was longer in patients treated between 1985 and 1993 compared to patients treated between 1975 and 1984, (2) survival was significantly longer in patients in whom induction chemotherapy was commenced before delivery compared to patients in whom chemotherapy was started after delivery, (3) treatment of acute leukemia during pregnancy should be started as soon as possible after establishing the diagnosis of leukemia with carefully selected chemotherapeutic regimens, and (4) the time of delivery should be selected considering maternal and fetal circumstances after consultation with obstetricians [42].

In a Canadian study, 7 patients with acute leukemia were included and 51 additional patients, reported between 1975 and 1987, were added [43]. Out of the 58 pregnant women reported, 53 patients received chemotherapy for acute leukemia during pregnancy. Forty nine pregnancies results in birth of 50 infants, 28 of them were prematurely delivered and 4 had low birth weights [43]. Cytopenias at birth were encountered in 39% of newborn infants who had been exposed to cytotoxic medications in the last month of pregnancy. One child had congenital malformations, neuroblastoma arising from the adrenal gland and papillary thyroid cancer

[43]. Long-term follow-up (ranging between 1 and 17 years) of the 7 Canadian patients showed normal growth of babies and no malignancies were encountered in the children born. The authors recommended having a central registry in order to document long-term complications in children exposed to chemotherapy in utero [43].

In a French retrospective study, 37 patients with acute leukemia (31 AML patients and 6 ALL patients) were reported [44]. The diagnosis of leukemia was made in: 9 patients in the first trimester, 10 patients in the second trimester and 18 patients in the third trimester of pregnancy. Cytogenetic analysis results were favorable in 10 patients, unfavorable in 6 patients and intermediate in 12 patients [44]. The outcomes of the pregnancies were as follows: 15 pregnancies ended in abortions (2 spontaneous and 13 therapeutic) and 22 deliveries (13 spontaneous vaginal deliveries and 9 cesarean sections) were reported. Out of the 23 healthy babies delivered, 22 of them had been exposed to chemotherapy during gestation [44]. Disease outcomes were as follows: 34 patients (92%) achieved complete remissions (CRs) of their leukemias, 2 patients (5.4%) had refractory disease, 1 patient (2.7%) had toxic death and 11 patients developed severe nonhematological complications [44]. HSCT was performed in 11 patients (6 autologous and 5 allogeneic). Disease-free survival was 65% at 3 years and 54% at 5 years, while overall survival was 64% at 3 years and 46% at 5 years. Follow-up showed death of 12 patients (32.4%) at 3.4 years and relapse of 10 patients (27%) at 11.9 months [44]. The authors concluded that: (1) although pregnancy, in general, does not affect the outcome of acute leukemia, relapse rate in pregnant ladies with acute leukemia is relatively high; (2) chemotherapy during the first trimester of pregnancy requires the termination of pregnancy to allow appropriate therapy to be administered; and (3) chemotherapy administration during the second and third trimesters of pregnancy does not require termination of pregnancy [44].

In a survey that had been performed at 24 institutions in Japan over 11 years, 11 cases of acute leukemia during pregnancy were reported [45]. Out of the 11 patients with acute leukemia, 8 patients had AML and 3 patients had ALL. The diagnosis of acute leukemia was made in 6 patients in the first trimester, 1 patient in the second and 4 patients in the third trimester [45]. Infant outcomes were as follows: 5 out of 6 patients had abortions before chemotherapy and 1 elective abortion was performed after chemotherapy, while all the patients diagnosed in the second and third trimester of pregnancy delivered live births. Four of the mothers diagnosed in the first trimester achieved CR of their leukemias, while 2 patients died of recurrent leukemia. Four of the mothers diagnosed in the second and third trimesters had CR and remained in remission, while 1 patient died of sepsis following cesarean section [45]. The authors concluded that careful surveillance and monitoring of the fetus in addition to close co-operation between hematologists, gynecologists and pediatricians are essential to successfully treat pregnant women with acute leukemia [45].

A retrospective study included 10 pregnancies in 8 patients with acute leukemia (6 patients with AML and 2 patients with ALL) [46]. The diagnoses of acute leukemia were made in 6 pregnancies in the first trimester, 3 pregnancies in the second trimester and 1 patient in the third trimester. Three pregnancies ended in spontaneous abortions, 3 in intra-uterine fetal death and 3 in therapeutic abortions [46]. One spontaneous abortion and one intrauterine fetal death were encountered during combination chemotherapy (cytarabine and daurorubicin) given for AML. Only 1 baby survived and that baby was never exposed to chemotherapy [46]. The conclusions from this study included the following: (1) while none of the mothers had obstetric complications, 5 out of 8 pregnant women with acute leukemia died because of primary disease, and (2) fetal outcome was very poor, thus the diagnosis of acute leukemia particularly during early pregnancy carries poor outcome for both the fetus and the mother [46].

8. AML in pregnancy

AML occurs more frequently in young adults and in elderly individuals. Consequently, more data are available on the management of AML in pregnancy [1,24]. As AML is an aggressive malignancy, delaying chemotherapy has adverse consequences on the mother so a balance between having the consequences of intensive chemotherapy on both the mother and the fetus as well as the negative impact of postponing chemotherapy on the mother must be carefully evaluated [1,24]. Also, the possibility of long-term consequences of cytotoxic chemotherapy on future fertility of the mother has to be taken into consideration [24,27]. Clinical studies and recent research suggest: (1) a similar prognosis for women treated during pregnancy as compared to nonpregnant patients, and (2) most modern remission induction chemotherapeutic regimens used in the treatment of acute leukemia do not induce sterility [24].

The existing therapeutic protocols or regimens including modern agents that are utilized in the management of AML include: anthracyclines such as daunorubicin, idarubicin and doxorubicin; antimetabolites such as cytarabine; topoisomerase II inhibitors such as etoposide; monoclonal antibodies such as gemtuzumab (myelotarg, anti-CD33 monoclonal antibody); and multikinase inhibitors [24]. The induction regimens of AML consist of a combination of cytarabine and an anthracycline, while various combinations of intensive chemotherapies are used in the consolidation therapy [1,2]. Enough data is available on the use of cytarabine and anthracyclines during pregnancy, except in the first trimester, but there is a lack of data on the use of modern therapies such as gemtuzumab and multikinase inhibitors in pregnant females having AML [1,24]. Cytarabine therapy in pregnancy carries a significant risk to the fetus, so its use is not advocated in the first trimester of pregnancy [2]. The administration of cytarabine, alone or in combination with other chemotherapeutic agents such as anthracyclines, during the first trimester is associated with the development of congenital malformations, miscarriage, low birth weight and fetal death, while embryonic exposure to etoposide is associated with genomic instability and mixed-lineage leukemia (MLL) rearrangement [2,24]. The unfavorable experiences of chemotherapy in the first trimester of pregnancy have resulted in the recommendation for therapeutic abortion and the decision to treat AML in the first trimester with a regimen containing an antimetabolite must be accompanied by careful counseling of the mother [1,24]. So, in pregnant females with AML presenting during the first trimester, termination of pregnancy is strongly recommended then intensive chemotherapeutic regimens that include cytaribine and anthracyclines should be commenced [1,2].

The experience with the use of anthracyclines during pregnancy is limited mostly to doxorubicin and daunorubicin as idarubicin which is more lipophilic may be associated with higher rates of fetal complications [2,27]. Three major studies that included more than 200 patients with various cancers including hematological malignancies (at least 60 of them were treated during the first trimester of pregnancy with doxorubicin, daunorubicin, cytarabine and other chemotherapeutic agents) reported the following complications: pre-eclampsia, premature deliveries, stillbirths, miscarriages, congenital malformations, intrauterine fetal death, growth retardation and neonatal sepsis. These studies confirmed that doxorubicin is more effective and safer than other anthracyclines in treating leukemia during pregnancy. However, it is still unknown whether exposure to anthracyclines is cardiotoxic to the developing fetus [2].

The administration of cytotoxic chemotherapy including cytarabine in the second and third trimesters of pregnancy is associated with intrauterine fetal death and growth retardation, preterm deliveries in addition to neonatal cytopenias that may cause deaths due to severe infections, but no increase in congenital malformations, unfavorable neurological development or childhood malignancy [1,24,27]. In patients presenting during the second or third trimesters of pregnancy, induction chemotherapy with cytarabine and either daunorubicin or doxorubicin should be instituted promptly [1,2,24]. In AML relapsing during pregnancy, the termination of pregnancy should be performed as treatment of AML in relapse includes: high dose chemotherapy followed by HSCT or experimental therapy all of which cannot be delivered during pregnancy [1,2].

Adequate supportive care should be given to mothers as aggressive chemotherapy may cause infections, nausea, vomiting and variable cytopenias [1]. Regular surveillance for the development of congenital abnormalities and monitoring of fetal cardiac function are essential [1,24]. Delivery should be electively planned after the 32nd week of gestation and it should be done 2-3 weeks after the last session of chemotherapy to allow recovery of bone marrow function [2].

In a large systematic review that included 83 pregnant females with AML diagnosed and treated between January 1969 and June 2014, 85 fetuses were exposed to cytotoxic chemotherapy during pregnancy [27]. During the first trimester of pregnancy 8 mothers were treated and all achieved CR, 61 mothers were treated during the second trimester and 81% of them achieved CR, while 14 patients with AML were treated during the third trimester and 67% of them achieved CR of their AML. Fetal deaths and/or spontaneous abortions occurred in 37.5% of cases in the first trimester, 9.7% of cases in the second trimester and 0.0% of cases in the third trimester of pregnancy [27]. All fetuses were exposed to cytarabine, 47 fetuses were exposed to daunorubicin and only 8 fetuses were exposed to idarubicin. In fetuses exposed to cytarabine and daunorubicin, fetal defects occurred in 8.5% of cases and fetal deaths were encountered in 6.4% of cases, while in fetuses exposed to cytarabine and idarubicin, fetal defects occurred in 28.6% of cases and fetal deaths occurred in 12.5% of cases [27]. The following conclusions were made: (1) treatment during the second and third trimesters of pregnancy resulted in fewer fetal complications than in the first trimester, (2) delaying treatment of AML may adversely affect the outcomes of pregnant mothers, (3) induction chemotherapy administered during pregnancy resulted in CR rates comparable to those obtained in nonpregnant females, and (4) the choice of anthracycline is unclear but the decision should be made with careful consideration, weighing the outcomes of both the mother and the fetus [27].

In a retrospective study that was published in 1977 the outcomes of 32 pregnant mothers with AML and their offspring were reported [47]. Out of the 32 pregnancies with AML reported between 1905 and 1976, the outcomes of 27 mothers were known and only 1 of these mothers was alive and the survival rate was 3.7% for 6 months postpartum. Approximately 43% of fetuses were either delivered normally or were premature live births, while 53% of them were dead due to abortion, stillbirth or intrauterine fetal death [47]. The chemotherapeutic regimens that were used to treat AML included: corticosteroids, adrenocorticotropic hormone and 6-mercaptopurine. Hence, the recent improvement in fetal and maternal outcomes of AML in pregnancy is due to improvements not only in supportive care, but also in specific anti-leukemic therapies [47].

There are numerous reports of the successful management of AML in pregnancy and few reports of vertical transmission of acute leukemia from the mother to the fetus [48-50]. The spontaneous remission of acute leukemia after the termination of pregnancy and the following rare forms of AML have been reported: erythroleukemia, t(8,21) AML with granulocytic sarcoma causing spinal cord compression, and AML mimicking HELLP (hemolysis, elevated liver enzymes and low platelet counts) syndrome [50-53].

Although acute leukemia is a rare event in pregnancy, it may be associated with life-threatening complications to both the mother and the fetus [49]. Therefore, acute leukemia diagnosed during pregnancy should be treated promptly as delay in treatment is associated with higher maternal mortality, but decision on the choice of treatment for acute leukemia during pregnancy should be case-dependent [50,54]. If AML is diagnosed during the first trimester of pregnancy, the immediate termination of pregnancy should be considered then standard induction chemotherapy should be commenced [48,55-57]. Without the termination of pregnancy, combination chemotherapy is associated with an unacceptable high incidence of fetal abnormalities and/or fetal loss [55]. The management of AML diagnosed during the second and third trimesters of pregnancy is often difficult because delay in administration of chemotherapy implies significant risk to the mother, and administration of chemotherapy may induce: fetal death, prematurity and congenital malformations [55]. There are reports that chemotherapy can be safely given during the second and third trimesters of pregnancy and that induction chemotherapy using cytarabine and idarubicin for AML in the second trimester of pregnancy may be associated with fetal abnormalities including cardiac malformations [48,57]. Close monitoring of the fetus and the mother should be considered when chemotherapy is administered during the second trimester of pregnancy, [58]. However, the administration of standard chemotherapy including idarubicin during the third trimester of pregnancy may increase the chances of CR of AML without adversely affecting fetal outcome or increasing the risk of leukemia in the offspring [55,59]. In selected AML patients presenting in late pregnancy, it is possible to offer leukapheresis and blood product transfusions and to plan early delivery [55].

As in utero exposure to chemotherapy carries a significant risk of unfavorable outcome including low birth weight, fetal death and intrauterine fetal death, the fetus should be regularly evaluated by sonograms and umbilical blood sampling through cordiocentesis [54,60]. Unfortunately, AML diagnosed during pregnancy may be associated with poor outcome including maternal death, even if chemotherapy or HSCT are offered [57].

http://dx.doi.org/10.5772/61290

9. APL in pregnancy

APL is recognized to occur infrequently during pregnancy. APL is characterized by an onset at young age and life-threatening bleeding diathesis attributed to disseminated intravascular coagulation (DIC)-like coagulopathy [61,62]. The discovery of all trans-retinoic acid (ATRA) has changed the course of APL treatment by reducing the onset of DIC and inducing complete and durable remissions in more than 90% of patients [61]. The prognosis is good for APL with modern treatment that includes ATRA which specifically targets the causative retinoid acid receptor oncoprotein (PML-RARA) [63].

The use of daunorubicin therapy in pregnancy was first reported in 1976. The patient was in the 23rd week of gestation and despite the use of daunorubicin, she gave birth to a normal full term baby [64]. Thereafter, daunorubicin has been successfully used in the second and third trimesters of pregnancy without adversely affecting the offspring of pregnancy. Additionally, there are reports of using daunorubicin in the first trimester of pregnancy without causing fetal adverse events [64].

ATRA alone or combined with chemotherapy has been safely and successfully used in the treatment of APL during the second and third trimesters of pregnancy [65-67]. ATRA has been reported to ameliorate coagulation parameters and to induce remissions of APL in pregnant females [65-67]. However, close monitoring for fetal cardiac complications throughout pregnancy is mandatory and long-term follow up of children born to mothers treated with ATRA during pregnancy is warranted [65].

The management of APL in pregnant females requires special considerations [68]. Patients diagnosed to have APL during pregnancy pose a distinct challenge requiring a team approach involving a hematologist, an obstetrician and a neonatologist [68]. Nevertheless, the management of APL depends to a large extent on the trimester of pregnancy during which APL is diagnosed [68,69].

During the first trimester of pregnancy, both ATRA and arsenic trioxide (ASO) are contraindicated as both of them are highly teratogenic [68,69]. The critical factor in determining the line of management in women with APL in the first trimester of pregnancy is whether the pregnancy will be electively terminated once the patient is hemodynamically stable [68]. If the patient plans to terminate the pregnancy then conventional treatment with ATRA and chemotherapy can be commenced. If the elective termination of the pregnancy is unacceptable to the patient, the only available therapeutic option is the administration of chemotherapy such as daunorubicin [68]. In patients with APL, chemotherapy alone compared to ATRA and chemotherapy is associated with inferior response rates and progression-free survival but higher relapse rates and risk of bleeding due to coagulopathy. If chemotherapy alone is chosen, daunorabicin is the anthracycline of choice in pregnant females as there is greater experience with it and there are concerns over the lipophilic nature of idarubicin that may increase its fetal transfer and consequently fetal toxicity [68]. If the remission of APL is achieved with chemotherapy alone, ATRA may then be added in the second and third trimesters. After delivery, breast feeding is contraindicated during treatment with chemotherapy or ATO [68].

During the second and third trimesters of pregnancy, ATRA can be used but arsenic derivatives are contraindicated as they are highly embryotoxic [68,69]. In women diagnosed to have APL in the second or third trimesters of pregnancy, two main options are available: (1) induction of remission with ATRA alone with postponement of chemotherapy administration until after delivery, and (2) simultaneous administration of ATRA and chemotherapy as given in patients who are not pregnant at the time of diagnosis [68]. The immediate administration of combined ATRA and chemotherapy offers the best chance of cure but is accompanied by an increased risk of spontaneous abortion, premature delivery, low birth weights, neonatal neutropenia and sepsis so induction of labor between cycles of chemotherapy should be considered [68,69]. Patients treated with ATRA alone, compared to patients treated with ATRA and chemotherapy, have similar rates of remission, but higher rates of hyperleukocytosis and higher rates of relapse [68]. Patients treated with ATRA alone require frequent monitoring by real time-quantitative-polymerase chain reaction (RT-q-PCR) after induction of remission to monitor them for relapse while awaiting delivery, but patients receiving combined therapy with ATRA and chemotherapy require stringent fetal monitoring with particular emphasis on cardiac function [68,69]. For deliveries before 36 weeks of gestation, antenatal corticosteroids before preterm delivery are recommended to reduce the risk of morbidity and mortality associated with respiratory distress syndrome [69]. Vaginal delivery is generally preferred since it is associated with a reduced risk of bleeding [68]. After successful delivery, breast feeding is contraindicated if chemotherapy or ATO are required [69]. Female patients with APL should be advised against conceiving whilst exposed to ATRA or ATO for consolidation or maintenance therapy [69].

In an English literature review on APL in pregnancy that included 35 studies, 42 females with APL were reported between January 1972 and May 2008 [70]. Twelve cases of APL in pregnancy were reported in the first trimester, 21 cases in the second trimester and 9 cases in the third trimester. Thirty five patients (83%) achieved CR and the most commonly administered drugs were ATRA, anthracyclines and antimetabolites [70]. Fetal outcomes with ATRA and chemotherapy were as follows: spontaneous abortions and fetal malformations were encountered during the first trimester, while relatively favorable outcomes were encountered in the second and third trimesters [70]. The following conclusions were made: (1) the management of pregnant patient with APL is a real challenge; (2) the immediate treatment of APL is critical as APL is an oncologic emergency associated with high risks of morbidity and mortality due to DIC; (3) the administration of chemotherapy and differentiating agents in pregnancy is controversial because of the potential teratogenic effects; (4) the management of a pregnant woman with APL should include discussion about pregnancy termination particularly if APL is diagnosed during the first trimester of pregnancy; (5) if the patient and her family refuse pregnancy termination, then appropriate chemotherapeutic regimens need to be determined; and (6) frequent fetal monitoring and aggressive management of potential APL-related complications are essential to allow for optimal maternal and fetal outcomes [70].

In another study that included literature review of 23 cases of APL in pregnancy, 8 patients received chemotherapy and 3 patients received ATRA in late pregnancy [62]. There was one spontaneous abortion and one therapeutic abortion. Eleven patients had spontaneous vaginal delivery, 8 patients required cesarean section and 1 patient needed low forceps delivery while the mode of delivery was unknown in 1 pregnancy [62]. Sixteen patients (72%) achieved CRs of their APLs, 1 patient achieved partial remission and 2 patients showed no response while no information was obtained on the treatment given to 2 patients. Ten mothers (43.5%) died, while outcomes of newborn infants were as follows: 19 infants were born alive, 1 infant was gravely ill at birth and 2 infants had intrauterine fetal death [62]. The following conclusions were made: (1) pregnancy in APL requires special consideration to maximize the probability of survival of both the mother and the fetus, and (2) proper management of a pregnant female with APL usually results in a live birth with CR of the mother's leukemia despite the potentially devastating consequences of DIC, which is present at the time of diagnosis of APL in most patients [62].

A third study performed in Russia between 1998 and 2013 included 9 patients with APL and 6 patients were having APL during pregnancy [71]. The diagnosis of APL was made in 1 patient in the first trimester, 3 patients in the second trimester and 2 patients in the third trimester. Management was tailored according to the trimester of pregnancy: the termination of pregnancy was performed for patients presenting in the first trimester, chemotherapy then delivery for patients presenting in the second trimester while delivery followed by chemotherapy was offered to patients presenting in the third trimester [71]. Out of the 6 patients of APL diagnosed in pregnancy, 5 received AIDA (ATRA and idarubicin) regimen of treatment while one patient received 3+7 chemotherapy in addition to ATRA. Late recurrences were encountered in 33% of patients with APL and 44.4% of patients were alive with a median overall survival of 26 months while the median relapse-free survival was 17.5 months. The authors concluded that APL treatment in pregnancy, which is aimed at saving lives of both mothers and infants, is effective and results in a reasonable outcome [71].

Three patients with APL in pregnancy were reported from Italy [61]. The authors concluded that despite the rare occurrence of APL in pregnancy, the management of these patients raises many therapeutic and ethical dilemmas and requires careful clinical case evaluation of fetal and maternal risk, coagulation status, parents' wishes and therapeutic options [61]. Another study that included 3 patients with APL diagnosed during pregnancy concluded that: (1) management of APL in during pregnancy is complex because there are a number of possible therapeutic strategies that have varying implications for the mother and the fetus, and (2) response to treatment is subject to stringent monitoring by RT-q-PCR for the PML-RARA transcript [63]. Finally, 2 cases of APL in pregnancy were reported in Japan [72]. The first patient was diagnosed in the 14th week of gestation and she presented with pancytopenia and bleeding diathesis. She was treated with a combination of chemotherapeutic drugs that included daunorubicin [72]. Pregnancy ended in intrauterine fetal death at week 19 of gestation and the baby was found to be anemic with hypoplastic bone marrow [72].

A number of rather exceptional cases of APL in pregnancy have been reported [73-78]. Pregnancy has been reported after successful treatment of secondary APL following multi-agent chemotherapy and radiotherapy for lymphoma [73]. ATRA or differentiation syndrome has been reported in a pregnant patient with APL treated with ATRA and the respiratory failure induced by ATRA was successfully treated with non-invasive ventilation and corticosteroid therapy

[74]. Cesarean section was performed for a pregnant woman with untreated APL having DIC after active treatment of coagulopathy and close collaboration between hematologists and obstetricians [75]. Fetal arrhythmias and fetal growth retardation have been reported following the use of ATRA in treating pregnant females having APL [76]. APL has been diagnosed after management of placental abruption causing prolonged DIC [77]. Also, APL with t (15,17) and variant PML-RARA fusion transcript has been reported in pregnancy [78].

10. ALL in pregnancy

ALL is relatively rare in adults [1,2]. Only 21 cases of ALL in pregnancy had been reported prior to the year 2009 [1,2]. Subsequently, limited data on the treatment of ALL in pregnancy impedes absolute recommendations on the management of ALL in pregnant females [1,24].

As ALL is a highly aggressive malignancy, it is essential to administer adequate and appropriate chemotherapy immediately after diagnosis of ALL to control the disease [1,2]. Worldwide, different induction regimens of chemotherapy are utilized in the treatment of ALL [79-81]. Even in the same country, various chemotherapeutic protocols may be used such as CALGB, CCG and DFCI in the United States of America and FRALLE, LALA and GRAALL protocols in France [79-81]. Also, these therapeutic regimens undergo modifications or total replacement as new data evolve or whenever results of large studies are published [79-82]. Despite the development of multiple induction regimens, still there is no best regimen for induction therapy in ALL. However, the constituents of these chemotherapeutic regimens are almost similar with different dosing and schedules [79-82]. Recently, the more intensified pediatric ALL treatment regimens have been used in patients belonging to the age-group 15 to 40 years having ALL because several studies had shown that adolescents and young adults treated with adult ALL regimens of chemotherapy have poorer outcome compared to patients belonging to the same age-group treated with pediatric protocols [79,81,83]. Certain cancer centers are currently treating ALL patients between 1 and 50 years of age with the same chemotherapeutic protocols and are incorporating novel agents such as nelarabine and rituximab in the treatment of ALL [80,81]. Thus, unlike the situation in AML, the use of different treatment regimens in ALL makes it very difficult to adopt strong recommendations or to establish strict guidelines for the management of ALL in pregnancy [79-83].

Studies have shown that in patients in whom induction chemotherapy is commenced before delivery, survival is longer than in those treated after delivery [2]. The risk of congenital malformations diminishes as pregnancy advances [1,2]. The absence of autopsy data on fetuses delivered by terminations could result in a decrease in the incidence of congenital malformations in the fetuses delivered [24]. High-dose methotrexate is a crucial component of most of the ALL intensification protocols of chemotherapy but unfortunately the drug is highly teratogenic and its administration during the first trimester of pregnancy is associated with the development of aminopterin syndrome and a high risk of miscarriage [1,2,24].

When the diagnosis of ALL is made during the first trimester of pregnancy, the termination of pregnancy is strongly recommended in order to commence standard induction chemotherapy [1]. Chemotherapeutic regimens have included: cytarabine, cyclophosphamide, L-asparaginase, anthracyclines, vincristine and corticosteroids [1,24]. The second trimester of pregnancy can be roughly divided into two parts: (1) part one, before the 20th week of gestation: management resembles that in the first trimester of pregnancy, so the termination of pregnancy should be considered, followed by the administration of adequate or standard ALL induction chemotherapy, and (2) part two, after the 20th week of gestation: bridging chemotherapy or modified ALL regimens of chemotherapy without methotrexate can be given till the third trimester of pregnancy, although possible damage to the fetus should be taken into consideration [1,2,24]. Several chemotherapeutic regimens that exclude the use of methotrexate have been suggested, but the experience with these modified therapies is extremely limited, so these therapeutic regimens should be used as short bridging treatments till the third trimester starts [1,2,24].

A brief period of treatment with prednisolone alone for 1-2 weeks may allow the patient to enter the period of gestation beyond the 20 weeks in order to receive more intensive chemotherapy thereafter. A similar approach with prednisolone alone can be recommended for patients presenting close to 32 weeks of gestation [24]. For patients presenting in the third trimester of pregnancy, they can be treated with the same chemotherapeutic protocols that are used to treat their nonpregnant counterparts [2,24]. The outcome of ALL is stratified according to a number of risk factors: (1) patients with a good prognosis can be treated with less intensive chemotherapeutic approaches, and (2) patients with more aggressive features will require interventions according to the pace of the underlying disease [24]. Close obstetric care and close monitoring of the mother and the fetus are essential to ensure the best possible outcome [2]. Elective delivery after 32 weeks of gestation should be planned but timing of delivery should avoid periods of pancytopenia to prevent further complications [2,24].

Acute leukemia develops in 1:750,000 pregnancies and ALL accounts for 11-28% of acute leukemia in pregnancy [84,85]. Although ALL is rare in pregnancy, it can be rapidly fatal if left untreated. Thus, it requires immediate therapy irrespective of the gestational age [85,86]. Advances in the management of leukemia have led to improved survival and emphasized the importance of initiation of cytotoxic chemotherapy in the antepartum period [85]. Several case reports, case series and retrospective studies have shown successful treatment of ALL in pregnancy using several combinations of the following cytotoxic agents: prednisolone, cytarabine, cyclophosphamide, vincristine, daunorubicin or doxorubicin, L-asparaginase, 6-mercaptopurine and intrathecal methotrexate [85]. However, the choice of specific chemotherapeutic regimen depends on the gestational age and clinical status of the pregnant female as well as the anticipated toxicities of the cytotoxic agents [85].

The basic principle of ALL treatment is combination chemotherapy with the sequential administration of induction, consolidation and maintenance therapy and this holds true for ALL in pregnancy [86]. Thus, the management of ALL during pregnancy requires high-dose chemotherapy that can pose risks to both the mother and the fetus [84]. In order to limit fetal exposure to chemotherapy and to provide optimal care to the mother, particular attention should be paid to: the chemotherapeutic regimen to be administered, the doses of the cytotoxic agents to be used and the gestational age at the time of chemotherapy administration [84].

During the first trimester of pregnancy, chemotherapy used in the treatment of ALL is associated with teratogenicity, stillbirths and abortions, so the termination of pregnancy should be considered and the risks of chemotherapy administered during this part of pregnancy should be discussed with the pregnant mother [84,86]. During the second and third trimesters of pregnancy, the administration of chemotherapy has been widely practiced, although the following adverse events have been reported: intrauterine fetal death and growth retardation, premature delivery, low birth weight, maternal as well as fetal myelosuppression and pre-eclampsia of pregnancy [84,86].

Some of the rather exceptional case reports include: (1) relapse of ALL in pregnant females; (2) presentation of ALL in pregnancy with extra-medullary disease involving the central nervous system, breast and ovaries; and (3) successful treatment of ALL during the second and third trimesters of pregnancy with combination therapy or single agents such as corticosteroids [87-97].

In a literature review that included 17 patients with ALL treated during pregnancy the following maternal and fetal outcomes were reported: 9 mothers (53%) achieved CRs of their ALLs while 8 patients (47%) either died (5 patients) or had relapse of their leukemia (3 patients) [84]. Thirteen babies (76%) were alive, 4 babies (24%) were dead and 6 babies were delivered by cesarean section. The authors also concluded that: doxorubicin was the safest anthracycline employed in pregnant females and they highlighted the importance of long-term follow up of children exposed to chemotherapy in utero [84].

Pregnant females can achieve CR of their leukemia but the decisions on future conception need to be individualized because of unpredictable outcome [98]. Although the literature is modestly positive on the prognosis of ALL in pregnancy, this may not be entirely true particularly in aggressive forms or high-risk ALL presenting during pregnancy where termination of pregnancy should be performed in order to allow the administration of intensive chemotherapy that may be followed by HSCT [86].

11. CML in pregnancy

CML accounts for 15% of adult leukemias, but only 10% of cases are diagnosed during childbearing age as the median age at the diagnosis of CML is the sixth decade of life [1,24]. CML occurs in 10% of all pregnancy-associated leukemias and the annual incidence ranges between 1 in 75000 and 1 in 100000 pregnancies [2,24]. The diagnosis of CML during pregnancy may be made more complicated as the physiological changes, including those in hematological parameters which accompany pregnancy, may mask the symptoms of CML [24]. However, the diagnostic approach of CML in pregnant females is identical to that in non-pregnant patients [2].

Previously, there was a suggestion of an increase in the rates of miscarriage, low birth weight and premature babies in mothers having CML, but this is no longer apparent in the more recent years. Reassuringly, the course of CML does not appear to be adversely affected by pregnancy

[24]. Due to the excellent clinical outcome with tyrosine kinase inhibitors (TKIs), the expectations of a relatively normal life style inclusive of parenting children in increasing. Therapeutic approaches to CML diagnosed during pregnancy include: leukapheresis, hydroxyurea, α-interferon and imatinib [24]. There are numerous case reports describing the use of leukapheresis and plateletpheresis in pregnant women having CML but unfortunately, apheresis technology is not universally available [24].

There are several studies and literature reviews including relatively large numbers of patients with CML diagnosed during pregnancy [29,99-101]. The studies and reviews that included the largest numbers of cases are described below. In a literature review that included 265 pregnant ladies with CML treated with imatinib, the outcomes of pregnancies were known in 210 pregnancies while the outcomes of 55 other pregnancies were unknown [99]. Pregnancies that ended in the delivery of normal live infants were 128 (60%), elective terminations of pregnancy were described in 43 patients (20%), spontaneous abortions occurred in 24 cases (11%) and fetal abnormalities were described in 15 cases (7%) [99]. A second study reported 217 pregnancies in 215 women with CML. The number of fetuses exposed to imatinib was 217 [29]. Out of the 217 pregnancies, 46 had therapeutic or elective abortions and 5 out of the 46 aborted fetuses had congenital malformations. Out of the 217 pregnant females, 171 women decided to continue pregnancy. Only 85 pregnancies were carried out till term after being exposed to imatinib for some time during pregnancy. One out of 85 pregnancies ended in a stillbirth with meningocele and 84 pregnancies ended in delivery of live births of these: 73 were normal healthy babies, 9 were having congenital malformations and 2 had low birth weights [29]. Regarding the outcome of pregnancies, 24 pregnancies ended in spontaneous abortion, 62 had unknown outcomes and 109 had known outcomes. Among the 109 pregnancies with known outcomes, 36 (33%) resulted in complications. Regarding the 43 out of 84 babies who were carried to term and were exposed to imatinib throughout pregnancy, 22 babies were born without abnormalities and 2 were reported to have low birth weights [29]. A third review, over 10 years, included 180 pregnant females who had been exposed to imatinib [100]. However, data on outcomes were available for 120 patients (69% of cases). In this review, 50% of pregnancies ended in delivery of normal infants and 28% of pregnancies underwent elective terminations, 3 of them were done after identification of fetal abnormalities of the delivered infants, 18 had abnormalities identified, 3 of them were complex malformations [100]. The authors concluded that although most pregnancies exposed to imatinib are likely to yield successful outcome, there remains a risk that imatinib exposure during pregnancy may result in spontaneous abortions and serious fetal malformations [100]. A fourth study from China reported 16 pregnancies in patients with CML [101]. Out of the 16 pregnancies, 7 ended in deliveries and 9 ended in therapeutic abortions during the first and second trimesters of pregnancy. Out of the 9 patients with CML who required therapeutic abortions: 4 lost follow-up, 1 died 3 years after the diagnosis of her disease and 4 were alive at 5-72 months. Out of the 4 patients alive, 1 had HSCT, 2 were back on imatinib and one was given hydroxyurea [101]. Maternal outcome for the 7 pregnancies that ended in deliveries: 2 lost follow-up, 2 died and 3 were still alive. In these 7 patients, fetal outcome was as follows: 2 lost follow-up, and 5 babies had normal development and they were reported to be alive at 4 months to 9 years of follow up [101].

11.1. Planning an elective pregnancy in CML patients

Female patients with CML who wish to become pregnant should be advised to wait until they have achieved major molecular response (MMR) or better responses and sustained these responses for at least 2 years [24,99,102]. Imatinib can be discontinued shortly before ovulation and perhaps at the onset of menstruation. The duration of interruption of imatinib therapy should be limited to 6 months. However, if the RT-q-PCR analyses of BCR-ABL transcripts do not show a rise from the baseline, the duration of interruption can be extended further. RT-q-PCR monitoring in addition to complete blood count (CBC) should be performed every 2-3 months while imatinib therapy is on hold [24,99]. In females with CML achieving complete hematological response (CHR) or better responses, oocytes should be collected for future assisted conception, TKIs should be stopped at the onset of the menstrual cycle, in vitro fertilization medications should be commenced 7 days after stopping TKIs and TKI therapy should be resumed after oocyte collection [24,99].

The interruption of imatinib therapy in pregnant patients having CML should be considered seriously and replacement of imatinib by alternative therapies such as interferon, hydroxyurea or leukapheresis can be taken into consideration [100,102,103]. There are different opinions regarding the use of interferon in pregnancy. Although it is generally safe during pregnancy, some believe that it should be avoided unless the potential benefits justify the potential risks to the fetus [1,100,102]. After cessation of imatinib, treatment with interferon-α is effective to sustain the complete molecular response achieved in CML patients with low Sokal score, while patients with high Sokal score usually fail interferon-α therapy, relapse quickly and lose their CHR [102]. Decisions on the interruption of TKI therapy, replacement by alternative treatments and planning of delivery should all be made after counseling the patient and her family and after involvement of obstetricians and neonatologists [100,103]. There is no evidence that a brief exposure to imatinib therapy during conception and pregnancy adversely affects the developing fetus. Unfortunately, after interruption of imatinib therapy, most patients lose their achieved responses particularly those with high Sokal score [99,102].

In a study which tested the interruption of imatinib therapy in pregnant females with CML that included 7 patients, the results were as follows: in patients who achieved optimal responses prior to interruption of imatinib therapy during pregnancy, maintenance of optimal responses was achieved after delivery and resumption of imatinib, while in patients who had suboptimal responses before the interruption of imatinib during pregnancy, failure to achieve optimal responses years after delivery and resumption of imatinib therapy was encountered [105]. Therefore, the interruption of imatinib treatment should be considered in patients who achieved optimal responses well before planned pregnancy or interruption of TKI therapy [24,102,105].

11.2. Imatinib in CML post-stem cell transplantation

A single report of a female patient with CML who received reduced intensity conditioning (RIC) allogeneic HSCT for her CML was documented [106]. The patient was resumed on imatinib on day 100 post-HSCT for 30 months. Seven months after withdrawal of imatinib and all transplant-related medications, the patient was found to be pregnant. She had uneventful pregnancy and she delivered 2 full-term babies. No relapse of her CML was reported till 5 years post-HSCT [106].

11.3. Experience with second generation TKIs

The experience with dasatinib and nilotinib in pregnant females having CML is very limited [107-110]. Three spontaneous abortions and 4 successful pregnancies in CML patients exposed to dasatinib have been reported. In one additional patient, CML was diagnosed during pregnancy and the patient was treated with dasatinib but unfortunately she developed serious complications that lead to the termination of pregnancy [107-109]. A patient with CML had 2 pregnancies; no treatment was required for the first one but nilotinib was used during the second pregnancy, which ended in a successful delivery without maternal or fetal complications [110].

11.4. The use of leukapheresis in pregnancy with CML

Leukapheresis has been successfully utilized in the upfront management of CML patients during the 3 trimesters of pregnancy [24,111,112]. At least 12 cases have been reported and in few cases it was used as the sole management of CML in pregnant females. It was successfully used for up to 15 sessions per pregnancy and no adverse outcomes were encountered in the vast majority of cases [24,111,112]. However, one baby was delivered with myelomeningocele and talipes equinovarus to a patient with CML who received leukapheresis in addition to hydroxyurea during pregnancy [24].

12. CLL in pregnancy

CLL is very rare in pregnancy and only 7 cases of CLL were reported between 1996 and 2014 [1,2,24,113-116]. The following complications of CLL have been reported in pregnant females: autoimmune phenomena, anemia requiring blood transfusions, hyperleukocytosis and repeated infections [1,2,35,115,117]. The following therapeutic modalities have been reported to be safe in pregnant females having CLL, at any stage of pregnancy: (1) leukapheresis for hyperleukocytosis, (2) corticosteroids for autoimmune hemolytic anemia and autoimmune thrombocytopenia, and (3) certain antimicrobials for the treatment of infectious complications of CLL [1,2,35].

Chlorambucil is contraindicated during the first trimester of pregnancy because of its teratogenic effects and fludarabine should be avoided in pregnancy and can be used to treat CLL after delivery [2]. During the second and third trimesters of pregnancy, the following drugs can be safely used: rituximab, chlorambucil and cyclophosphamide [2].

13. HCL in pregnancy

Hairy cell leukemia (HCL) is rare in young women and it is exceptional in pregnancy [1,2,39]. Only 6 cases of HCL were reported in pregnant females between 1987 and 2008 and few additional cases have been added since the year 2008 [1.2,38,39]. All the reported cases of HCL in pregnancy ended in uncomplicated deliveries [2]. If HCL is diagnosed during pregnancy, management depends on whether the termination of pregnancy is considered or not. In case the termination of pregnancy is done or treatment is postponed till after delivery, the following therapeutic options are safe: splenectomy, interferon, cladrabine, rituximab and other new therapeutic modalities [1,2,36-39]. If the termination of pregnancy is not undertaken, the following options are available: (1) splenectomy and interferon have been safely reported in all trimesters of pregnancy, and (2) cladrabine can be safely used in the second and third trimesters [1,2,36-39]. However, due to the limited number of HCL in pregnancy reported, no definitive conclusions should be made [1,2,36-39].

14. Other therapeutic measures during pregnancy

14.1. Corticosteroids in pregnancy

Prednisolone, methylprednisolone and hydrocortisone are extensively metabolized in the placenta; therefore; they are preferred over dexamethasone and betamethasone [1,2]. Conti-costeroids are indicated for treating: (1) ALL in pregnancy, and (2) autoimmune complications of CLL during pregnancy. In animal studies, steroids are associated with development of cleft palate and altered neurological development resulting in complex behavioral abnormalities [1]. Corticosteroids have the following effects on pregnant women: (1) premature rupture of membranes, and (2) exacerbation of gestational diabetes mellitus and hypertension [1]. They also have the following effects on newborn infants: (1) intrauterine growth retardation, (2) low birth weight, (3) increased infant morbidity, (4) hyperactivity in the newborn infant, and (5) risk of adrenal insufficiency and infectious complications [1].

14.2. Growth factors in pregnancy

Granulocyte-colony-stimulating factor (G-CSF, filgrastim) is the most commonly used colony stimulating factor. It is usually used (1) in patients with neutropenia to reduce the incidence of infectious complications, and (2) for mobilization of stem cells in donors of autologous and allogeneic HSCT [118]. The administration of G-CSF in pregnant women who serve as donors for HSCT is generally safe as data from 5 studies that included HSCT donors including pregnant females did not show any evidence of increased risk of leukemogenicity [118]. Also, data from 8 studies that included 96 pregnant females having hematological malignancies showed delivery of 94 healthy babies, but one fetal death as the mother was exposed to idarubicin and cytarabine during pregnancy in addition to one birth of a child with low intelligence and malignancy [118].

14.3. Leukapheresis in pregnancy

Leukapheresis has been used in both acute and chronic leukemia in order to rapidly reduce high while blood counts (WBCs) in patients with an impending vascular occlusion due to leukostasis induced by hyperleukocytosis [2]. Although the experience is limited, the procedure has been successfully used as a short-term measure to rapidly control hyperleukocytosis at the presentation of acute and chronic leukemia [1,2,40].

14.4. Drugs and breast feeding after delivery

Chemotherapeutic agents differ in their concentrations that are found in breast milk [1,24]. Definitive neonatal toxicity during lactation has not been precisely delineated. However, it is advisable to avoid breast feeding for at least 2 weeks after the administration of cytotoxic chemotherapy [1,24]. Hydroxocobalamine is excreted in breast milk and should be avoided during lactation. Interferon-α is probably excreted in breast milk and should be avoided during lactation. TKIs such as imatinib are actively excreted in breast milk in animal studies. Although several reports show no harm, generally TKIs should be avoided during lactation as they have been reported to cause arrhythmias and cardiac toxicity [24].

Ciprofloxacin is excreted in breast milk and it has been reported to cause pseudomembranous colitis, arthropathies and cartilage erosions so the drug should be used with extreme caution, while fluconazole, itraconazole, voriconazole and posaconazole should be avoided during lactation [24]. However, there are no published data on the use of caspofungin and liposomal amphotericin-B in breast feeding women so they should be avoided in lactating women [24].

15. Fertility in patients with leukemia

Cytotoxic drugs, administered to premenstrual females having leukemia, may have adverse effects on ovarian reserve even in the setting of regular menses [119]. Hemato-oncologists, infertility specialists and patients should be aware of the potential risks of chemotherapy on ovarian function and should consider the available options for fertility preservation [119]. Options for fertility preservation in cancer patients include: (1) ovarian suppression during chemotherapy by hormonal therapy, (2) embryo cryopreservation, (3) oocyte cryopreservation, (4) ovarian tissue cryopreservation or gonadal tissue banking, (5) recent developments of in vitro fertilization for cancer patients and development of gonadotropin releasing hormone antagonists, (6) ovarian transposition during radiotherapy, and (7) additional considerations such as third party reproduction and adoption of children [120-122].

16. Conclusions and future directions

Leukemia is a rare event in pregnancy. Acute leukemia represents 90% of leukemias coexisting with pregnancy with AML accounting for two thirds of acute leukemias in pregnant mothers.

Vertical transmission of leukemic cells from the mother to her offspring is possible but very rare. During the first trimester of pregnancy, standard chemotherapy has a teratogenicity rate of 10-20% depending on the specific agent employed. Exposure to cytotoxic agents during the second and third trimesters is not teratogenic but carries the following risks: fetal growth retardation, premature delivery, fetal myelosuppression in addition to fetal and maternal exposure to malignancy and therapy-related toxicities such as thromboembolism and sepsis. Only absolutely necessary radiologic work-up is justified during the first trimester of pregnancy. Exposure to radiation during the first 2 weeks of pregnancy is usually lethal. Thereafter, radiation predisposes to congenital malformations, growth retardation and malignancy in the newborn. Few studies have demonstrated the potential risk of adult cancer after intrauterine exposure to radiation. Cytotoxic chemotherapy and radiotherapy increase genetic defects in germ cells. Although most infants exposed to multi-agent chemotherapy seem to suffer no long-term detrimental consequences, cytotoxic chemotherapy can cross the placenta and cause teratogenic effects.

The management of each pregnant patient with leukemia has to be highly individualized and should have a multidisciplinary approach. In the first trimester, the termination of pregnancy should seriously be considered if the disease is aggressive and if intensive chemotherapy is needed. In the second and third trimesters, standard chemotherapy can safely be administered without resorting to pregnancy termination. The choice of specific regimens depends upon: the gestational age, the clinical status of the patient, the specific type of leukemia and the anticipated toxic effects of the cytotoxic agents employed. The decision is often difficult and confounded by heightened emotions, ethical concerns and religious beliefs. Vaginal delivery is preferable while caesarean section is reserved for certain obstetric complications. The timing of delivery is essential. It is preferable between 32 and 36 weeks of gestation to ensure optimal fetal maturation, and it is advisable to avoid maternal myelosuppression prior to delivery.

Leukemia diagnosed during pregnancy can be considered a poor clinical prognostic factor owing to the less than average long-term disease free survival due to high relapse rates and high incidence of refractoriness to chemotherapy, particularly in young patients. Countries should have registries for mothers and children exposed to chemotherapy and radiotherapy. Also, it is essential to have guidelines on the management of various types of leukemia during pregnancy.

Author details

Khalid Ahmed Al-Anazi*

Address all correspondence to: kaa_alanazi@yahoo.com

Department of Hematology and Hematopoietic Stem Cell Transplantation, Cancer Center, King Fahad Specialist Hospital, Dammam, Saudi Arabia.

References

[1] Shapira T, Pereg D, Lishner M. How I treat acute and chronic leukemia in pregnancy. Blood Rev. 2008; 22: 247-259.

[2] Vandenbriele C, Vassou A, Pentheroudakis G, Van Calsteren K, Amant F. Hematologic malignancies in pregnancies. In Tech 2011. Acute leukemia-the scientist's perspective and challenge, Prof. Mariastefania Actina (Ed.). ISBN: 978-953-307-553-2.

[3] Vandenbriele C, Dierikx D, Amant F, Delforge M. The treatment of hematologic malignancies in pregnancy. Facts Views Vis Obgyn. 2010; 2 (2): 74-87.

[4] Townsley DM. Hematologic complications of pregnancy. Sem Hematol. 2013; 50 (3): 222-231.

[5] Koh MB, Lao ZT, Rhodes E. Managing haematological disorders during pregnancy. Best Pract Res Clin Obstet Gynecol. 2013; doi. org/10.1016/jbpogyn. 2013.08.002.

[6] Mims MP, Prchal JT. Hematology during pregnancy. In: Beutler E, et al. Williams Hematology, 7th edition. New York: McGraw-Hill; 2005.

[7] Latino-Martel P, Chan DSM, Druesne-Pecollo N, Barrandon E, Hercberg S, Norat T. Maternal alcohol consumption during pregnancy and risk of childhood leukemia: systematic review and meta-analysis. Cancer Epidemiol Biomarkers Prev. 2010; 19 (5): 1238-1260.

[8] Sasco AJ, Vainio H. From in utero and childhood exposure to parental smoking to childhood cancer: a possible link and the need for action. Human Exp Toxicol. 1999; 18 (4): 192-201.

[9] Lehtinen M, Ögmundsdottr HM, Bloigu A, Hakulinen T, Hemmin Ki E, Gudnadottr M, et al. Associations between three types of maternal bacterial infection and risk of leukemia in the offspring. Am J Epidemiol. 2005; 162 (7): 662-667.

[10] Kaatsch P, Scheidemann-Wesp U, Schüz J. Maternal use of antibiotics and cancer in the offspring: results of a case control study in Germany. Cancer Causes Control 2010; 21 (8): 1335-1345.

[11] Pambo-de-Oliveira MS, Koifman S, and the Brazilian Collaborative Study Group. Infant acute leukemia and maternal exposures during pregnancy. Cancer Epidemiol Biomarkers Prev. 2006; 15 (12): 2336-2341.

[12] Chantrain CF, Sauvage D, Brichard D, Dupont S, Poirel HA, Ameye G, et al. Neonatal acute myeloid leukemia in an infant whose mother was exposed to diethylstilboestrol in utero. Pediatr Blood Cancer 2009; 53 (2): 220-222.

[13] Zhou Y, Zhang S, Li Z, Zhu J, Bi Y, Bai Y, et al. Maternal benzene exposure during pregnancy and risk of childhood acute lymphoblastic leukemia: a meta-analysis of epidemiologic studies. PLOS One 2014; 9 (10): e 11 04 66.

[14] Chang JS, Buffler PA, Metayer C, Chokkaligam AP, Patoka J, Kronish D, et al. Maternal immunoglobulin E and childhood leukemia. Cancer Epidemiol Biomarkers Prev. 2009; 18 (8): 2221-2227.

[15] Dockerty JD, Herbison P, Skegg DCG, Elwood M. Vitamin and mineral supplements in pregnancy and the risk of childhood acute lymphoblastic leukemia: a case-control study. BMC Public Health 2007; 7: 136.

[16] Kwan ML, Jensen CD, Block G, Hudes ML, Chu LW, Buffler PA. Maternal diet and risk of childhood acute lymphoblastic leukemia. Public Health Rep. 2009; 124 (4): 503-514.

[17] Milne E, Royle JA, Miller M, Bower C, de Klerk NH, Baily HD, et al. Maternal folate and other vitamin supplementation during pregnancy and risk of acute lymphoblastic leukemia in the offspring. Int J Cancer 2010; 126 (11): 2690-2699.

[18] Franco EL, Turgeon G-A. Radiodiagnostic imaging in pregnancy and the risk of childhood malignancy: raising the bar. PLOS Med. 2010; 7 (9): e100038.

[19] Kruskal JB, Diagnostic imaging procedures drying pregnancy. UpToDate 2013. Edited by: Wilkins-Haug L, Levine D and Barss VA. Topic last updated: September 13, 2013.

[20] Lavi N, Horowitz NA, Brenner B. An update on the management of hematologic malignancies in pregnancy. Women's Health 2014; 10 (3): 255-266.

[21] Shu X-O, Jin F, Linet MS, Zheng W, Clements J, Mills J, et al. Diagnostic X-ray and ultrasound exposure and risk of childhood cancer. Br J Cancer 1994; 70: 531-536.

[22] Bailey HD, Armstrong BK, de Klerk NH, Fritschi L, Attia J, Lock wood L, et al. Exposure to diagnostic radiological procedures and the risk of childhood acute lymphoblastic leukemia. Cancer Epidemio Biomarkers Prev. 2010; 19 (11): 2897-2909.

[23] Brenner B, Avivi I, Lishner M. Hematological cancers in pregnancy. Lancet 2012; 580-587.

[24] Milojkovic D, Apperley JF. How I treat leukemia during pregnancy. Blood 2014, 123: 974-984.

[25] Aviles A, Neri N. Hematological malignancies and pregnancy: a final report of 84 children who received chemotherapy in utero. Clin Lymphoma 2001; 2 (3): 173-177.

[26] Dilek I, Topcu N, Demir C, Bay A, Uzun K, Gul A, et al. Hematological malignancy and pregnancy: a single institution experience of 21 cases. Clin Lab Haematol. 2006; 28 (3): 170-176.

[27] Chang A, Patel S. Treatment of acute myeloid leukemia in pregnancy. Ann Pharmacother. 2015; 49 (1): 48-68.

[28] Rizack T, Mega A, Legare R, Castillo J. Management of hematological malignancies during pregnancy. Am J Hematol. 2009; 84 (12): 830-841.

[29] Cole S, Kantarjian H, Ault P, Cortes JE. Successful completion of pregnancy in a patient with chronic myeloid leukemia without active intervention: a case report and review of the literature. Clin Lymphoma Myeloma 2009; 9 (4): 324-327.

[30] Pavilis NA. Coexistence of pregnancy and malignancy. The Oncologist 2002; 7: 279-287.

[31] Shepard TH. Agents that cause birth defects. Yonsei Med J. 1995; 36 (5): 393-396.

[32] Pentheroudakis G, Pavilis N, Castiglione M, on behalf of the ESMO Guidelines Working Group. Cancer, fertility and pregnancy: ESMO clinical recommendations for diagnosis, treatment and follow-up. Ann Oncol. 2009; Suppl 4: iv178-iv181.

[33] Arnon J, Lewis-Meiro D, Lewis-Roness H, Ornoy A. Genetic and teratogenic effects of cancer treatment on gametes and embryos. Hum Reprod Update 2001; 7 (4): 394-403.

[34] Peccatori FA, Azim HA, Orecchia R, Hoekstra HJ, Pavilis N, Kesic V, et al. Cancer, pregnancy, and fertility: ESMO clinical practice guidelines for diagnosis, treatment and follow-up. Ann Oncol. 2013; Suppl 6: vi160-vi170.

[35] Ali R, Özkalemkas F, Özkocaman V, Büllbül-Baskan E, Özcelik T, Ozan U, et al. Successful labor in the course of chronic lymphocytic leukemia (CLL) and managment of CLL during pregnancy with leukapheresis. Ann Hematol. 2004; 83 (1): 61-63.

[36] Ainoon O, Megat R, Cheong SK, Halimah Y. Hairy cell leukemia: a case report. Med J Malaysia 1988; 43 (1): 62-64.

[37] Williams JK. Hairy cell leukemia in pregnancy: a case report. Am J Obstet Gynecol. 1987; 156 (1): 210-211.

[38] Daver N, Nazha A, Kantarjian HM, Haltom R, Ravandi F. Treatment of hairy cell leukemia during pregnancy: are purine analogues and rituximab therapeutic options? Clin Lymphoma Myeloma Leuk. 2013; 13 (1): 86-89.

[39] Bustamante A, Rodriguez MA, Ocqueteau M, Bertin P, Lira P, Valbuena J. Hairy cell leukemia during pregnancy: report of one case. Rev Med Chil. 2010; 138 (11): 1422-1426.

[40] Saleh AJM, Alhejazi A, Ahmed SO, Al Mohareb F, AlSharif F, AlZahrani H, et al. Leukemia during pregnancy: long term follow up of 32 cases from a single institution. Hematol Oncol Stem Cell Ther. 2014; 7 (2): 63-68.

[41] Nomura RM, Igai AM, Faciroli NC, Aguiar IN, Zugaib M. Maternal and perinatal outcomes in pregnant women with leukemia. Rev Bras Ginecol Obstet. 2011; 33 (8): 174-181.

[42] Kawamura S, Yoshiike M, Shimoyama T, Suzuki Y, Itoh J, Yamagata K, et al. Management of acute leukemia during pregnancy: from the results of a nationwide questionnaire and literature review. Tohoku J Exp Med. 1994; 174: 167-175.

[43] Reynoso EE, Shepard FA, Messner HA, Farquharson HA, Garvey MB, Baker MA. Acute leukemia during pregnancy: the Toronto Leukemia Study Group experience with long-term follow-up of children exposed in utero to chemotherapeutic agents. J Clin Oncol. 1987; 5 (7): 1098-1106.

[44] Chelghoum Y, Vey N, Raffoux E, Huguet F, Pigneux A, Witz B, et al. Acute leukemia during pregnancy. Cancer 2005; 104: 110-117.

[45] Nakajima Y, Hattori Y, Ito S, Ohshima R, Kuwabara H, Machida S, et al. Acute leukemia during pregnancy: an investigative survey of the past 11 years. Int J Lab Hematol. 2014; doi: 10.1111/ijlh.12256.

[46] Ali R, Ozkalemkas F, Kimya Y, Kokasal N, Ozkocaman V, Yorulmaz H, et al. Pregnancy in chronic lymphocytic leukemia: experience with fetal exposure to chlorambucil. Leuk Res. 2009; 33 (4): 567-569.

[47] Lilleyman JS, Hill AS, Anderton KJ. Consequences of acute myelogenous leukemia in early pregnancy. Cancer 1977; 40: 1300-1303.

[48] Jeelani S, Rasool J, Jan A, Sajad A, Khan JAA, Lone AR. Pregnancy with acute myeloid leukemia. Indian J Med Paediatr Oncol 2008; 29 (4): 47-48.

[49] Menezes J, Emerenciano M, Pimenta F, Filho GG, Magalhaes IQ, Saut' Ana M, et al. Occurrence of acute myeloid leukemia in young pregnant women. Clin Med Blood Dis 2008; 1: 27-31.

[50] Yalcin AD, Aydemir N, Erbay H, Bir F. A case of acute myelomonocytic leukemia in a parturient whom refused the therapy. Internet J Hematol. 2003; 1 (1): 1-4.

[51] Tomizuka H, Yatabe M, Okudera K, Hatake K, Miwa T, Sakamoto S, et al. Erythroleukemia in pregnancy with successful outcome of delivery. Rinsho Ketsueki 1992; 33: 194-199.

[52] Al-Sobhi EM, Jeha TM, Al-Taher MI. Granulocytic sarcoma causing cord compression in a pregnant woman with acute myeloid leukemia and t (8;21). Saudi Med J. 2008; 29 (11): 1658-1661.

[53] Biener DM, Gossing G, Kuehnl A, Cremer M, Dudenhausen JW. Diagnosis and treatment of maternal acute myeloid leukemia during pregnancy imitating HELLP syndrome. J Perinat Med. 2009; 37 (6): 713-714.

[54] Tashiro H, Umezawa K, Shirota M, Oka Y, Shirasaka R, Nishi R, et al. Acute myelogenous leukemia developed at the 26th week of gestation. Rinsho Ketsueki 2011; 52 (11): 18-22.

[55] Larson RA. Induction therapy for acute myeloid leukemia in young adults. UpToDate 2014. Edited by Lowenberg B and Connor RF. Topic last updated: September 04, 2014.

[56] Avivi I, Brenner B. Management of acute myeloid leukemia during pregnancy. Future Oncol 2014; 10 (8): 1407-1415.

[57] Niedermeier DM, Frei-Lahr DA, Hall PD. Treatment of acute myeloid leukemia during the second and third trimesters of pregnancy. Pharmacotherapy 2005; 25 (8): 1134-1140.

[58] Baumgärtner AK, Oberhoffer R, Jacobs VR, Ostermayer E, Menzel H, Voigt M, et al. Reversible fetal cerebral ventriculomegaly and cardiomyopathy under chemotherapy for maternal AML. Onkologie 2009; 32: 40-43.

[59] Matsuo K, Shimoya K, Ueda S, Wada K, Koyama M, Murata Y. Idarubicin administered during pregnancy: its effects on the fetus. Gynecol Obstet Investing 2004; 58 (4): 186-188.

[60] Morishita S, Imai A, Kawabata I, Tamaya T. Acute myelogenous leukemia in pregnancy. Fetal blood sampling and early effects of chemotherapy. Int J Gynecol Obstet. 1994; 44 (3): 273-277.

[61] Consoli U, Figuera A, Milone G, Meli CR, Guido G, idelicato F, et al. Acute promyelocytic leukemia during pregnancy: report of 3 cases. Int J Lab Hematol. 2004; 79 (1): 31-36.

[62] Hoffman MA, Weirnik PH, Kleiner GJ. Acute promyelocytic leukemia and pregnancy: a case report. Cancer 1995; 76: 2237-2241.

[63] Culligan DJ, Merriman L, Kell J, Parker J, Jovanovic JV, Smith N, et al. The management of acute promyelocytic leukemia presenting during pregnancy. Clin Leuk. 2007; 1 (3): 183-191.

[64] Alegre A, Chunchurreta R, Rodriguez-Alarcon J, Cruz E, Prada M. Successful pregnancy in acute promyelocytic leukemia. Cancer 1982; 49: 152-153.

[65] Fadilah SAW, Hatta AZ, Keng CS, Jamil MA, Singh S. Successful treatment of acute promyelocytic leukemia in pregnancy with all-trans retinoic acid. Leukemia 2001; 1665-1666.

[66] Nakamura K, Dan K, Iwakiri R, Gomi S, Nomura T. Successful treatment of acute promyelocytic leukemia in pregnancy with all-trans retinoic acid. Ann Hematol 1995; 71:263-264.

[67] Breccia M, Cimino G, Alimena G, De Carolis S, Lo Coco F, Mandelli F. AIDA treatment for high-risk acute promyelocytic leukemia in a pregnant woman at 21 weeks of gestation. Haematologica 2002; 87 (02) ELT 12.

[68] Larson RA. Initial treatment of acute promyelocytic leukemia in adults. UpToDate 2014. Edited by: Lowenberg B and Connor RF. Topic last updated: April 29, 2014.

[69] Sanz MA, Grimwade D, Tallman MS, Lowenberg B, Fenaux P, Estey EH, et al. Management of acute promyelocytic leukemia: recommendation from an expert panel on behalf of the European Leukemia Net. Blood 2009; 113: 1875-1891.

[70] Yang D, Hladnik L. Treatment of acute promyelocytic leukemia during pregnancy. Pharmacotherapy 2009; 29 (6): 709-724.

[71] Troitskaia VV, Parovichnikova EN, Sokolov AN, Kokhno AV, Makhinia SA, Galstian GM, et al. Treatment of acute promyelocytic leukemia during pregnancy. Ter Arkh. 2013; 85 (10): 56-63.

[72] Takatsuki H, Abe Y, Goto T, Sadamura S, Taguchi F, Muta K, et al. Two cases of acute promyelocytic leukemia pregnancy and the effect of anthracyclines on fetal development. Rinsho Ketsueki 1992; 33 (11): 1736-1740.

[73] Elezovic I, Colovic M, Tomin D, Boskovic D. Pregnancy after treatment of secondary acute promyelocytic leukemia following Hodgkin's disease: a case report. Med Oncol 2000; 17 (3): 222-224.

[74] Bassani MA, de Oliveira AB, Oliveira Neto AF. Noninvasive ventilation in a pregnant patient with respiratory failure from all-trans retinoic acid (ATRA) syndrome. Respir Care 2009; 54 (7): 969-972.

[75] Celsing F, Ekman G, Granström L, Johnsson H, Björkholm M. Caesarean section in previously untreated acute promyelocytic leukemia: report of two patients. Eur J Obstet Gynecol Reprod Biol. 2000; 91 (1): 41-42.

[76] Terada Y, Shindo T, Endoh A, Watanabe M, Fukaya T, Yajima A. Fetal arrhythmia during treatment of pregnancy-associated acute promyelocytic leukemia with all-trans retinoic acid and favorable outcome. Leukemia 1997; 11(3): 454.

[77] Morimatsu Y, Matsubara S, Hirose N, Ohkuchi A, Izumi A, Ozaki K, et al. Acute promyelocytic leukemia: an unusual cause showing prolonged disseminated intravascular coagulation after placental abruption. Arch Gynecol Obstet. 2008; 277: 267-270.

[78] Park TS, Lee ST, Kim JS, Song J, Lee K-A, Kim SJ, et al. Acute promyelocytic leukemia in early pregnancy with translocation t (15,17) and variant PML-RARA fusion transcripts. Cancer Genet Cytogenet 2008; 188 (1): 48-51.

[79] Ribera J-M, Ribera J, Genesca E. Treatment of adolescents and young adults with acute lymphoblastic leukemia. Mediterr J Hematol Infect Dis. 2014; 6 (1); e2014052.

[80] DeAngelo DJ. The treatment of adolescent and young adults with acute lymphoblastic leukemia. Hematology Am Soc Hematol Educ Program 2005; 123-130.

[81] Larson RA. Induction therapy for Philadelphia chromosome negative acute lymphoblastic leukemia in adults. Up To Date; Topic 4524; Version 28.0; Topic edited by Lowenberg B, Connor RF. Topic last updated Dec. 23, 2014.

[82] Rowe JM, Buck G, Burnett AK, Chopra R, Wiernik PH, Richards SM, et al. Induction therapy for adults with acute lymphoblastic leukemia: results of more than 1500 patients from the international ALL trial: MRC UKALL XII/ECOG E2993. Blood 2005; 106: 3760-3767.

[83] Nachman JB, La MK, Hunger SP, Heerema NA, Gaynon PS, Hastings C, et al. Young adults with acute lymphoblastic leukemia have an excellent outcome with chemotherapy alone and benefit from intensive postinduction treatment: a report from the Children's Oncology Group. J Clin Oncol. 2009; 27 (31): 5189-5194.

[84] Ticku J, Oberoi S, Friend S, Busowski J, Langenstroer M, Baidas S. Acute lymphoblastic leukemia in pregnancy: a case report with literature review. Ther Adv Hematol. 2013; 4 (5): 313-319.

[85] Bottsford-Miller J, Haeri S, Baker AM, Boles j, Brown M. B-cell acute lymphocytic leukemia in pregnancy. Arch Gynecol Obstet 2010; doi: 10. 1007/s 00404-010-1647-2.

[86] Molkenboer JFM, Vos AH, Shouten HC, Vos MC. Acute lymphoblastic leukemia in pregnancy. Neth J Med. 2005; 63 (5): 361-363.

[87] Tewari K, Cappuccini F, Rosen RB, Brsenthal J, Asrat T, Kohler MF. Relapse of acute lymphoblastic leukemia in pregnancy: survival following chemoirradiation and autologous transfer of interleukin-2-activated stem cells. Gynecol Oncol 1999; 74 (1): 143-148.

[88] Camera A, Campanile M, Catalano D, Mattace Raso A, Rotoli B. Relapse of acute lymphoblastic leukemia during pregnancy. Eur J Gynaecol Oncol 1996; 17 (4): 303-305.

[89] Bohgaki T, Notoya A, Mukai M, Kohno M. Acute lymphoblastic leukemia with breast infiltration during the second trimester of pregnancy and followed by successful delivery. Rinsho Ketsueki 1999; 40 (8): 652-657.

[90] Terek MC, Ozkinay E, Zekioglu O, Erhan Y, Cagirgan S, Pahilvan M, et al. Acute leukemia in pregnancy with ovarian metastasis: a case report and review of the literature. Int J Gynecol Cancer 2003; 13 (6): 904-908.

[91] Yucibilgin MS, Cagirgan S, Donmez A, Ozkinay E, Akercan F, Mgoyi L, et al. Acute myeloblastic leukemia in pregnancy: a case report and review of the literature. Eur J Gynaecol Oncol 2004; 25 (1): 126-128.

[92] Okun DB, Groncy PK, Sieger L, Tanaka KR. Acute leukemia in pregnancy: transient neonatal myelosuppression after combination chemotherapy in the mother. Med Pediatr Oncol. 1979; 7 (4): 315-319.

[93] Choi HJ, Park YW, Cheong JW, Min YH, Kwon JY, Kwon HS; et al. A case of acute lymphocytic leukemia in pregnancy. Korean J Obstet Gynecol 2005; 48 (2): 467-472.

[94] Dara P, Slater LM, Armentrout SA. Successful pregnancy during chemotherapy for acute leukemia. Cancer 1981; 47 (6): 845-846.

[95] Matsouka C, Marinopoulos S, Barbaroussi D, Antsaklis A. Acute lymphoblastic leukemia during gestation. Med Oncol 2008; 25 (2): 190-193.

[96] Panatoniou N, Daskalakis G, Marinopoulos S, Anastasakis E, Mesogitis S, Antsaklis A. Management of pregnancy in adolescence complicated by acute lymphoblastic leukemia. Fetal Diagn Ther. 2008; 23 (2): 164-167.

[97] Cutting HO, Collier TM. Acute lymphocytic leukemia during pregnancy. Obstet Gynecol. 1964; 24: 941-945.

[98] Avasthi R, Agarwal MP. Acute lymphatic leukemia and pregnancy. Indian J Cancer 1993; 30 (3): 143-145.

[99] Abruzzese E, Trawinska MM, Perrotti AP, De Fabritiis P. Tyrosine kinase inhibitors and pregnancy. Mediterr J Hematol Infect Dis. 2014; 6 (1): ė 2014028.

[100] Pye SM, Cortes J, Ault P, Hatfield A, Kantarjian H, Pilot R, et al. The effects of imatinib on pregnancy outcome. Blood 2008; 111: 5505-5508.

[101] Wang DP, Liang My, Zhang XH, Wang SM. Clinical analysis about the management and the perinatal outcomes of pregnancy with chronic myeloid leukemia. Zhonghua Fu Chan Ke Za Zhi. 2010; 45 (10): 735-739.

[102] Usui N. Discontinuation of tyrosine kinase inhibitors and pregnancy for female patients with chronic myeloid leukemia. J Hematol Transfus. 2014; 2 (3): 1023.

[103] Negrin RS, Schiffer CA. Clinical use of tyrosine kinase inhibitors for chronic myeloid leukemia. UpToDate 2014, Edited by Larson RA and Connor RF. Topic last updated: October 22, 2014.

[104] Ault P, Kantarjian H, O' Brien S, Faderl S, Beran M, Rios MB, et al. Pregnancy among patients with chronic myeloid leukemia treated with imatinib. J Clin Oncol. 2008; 24 (7): 1204-1208.

[105] Kuwabara A, Babb A, Ibrahim A, Milojkovic D, Apperley J, Bua M, et al. Poor outcome after reintroduction of imatinib in patients with chronic myeloid leukemia who interrupt therapy on account of pregnancy without having achieved an optimal response. Blood 2010; 116 (6): 1014-1016.

[106] Wu K-N, LuoY, Liu L-Z, Zhao Y-M, Hu Y-X, Tan Y-M, et al. Twin pregnancy and childbirth after reduced-intensity conditioning allogeneic hematopoietic stem cell transplantation combined with imatinib mesylate for chronic myeloid leukemia: case report and literature review. J Int Med Res. 2012; 40: 2409-2415.

[107] Oweini H, Otrock ZK, Mahfouz RA, Bazarbachi A. Successful pregnancy involving a man with chronic myeloid leukemia on dasatinib. Arch Gynecol Obstet. 2011; 283 (1): 133-134.

[108] Bayraktar S, Morency B, Escalon MP. Successful pregnancy in a patient with chronic myeloid leukemia exposed to dasatinib during the first trimester. BMJ Case Rep. 2010; doi: 10.1136/bcr. 05.2010.2975.

[109] Berveiller P, Andreoli A, Mir O, Anselem O, Delezoide AL, Sauvageon H, et al. A dramatic fetal outcome following transplacental transfer of dasatinib. Anticancer Drugs 2012; 23 (7): 754-757.

[110] Conchon M, Sanabani SS, Bendit I, Santos FM, Serpa M, Dorliac-Llacer PE. Two successful pregnancies in a woman with chronic myeloid leukemia exposed to nilotinib during the first trimester of her second pregnancy: case study. J Hematol Oncol. 2009; 2: 42.

[111] Klaasen R, de Jong P, Wijermans PW. Successful management of chronic myeloid leukemia with leukapheresis during a twin pregnancy. Neth J Med. 2007; 65 (4): 147-149.

[112] Ali R, Özkalemkas F, Özkocaman, Özcelik T, Ozan U, Kimya Y, et al. Successful pregnancy and delivery in a patient with chronic myelogenous leukemia (CML) and management of CML with leukemia during pregnancy: a case report and review of the literature. Jpn J Clin Oncol. 2014; 34 (4): 215-217.

[113] Hamad N, Kliman D, Best OG, Caramins M, Hertzberg M, Linderman R, etal. Chronic lymphocytic leukemia, monoclonal *B*- Lymphocytosis and pregnancy: five cases, a literature review and discussion of management: Br J Haematol. 2014; doi: 10.1111/bjh. 13134.

[114] Welsh TM, Thompson J, Lim S. Chronic lymphocytic leukemia in pregnancy. Leukemia 2000; 14(6): 1155.

[115] Chrisomalis L, Boxi LV, Heller D. Chronic lymphocytic leukemia in pregnancy. Am J Obstet Gynecol. 1996; 175(5): 1381-1382.

[116] Gürman G. Pregnancy and successful labor in the course of chronic lymphocytic leukemia. Am J Hematol. 2002; 71 (3): 208-210.

[117] Jonsson V, Bock JE, Hilder J, Houlston RS, Wiik A. The influence of pregnancy on the development of autoimmunity in chronic lymphocytic leukemia. Leukemia. Leuk lymphoma 2006; 47 (8): 1481-1487.

[118] Pessach I, Shimoni A, Nagler A. Granulocyte-colony stimulating factor for hematopoietic stem cell donation from healthy female donors during pregnancy and lactation: what do we know? Human Reprod Update 2013; 19 (3): 259-267.

[119] Rossi BV, Missmer S, Correia KE, Wadleigh M, Ginsburg ES. Ovarian reserve in women treated for acute lymphocytic leukemia in women treated for acute lymphocytic leukemia or acute myeloid leukemia with chemotherapy but not stem cell transplantation. ISRN Oncol 2012; 956190-2012.

[120] Jadoul P, Kim S, on behalf of ISFP Practice Committee. Fertility considerations in young women with hematological malignancies. J Assist Reprod Genet. 2012; 29: 479-487.

[121] Joshi S, Savani BN, Chow EJ, Gilleece MH, Halter J, Jacobsohn DA, et al. Clinical guide to fertility preservations in hematopoietic stem cell transplant recipients. Bone Marrow Transplant. 2014; 49: 477-484.

[122] Mathews ML, Hurst BS, Marshburn PB, Usadi RS. Papadakis MA, Sarantou T. Cancer, fertility preservation and future pregnancy: a comprehensive review. Obstet Gynecol Int. 2012; 953937-2012.